M. D. ANDERSON
CANCER CARE
SERIES

Series Editors

Aman U. Buzdar, MD   Ralph S. Freedman, MD, PhD

M. D. ANDERSON CANCER CARE SERIES

Series Editors: Aman U. Buzdar, MD, and
Ralph S. Freedman, MD, PhD

K.K. Hunt, G.L. Robb, E.A. Strom, and N.T. Ueno, Eds., *Breast Cancer*

F.V. Fossella, R. Komaki, and J.B. Putnam, Jr., Eds., *Lung Cancer*

J.A. Ajani, S.A. Curley, N.A. Janjan, and P.M. Lynch, Eds.,
Gastrointestinal Cancer

K.W. Chan and R.B. Raney, Jr., Eds., *Pediatric Oncology*

P.J. Eifel, D.M. Gershenson, John J. Kavanagh, and Elvio G. Silva, Eds.,
Gynecologic Cancer

F. DeMonte, M.R. Gilbert, A. Mahajan, and I.E. McCutcheon, Eds.,
Tumors of the Brain and Spine

Franco DeMonte, MD, Mark R. Gilbert, MD,
Anita Mahajan, MD, and Ian E. McCutcheon, MD
Editors

The University of Texas M. D. Anderson Cancer Center, Houston, Texas

Tumors of the Brain and Spine

Foreword by Raymond Sawaya, MD, and
W. K. Alfred Yung, MD

With 73 Illustrations and 32 Tables

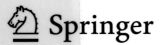 Springer

Franco DeMonte, MD
The University of Texas
Department of Neurosurgery
M. D. Anderson Cancer Center
1515 Holcombe Blvd., Unit 442
Houston, TX 77030-4009, USA

Mark R. Gilbert, MD
The University of Texas
Department of Neuro-Oncology
M. D. Anderson Cancer Center
1515 Holcombe Blvd., Unit 431
Houston, TX 77030-4009, USA

Anita Mahajan, MD
The University of Texas
Department of Radiation Oncology
M. D. Anderson Cancer Center
1515 Holcombe Blvd., Unit 97
Houston, TX 77030-4009, USA

Ian E. McCutcheon, MD
The University of Texas
Department of Neurosurgery
M. D. Anderson Cancer Center
1515 Holcombe Blvd., Unit 442
Houston, TX 77030-4009, USA

Series Editors:
Aman U. Buzdar, MD
Department of Breast Medical Oncology
The University of Texas
M. D. Anderson Cancer Center
Houston, TX 77030-4009, USA

Ralph S. Freedman, MD, PhD
Department of Gynecologic Oncology
The University of Texas
M. D. Anderson Cancer Center
Houston, TX 77030-4009, USA

TUMORS OF THE BRAIN AND SPINE

Library of Congress Control Number: 2006939206

ISBN-13: 978-0387-29201-4   e-ISBN-13: 978-0387-29202-1

Printed on acid-free paper.

Printed in the United States of America.

9 8 7 6 5 4 3 2 1

springer.com

FOREWORD

It is frequently stated that progress in the management of tumors of the brain and spine has not occurred in the past 25 years. Such statements seriously underestimate and misrepresent progress in managing various central nervous system tumors, the tremendous technologic enhancements that have revolutionized the imaging of the tumors and the host organ, the multitude of surgical adjuncts such as computerized imaging guidance and functional mapping of the brain and its tracts that are routinely used in the modern neurosurgical operating room, and the highly conformal delivery of radiation to the tumor mass with remarkable sparing of the surrounding nervous tissue. Underlying these technologic improvements are the changes in philosophy that have resulted in a true multidisciplinary approach.

Equally significant is the molecular revolution that is identifying key markers behind the genesis of brain tumors, their proliferation, and their resistance to therapy. These molecular discoveries have ushered in the era of molecular targeted therapy, as first demonstrated by the extraordinary success story in chronic myelogenous leukemia of imatinib (Gleevec). The rational combination of targeted agents will revolutionize the way chemotherapy is given, either alone or in conjunction with radiotherapy.

Lastly, focused attention to patients' well-being has emphasized all measures of quality of life, has encouraged greater participation by patients and their caregivers in the decision-making process, and has encouraged the development of a variety of quality-of-life measurement tools to ensure that adverse effects of treatment are recognized and addressed.

In this monograph of the M. D. Anderson Cancer Care Series, the authors have captured the essence of the progress experienced to date and, in the most appropriate multidisciplinary fashion, they have outlined the principles behind patient assessment, decision making, and management of tumors of the brain and spine. Their expertise and commitment to their patients are evident throughout.

Raymond Sawaya, MD
W. K. Alfred Yung, MD

PREFACE

Although the annual incidence of intrinsic tumors of the central nervous system (CNS)—about 17,000 to 20,000 in the United States—is much lower than that of more common cancers arising in the lung, breast, or other sites, CNS tumors are prominent in oncology for several reasons. First, they attack the very structure of our personhood and in so doing, create fear and functional deficits as profound as they are disturbing to patients and their families alike. Second, CNS tumors can be difficult to cure when they are infiltrative or located in places that are difficult to access surgically without putting patients at some risk. Third, since tumors originating in any organ system can secondarily affect the brain or spine, much crossover exists between neuro-oncology and general oncology. And finally, CNS tumors are prominent in oncology because of the great strides being made in our understanding of these tumors on a molecular and genetic level and because treatments can now be based on hitherto unrecognized genetic alterations, advances that go hand in hand with similar knowledge being gathered in all the subspecialties of oncology.

Because of our rapidly increasing knowledge about tumors of the brain and spine, these tumors are becoming more treatable—either for palliation or for cure—than ever before. The effects of environmental exposures on tumor formation are coming more into focus, and epidemiologic knowledge is now linking nicely with molecular genetic alterations derived from kindreds susceptible to brain tumor formation. Such alterations have been correlated with a progression from benign to malignant forms of several tumor types, most notably the astrocytoma; and although an initiating genetic mutation cannot yet be traced for most tumors, molecular genetics is now being used in neuropathologic diagnoses to supplement more traditional histologic approaches. Diagnostic tools such as magnetic resonance imaging continue to develop and have become quite sensitive, albeit less than perfectly specific, in revealing CNS tumors at earlier and earlier stages. Surgical procedures too are advancing through a combination of more complex technologies and the development of a cadre of neurosurgeons specialized in the nuances of tumor care.

In the new world of CNS oncology, maximally complete resection is followed by conformal radiotherapy and often by chemotherapy, the selection of which is based on the tumor's susceptibility to drugs that have biological actions known to interact with the tumor's particular molecular signature. For example, oral temozolomide is better tolerated by patients than predecessor intravenous chemotherapeutic agents and is more effective in patients with epigenetic silencing of the *MGMT* gene associated with DNA repair. This agent has become the standard of care for patients with anaplastic or malignant astrocytomas after resection and irradiation. In the future, we may find that today's groundwork in immunotherapy or in stem cell biology will further improve our therapeutic reach.

The chapters of this book collectively weave a tapestry that depicts the broad range of medical, surgical, and radiotherapeutic approaches to neuro-oncology as it is practiced at M. D. Anderson Cancer Center, along with the diversity of disciplines needed for effective therapy. This is now the sixth book in the M. D. Anderson Cancer Care Series. The first of these was published in 2001 and was devoted to breast cancer. This book, like the others, highlights integrated care and focuses on treating the patient through the entire spectrum of a disease.

We thank Walter Pagel for shepherding the Cancer Care Series since its inception and Elizabeth Hess, Manuel Gonzales, and Tamara Locke of the Department of Scientific Publications for their dedication to producing this book. And we thank you, the reader, for your interest in this most intricate and fascinating corner of oncology in which we practice our art and our science.

Franco DeMonte, MD
Mark R. Gilbert, MD
Anita Mahajan, MD
Ian E. McCutcheon, MD

CONTENTS

Foreword   v
Raymond Sawaya and W. K. Alfred Yung

Preface   vii

Contributors   xi

Chapter 1
Epidemiology of Brain Tumors   1
Melissa L. Bondy, Randa El-Zein, and Michael E. Scheurer

Chapter 2
Neuropathology and Molecular Biology of Intracranial Tumors   23
Gregory N. Fuller and Kenneth D. Aldape

Chapter 3
Radiology of Brain Tumors: Structure and Physiology   37
*J. Matthew Debnam, Leena Ketonen, Leena M. Hamberg,
and George J. Hunter*

Chapter 4
Surgically Curable Brain Tumors of Adults   53
Franco DeMonte

Chapter 5
Low-Grade Gliomas: Evidence-Based Treatment Options   93
Frederick F. Lang

Chapter 6
Surgical Strategies for High-Grade Gliomas   121
Sujit S. Prabhu

Chapter 7
Radiation Oncology for Tumors of the Central Nervous System:
Improving the Therapeutic Index   135
Shiao Y. Woo

Chapter 8
Cytotoxic Chemotherapy for Diffuse Gliomas   153
Ivo W. Tremont-Lukats and Mark R. Gilbert

Chapter 9
Innovative Treatment Strategies for High-Grade Gliomas   171
Charles A. Conrad and Amy B. Heimberger

Chapter 10
Pituitary Tumors in Oncology   191
Ian E. McCutcheon

Chapter 11
Management of Lung Cancer, Breast Cancer,
and Melanoma Metastatic to the Brain   225
Jeffrey S. Weinberg

Chapter 12
Neoplastic Meningitis   245
Morris D. Groves

Chapter 13
Lymphoma Affecting the Central Nervous System   263
Barbara Pro

Chapter 14
Tumors of the Extradural Spine   273
Ehud Mendel

Chapter 15
Tumors of the Spinal Cord and Intradural Space   295
Laurence D. Rhines and Morris D. Groves

Chapter 16
Symptom Management for Patients with Brain Tumors:
Improving Quality of Life   329
Allen W. Burton, Tracy L. Veramonti, Phillip C. Phan,
and Jeffrey S. Wefel

Index   353

CONTRIBUTORS

Kenneth D. Aldape, MD, Associate Professor, Department of Pathology

Melissa L. Bondy, PhD, Professor, Department of Epidemiology

Allen W. Burton, MD, Section Chief, Cancer Pain Management; Associate Professor, Department of Anesthesiology and Pain Medicine

Charles A. Conrad, MD, Associate Professor, Department of Neuro-Oncology

J. Matthew Debnam, MD, Assistant Professor, Department of Diagnostic Radiology

Franco DeMonte, MD, FRCSC, FACS, Professor, Departments of Neurosurgery and Head and Neck Surgery

Randa El-Zein, MD, PhD, Assistant Professor, Department of Epidemiology

Gregory N. Fuller, MD, PhD, Chief, Section of Neuropathology; Professor, Department of Pathology

Mark R. Gilbert, MD, Deputy Chair and Professor, Department of Neuro-Oncology

Morris D. Groves, MD, JD, Associate Professor, Department of Neuro-Oncology

Leena M. Hamberg, PhD, Associate Professor, Department of Diagnostic Radiology

Amy B. Heimberger, MD, Assistant Professor, Department of Neurosurgery

George J. Hunter, MD, PhD, Head, Section of Neuroradiology; Associate Professor, Department of Diagnostic Radiology

Leena Ketonen, MD, PhD, Professor, Department of Diagnostic Radiology

Frederick F. Lang, MD, Professor and Director of Clinical Research, Department of Neurosurgery

Ian E. McCutcheon, MD, FRCS(C), Professor, Department of Neurosurgery

Ehud Mendel, MD, FACS, Co-Director, Spine Program; Associate Professor, Department of Neurosurgery

Phillip C. Phan, MD, Assistant Professor, Department of Anesthesiology and Pain Medicine

Sujit S. Prabhu, MD, FRCS (Edin), Assistant Professor, Department of Neurosurgery

Barbara Pro, MD, Associate Professor of Medicine, Department of Lymphoma-Myeloma

Laurence D. Rhines, MD, Associate Professor, Department of Neurosurgery

Michael E. Scheurer, PhD, MPH, Instructor, Department of Epidemiology

Ivo W. Tremont-Lukats, MD, Fellow, Department of Neuro-Oncology

Tracy L. Veramonti, PhD, Postdoctoral Fellow, Department of Neuro-Oncology

Jeffrey S. Wefel, PhD, Assistant Professor, Department of Neuro-Oncology

Jeffrey S. Weinberg, MD, Assistant Professor, Department of Neuro-surgery

Shiao Y. Woo, MD, Professor, Department of Radiation Oncology

1 EPIDEMIOLOGY OF BRAIN TUMORS

Melissa L. Bondy, Randa El-Zein,
and Michael E. Scheurer

Chapter Overview 2
Introduction 2
Descriptive Epidemiology 3
 Incidence 3
 Mortality and Survival 4
 Trends in Incidence and Mortality 5
 Differences by Age, Sex, and Ethnicity 6
  Age 6
  Sex 8
  Ethnicity 8
 Differences in Histologic Characteristics as Determined
  by Molecular Genetics 10
 Gliomas (Astrocytic Tumors) 10
 Oligodendrogliomas 10
 Gangliogliomas 11
 Medulloblastomas 11
 Ependymomas 11
 Meningiomas 11
 Schwannomas 11
 Chordomas 12
Analytic Epidemiology of Risk Factors 12
 Genetic Susceptibility and Familial Aggregation 12
 Ionizing and Non-ionizing Radiation 15
  Ionizing Radiation 15
  Electromagnetic Fields 16
  Cellular Telephones 16
 Occupational Exposure 17
 Parental Occupational Exposure 18
 Lifestyle Factors 18
  Diet 18
  Tobacco and Alcohol Use 19
 Medical History and Medication Use 19
  Head Trauma and Seizure 19
  Medications 20

Infectious Agents and Immunologic Response 20
Key Practice Points 21
Suggested Readings 21

CHAPTER OVERVIEW

Brain tumors are rare compared with other fatal and life-diminishing diseases. However, rarity is a relative term: more than 18,000 persons in the United States are diagnosed each year with brain tumors. Two thirds of them will die, and the others will survive but with severe restrictions in function. The etiology of brain tumors is poorly characterized, and the relationship between and contribution of heritable and environmental conditions are unclear. Traditional descriptive epidemiology has been able to accurately show the incidence and outcome differences of these tumors according to ethnic, geographic, occupational, and histologic factors. However, the investigation of risk factors (analytic epidemiology) has been hampered because of inconsistencies in reporting, diagnosis, study subject selection, and tumor classification. Despite these limitations, analytic epidemiology is becoming more penetrating because of the many studies that have associated brain tumors with genetic alterations and because of the earlier supporting studies on familial cancer syndromes, ionizing radiation, occupational exposure, and consumption of nitrosamines that link these factors to genetic change and higher risk. Genetic studies at the molecular level offer a new means of diagnosing, treating, and preventing cancers of the brain, and they will help explain who is at elevated risk and, through studies of such patients, identify more precisely the genetic and environmental risk factors.

INTRODUCTION

Brain tumors account for a small proportion of all cancers (1.4%) and cancer-related deaths (2.4%). However, most of these tumors are fatal, and even benign brain tumors can interfere with brain functions that are essential for daily living. The American Cancer Society (2006) estimated that 18,820 individuals in the United States would be diagnosed with a malignant brain tumor in 2006 and that 12,820 would die from a brain tumor that year. Brain tumors are the 10th-leading cause of overall cancer deaths in women and the 5th-leading cause of cancer deaths in women aged 20 to 39 years. In addition, among persons younger than 20 years old, brain tumors are the most frequent solid tumor and the 2nd-leading cause of cancer death, behind leukemia (Jemal et al, 2005).

Because of the extremely high mortality—especially among patients diagnosed with glioblastomas—and significant morbidity due to brain tumors, there is an ever-intensifying interest in understanding their etiology. Epidemiologic studies enhance this understanding in 2 ways. First, descriptive studies characterize the incidence of brain tumors and the mortality and survival rates associated with them with respect to histologic tumor type and demographic characteristics (e.g., age, sex, and geographic region). Second, analytic studies compare the risk of brain tumors in people with and without certain characteristics (cohort studies) or compare the histories of people with and without brain tumors (case-control studies) to provide information on a wide range of possible risk factors, including inherited and acquired alterations in genes related to carcinogenesis, exposures to ionizing or non-ionizing radiation, occupation and industry, diet, smoking, alcohol, personal medical history, and certain common infections. In addition to epidemiologic analyses, the molecular classification of brain tumors could provide greater insight into genetic roles in disease progression and sensitivity to radiotherapy and chemotherapy. The hope is that this knowledge will result in better, and possibly individualized, treatment regimens and eventually feasible strategies for preventing brain tumors.

DESCRIPTIVE EPIDEMIOLOGY

Data on the occurrence of brain tumors in the United States are gathered primarily by 2 agencies, the Surveillance, Epidemiology, and End Results (SEER) program of the National Cancer Institute (http://seer.cancer.gov) and the Central Brain Tumor Registry of the United States (CBTRUS) (http://www.cbtrus.org). Both sources are important because they contain different types of data: the SEER program reports on malignant primary brain tumors, whereas the CBTRUS reports on both malignant and nonmalignant tumors. The data on nonmalignant tumors are important because of the morbidity caused by the presence of these tumors in the brain. The data from both programs allow us to estimate the incidence and mortality of brain tumors in the United States.

Incidence

The most recent statistical report (data collected from 1998 through 2002) from CBTRUS estimated the incidence of all primary nonmalignant and malignant brain and central nervous system (CNS) tumors to be 14.8 per 100,000 person-years. This figure can be separated by malignancy: 7.438 per 100,000 person-years for benign and borderline tumors and 7.37 per 100,000 person-years for malignant tumors. The most recent SEER program data (collected from 1994 through 2003) indicated an annual incidence of primary malignant brain and CNS tumors of 6.4 per 100,000 person-years. This rate is higher in males (7.6 per 100,000 person-years) than females (5.3 per 100,000 person-years).

CBTRUS also reports incidence separately for pediatric brain tumors. For children aged 0 to 19 years, the incidence of primary nonmalignant and malignant brain and CNS tumors is 4.28 per 100,000 person-years.

Again, this rate is higher among males (4.49 per 100,000 person-years) than females (4.04 per 100,000 person-years).

Mortality and Survival

The American Cancer Society estimated 12,820 deaths due to primary malignant brain and CNS tumors for 2006. This value corresponds to an annual incidence of 4.60 per 100,000 persons (based on the 2000 U.S. population) as reported by the SEER program.

Data from the SEER program also estimated an overall 5-year survival rate of 33.2% for males and 36.0% for females. This rate decreases markedly with age. Children under the age of 20 experience a 5-year survival rate of approximately 65%. That value drops dramatically to 28.1% among adults 45 to 54 years of age and to only 4.0% for adults aged 75 years or older.

Of all the histologic types of brain cancer, glioblastoma has the lowest 2- and 5-year survival rates for all age groups. The 2-year survival rate is approximately 30% for those diagnosed before 45 years of age, and it decreases dramatically as age increases, to less than 2% for those aged 75 years or older (Figure 1–1). The 5-year survival rate of patients with

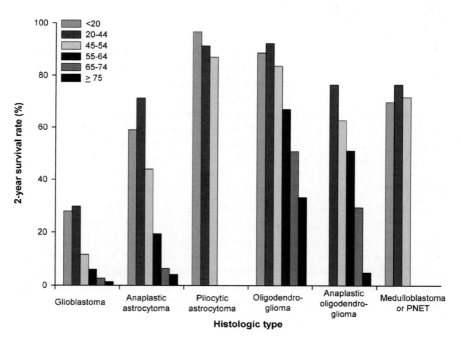

Figure 1–1.   Two-year survival rates for selected brain tumors, by age group and histologic type. Age at diagnosis is given in years. Blank entries indicate that too few cases were available to calculate a survival rate. Source: SEER program, 1973–2002, as reported by CBTRUS.

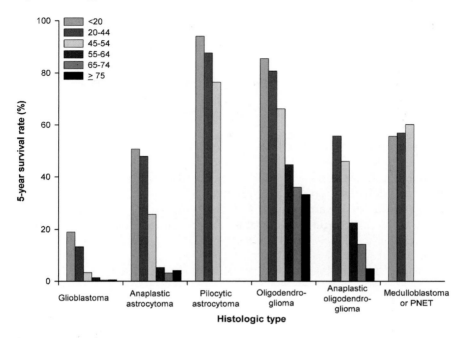

Figure 1–2. Five-year survival rates for selected brain tumors, by age group and histologic type. Age at diagnosis is given in years. Blank entries indicate that too few cases were available to calculate a survival rate. Source: SEER program, 1973–2002, as reported by CBTRUS.

glioblastomas and most other histologic types of brain cancer is even worse, especially for older patients (Figure 1–2). Although the survival rates are bleak, the lifetime risk of being diagnosed with a primary malignant tumor of the brain or CNS is very low: 0.67% for males and 0.51% for females. Even lower is the lifetime risk of dying from a primary brain or CNS tumor, which is 0.49% for males and 0.39% for females.

Trends in Incidence and Mortality

Assessing the trends in the incidence and mortality of any disease is important for determining the effectiveness of prevention and treatment efforts, especially for fatal diseases such as brain cancer. Trend information is conveniently on hand: the SEER program and CBTRUS have reports and data accessible on their Web sites, and several reviews of epidemiologic trends for brain and CNS tumors have been published (Davis and McCarthy, 2001; Gurney and Kadan-Lottick, 2001; Minn et al, 2002).

The incidence and mortality rates of brain tumors have increased since the late 1960s. The largest increases, a near doubling for both incidence and mortality, have been noted among the elderly (Figure 1–3). The incidence

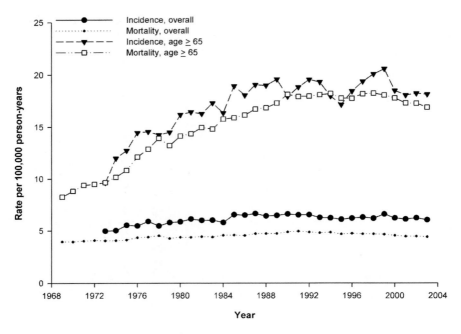

Figure 1–3.   Overall age-adjusted incidence and mortality rates for brain and other CNS malignancies, 1969–2003. Rates are age adjusted to the 2000 U.S. standard population. Source: SEER program, 1973–2003 (incidence) and 1969–2003 (mortality).

and mortality rates of primary malignant brain tumors have also increased in children, although to a lesser extent, by about 35%. Much of the reported increases, especially among the elderly, can be attributed to the introduction of diagnostic technologies such as computed tomography and magnetic resonance imaging. Other contributing factors are a longer life expectancy, changing medical practices among the elderly, and a greater availability of neurosurgeons. The idea that some of the increased incidence and mortality rates could be due to increased exposure to causal factors is supported by the increased rates seen with brain tumors in children. However, few environmental factors have been consistently associated with temporal trends in the incidence of brain tumors. In addition, 3 key factors must be noted when comparing rates and studies of trends in brain cancer: the reference population used for age adjustment, the inclusion of nonmalignant tumors, and methodologic differences. All of these factors can greatly affect trend analyses.

Differences by Age, Sex, and Ethnicity

Age

According to CBTRUS, the mean age of onset for all primary brain tumors is 53 years. However, the average age of onset for glioblastoma and meningioma, the 2 most common types of tumors among adults (Table 1–1), is about 62 years. More important, the age distribution varies greatly by tumor site and histologic type (Figure 1–4). For example, the incidences of glioblastoma and astrocytoma peak at ages 65 to 74 years and then decline, whereas the incidence of meningioma continues to increase with increasing age. Because cancers are generally thought of as diseases of

Table 1–1. **Most Common Brain and CNS Tumor Histologic Types, by Age Group, 1998–2002**

Age Group* (Years)	Most Common Histologic Type	Second Most Common Histologic Type
0–4	Medulloblastoma or PNET	Pilocytic astrocytoma
5–19	Pilocytic astrocytoma	Medulloblastoma or PNET
20–34	Meningioma	Pituitary tumor
35–44	Meningioma	Nerve sheath tumor and glioblastoma
≥45	Meningioma	Glioblastoma

*Age at diagnosis.
Source: CBTRUS.

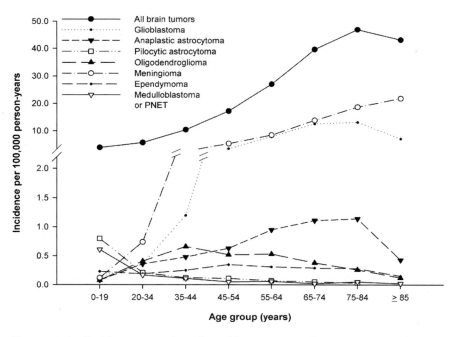

Figure 1–4. Incidence rates for selected brain tumors, by age group and histologic type. Age is at diagnosis. Note that the y-axis scale changes between 2.0 and 10.0. Source: SEER program, 1973–2003.

older age, the increasing incidence of most types of brain tumors with age could be due to the length of exposure to causal factors required for malignant transformation, the necessity of many genetic alterations before clinical disease, or poorer immune surveillance. An intriguing feature of brain tumor epidemiology is the peak in incidence of medulloblastoma and other primitive neuroectodermal tumors (PNETs) in young children.

Sex

The most consistent epidemiologic finding for brain tumors is that neuroepithelial tumors are more common among men, whereas meningeal tumors are more common among women (Counsell and Grant, 1998; Surawicz et al, 1999). For example, the incidence of glioma is 40% higher among men than women, whereas the incidence of meningioma is 80% higher among women. Biologic or social factors may account for these consistently observed sex differences, and although they are not well understood, these factors must be considered in the etiology of brain tumors.

Ethnicity

The interpretation of geographic and ethnic variations in the incidence of brain tumors is often confounded not only by ascertainment bias due to lack of access to health care by some populations but also by inconsistencies in reporting. Differential access to health care means that reported rates for primary malignant brain tumors tend to be higher in countries with better developed and generally accessible medical care (Inskip et al, 1995; Preston-Martin and Mack, 1996). In addition, reporting is likely more consistent in countries with nearly universal access than in areas where health care and surveillance may be spotty.

Cultural, ethnic, and geographic differences in risk factors may also influence differences in tumor incidence. The incidence of malignant brain tumors in Japan is less than half that in Northern Europe. In the United States, gliomas affect a greater proportion of whites than blacks, but the incidence of meningioma is nearly equal (Figure 1–5). These differences cannot be attributed only to differences in access to health care or in diagnostic practices between whites and blacks (Surawicz et al, 1999).

The geographic variation in brain tumor incidence from high-risk to low-risk areas in both the United States and throughout the world is about 4- to 5-fold. In contrast, 20-fold geographic differences have been observed for lung cancer and 150-fold differences for melanoma (Inskip et al, 1995).

The *Atlas of Cancer Mortality in the United States* (Devesa et al, 1999) shows higher death rates from malignant brain tumors from 1970 through 1994 among whites in the South and parts of the Midwest and Pacific Northwest and lower rates in most of New England and the Southwest. As with international comparisons, interpretation of these

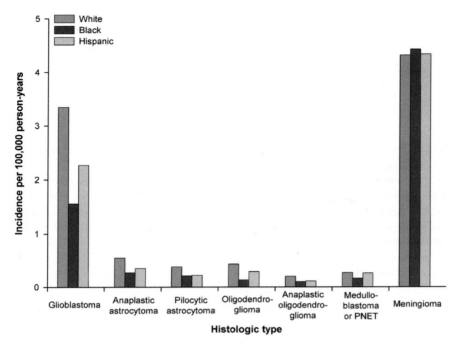

Figure 1–5. Incidence rates for selected brain tumors, by ethnicity and histologic type. Rates are age adjusted to the 2000 U.S. standard population. Hispanic category includes all subjects of Hispanic origin regardless of race. Source: SEER program, 1973–2003.

geographic differences is complicated by variations in diagnostic and reporting practices.

Numerous studies of cancer risk have shown differences between U.S.-born and foreign-born Americans (reviewed in Wrensch et al, 2002). For example, U.S.-born men and women have lower mortality rates for brain cancer, stomach cancer, and infection than foreign-born Americans do. It has also been shown that non-Hispanic whites (male and female) exhibit a higher incidence of brain malignancies than do Hispanic whites, blacks, Chinese, Japanese, and Filipinos. There is also some evidence of ethnic variation in molecular subtypes of tumors (reviewed in Wrensch et al, 2002); however, these findings need to be validated in future research. One study showed that whites were about 3 times more likely than non-whites to have astrocytic gliomas with mutations in the *p53* gene, and another study found more deletions and mutations of *p16^{ink4a}* among Japanese patients than white patients with gliomas. Although other explanations could exist for these ethnic differences, further research into ethnic variation in molecular subtypes of gliomas is justified.

Differences in Histologic Characteristics as Determined by Molecular Genetics

Primary brain tumors are classified by their histologic characteristics and their location and are often further classified on the basis of their invasiveness or malignancy. More invasive forms (which often have more gene mutations) are classified as higher grades. The relevant research findings on individual brain tumors have previously been reviewed (El-Zein et al, 2002), and the major findings are summarized next. Briefly, recent cytogenetic and molecular studies have identified subtypes of tumors and tumor patterns within the larger homogeneous histologic categories, such as glioblastoma (also called astrocytoma). The ability to categorize brain tumors according to these alterations may help us form groupings that are more etiologically homogeneous than standard histologic groupings are. For more information about the molecular biology of brain tumors, see chapter 2.

Gliomas (Astrocytic Tumors)

Astrocytic tumors encompass a wide range of neoplasms that differ by morphologic characteristics, location within the CNS, growth potential, extent of invasiveness, tendency for progression, and age and sex distribution. Increasing evidence suggests that these differences reflect the type and sequence of genetic alterations acquired during carcinogenesis. Several chromosomal abnormalities have been noted in astrocytomas. Mutations in the *p53* gene have been reported in 40% of astrocytic tumors of all grades and occur primarily in young adults rather than children. Deletion of both copies of and rearrangements of the *p16* gene are common in high-grade but not low-grade astrocytomas. Deletions of chromosome 10 (which harbors several tumor-suppressor genes) also commonly occur in higher grade astrocytic tumors. Phosphatase and tensin homolog (*PTEN*), a tumor-suppressor gene mutated in 40% of glioblastomas, has been suggested as a promoter of progression from low-grade to high-grade glioma. Last, amplification of a mutated epidermal growth factor receptor (*EGFR*) allele has been found in approximately one third of glioblastomas but is absent in low-grade astrocytomas.

Oligodendrogliomas

Oligodendrogliomas typically occur in the cerebrum and are more common in adults than children and in men than women. These tumors can metastasize via the cerebrospinal fluid; however, prognosis and survival are generally better for patients with oligodendrogliomas than other gliomas. Oligodendrogliomas exhibit characteristic losses of regions on chromosomes 1, 9, 19, and 22. Homozygous deletion of the *p16* gene, loss of heterozygosity (LOH) on chromosome 10, and amplification of *EGFR* have also been shown in these tumors. In particular, LOH on chromosome

10q and amplification of *EGFR* have been shown to be significant predictors of shorter progression-free survival, whereas LOH on chromosome 1p has been associated with longer progression-free survival.

Gangliogliomas

Gangliogliomas are highly curable by surgery alone, with radiotherapy generally reserved for subtotally resected or recurrent cases (see chapter 5). CNS gangliogliomas occur more frequently in children than adults but show no sex or ethnic differences in incidence. Most cases occur in patients younger than 30 years. It has also been shown that a mutation in the tuberous sclerosis 2 (*TSC2*) gene may predispose an individual to the development of sporadic gangliogliomas. In addition, genetic alterations in chromosomes 7 and 9 are associated with these tumors.

Medulloblastomas

Medulloblastomas constitute 3% to 5% of all brain tumors but 25% of all childhood brain tumors. They can be found in adults but most commonly occur in children aged 3 to 8 years. Little is known about the long-term survivorship of patients with childhood medulloblastomas, but treatment with radiation has been implicated in the development of secondary malignancies. Deletions in chromosome 17p and, less frequently, deletions in chromosomes 2p, 6q, 10q, 11p, 11q, and 16q are associated with these tumors.

Ependymomas

Ependymomas occur primarily in children younger than 20 years. Thirty percent of childhood ependymomas occur before the age of 3 years, and these tumors are more aggressive than adulthood ependymomas. The most common genetic alterations in these tumors are deletions of chromosome 17p and monosomy of chromosome 22.

Meningiomas

Benign tumors of the meninges account for 10% to 20% of all brain tumors. Meningiomas have a fairly uniform age distribution, which peaks in midlife, but are very infrequent in children (less than 2%). Meningiomas occur twice as frequently in women than men. High-grade meningiomas are associated with deletions on chromosome 1 and, to a lesser extent, deletions on chromosomes 6p, 9q, and 17p and mutations in *p53*.

Schwannomas

Schwannomas are typically benign tumors of cranial nerves and account for 8% of primary brain tumors. They are twice as common in women than men and are most often seen in middle-aged patients. Malignant schwannomas originate from peripheral nerves, and recurrent disease and metastases develop early. Losses on chromosome 1p and gains on chromosome 11q have been detected in a few schwannomas, but no single consistent genetic alteration has been found other than a loss on chromosome 22q.

Chordomas

Chordomas are rare neoplasms that arise from embryonic notochordal remnants and comprise less than 1% of intracranial neoplasms. Chordomas occur predominately in patients 30 to 50 years old and show a slight predominance in men. Genetic research is lacking for these tumors; however, 1 study has shown chromosomal imbalances in tumor-suppressor genes or mismatch repair genes, and oncogenes might be involved in chordoma genesis.

ANALYTIC EPIDEMIOLOGY OF RISK FACTORS

Despite the increasing number of epidemiologic studies, there is no consensus on the nature and magnitude of the risk factors for primary brain tumors. Several aspects of the epidemiologic study of these tumors hinder the comparison of studies and the formation of precise estimates of association. These factors include methodologic differences in eligibility; lack of representativeness of the patients studied; use of proxies to report information about the cases; use of inappropriate control groups; substantial heterogeneity of primary brain tumors; inconsistencies in histologic diagnoses, definitions, and groupings; difficulties in retrospective exposure assessment; and undefined latency periods. Table 1–2 summarizes the categories of potential risk factors for primary brain tumors and the current findings detailed in the following sections. Most studies have been conducted on gliomas, but more recent studies have reported findings for meningiomas as well.

Genetic Susceptibility and Familial Aggregation

The examination of genetics is playing an ever-expanding role in explicating the pathogenesis of primary brain tumors and other cancers. Cancers are believed to develop through accumulation of genetic alterations that allow the cells to grow out of the control of normal regulatory mechanisms and escape destruction by the immune system. Inherited or acquired alterations in crucial cell cycle control genes such as *p53* are therefore considered candidate carcinogens. Genetic and familial factors implicated in the formation of brain tumors have been reviewed previously (Bondy et al, 1994; Minn et al, 2002; Wrensch et al, 2002). Because of the results of numerous studies and substantiating biologic plausibility, it is generally accepted that certain inherited genes may contribute to primary brain tumors.

Table 1–2.   Established and Potential Risk Factors for Primary Brain Tumors of the Neuroepithelium or Meninges

Risk Factor	Summary of Current Findings
Genetic susceptibility and familial aggregation: hereditary syndromes and family history of brain tumors (tuberous sclerosis, neurofibromatosis types 1 and 2, nevoid basal cell carcinoma syndrome, adenomatous polyposis syndromes, Li-Fraumeni cancer family syndrome [inherited *p53* mutations]); constitutive polymorphisms in DNA repair, cell cycle regulation, carcinogen metabolization, and immune function genes	• Mutations in *p53* or other cell cycle regulatory genes (e.g., *p16, RB,* and *MDM2*) are likely responsible for increased risk in families • Common exposure to environmental agents or gene–environment interactions are a more likely explanation for increased risk in families • Multiple polymorphisms in these genes (e.g., glutathione transferases, cytochrome p450, *N*-acetyltransferase, ERCC1, and ERCC2) are probably responsible for the increased familial risk
Ionizing and non-ionizing radiation: ionizing radiation (therapeutic or diagnostic), electromagnetic fields, and cellular telephones	• Low-dose therapeutic radiation is the only established risk factor for gliomas, meningiomas, and nerve sheath tumors • Exposure to diagnostic radiation has yielded mixed results • Electromagnetic field studies have yielded mixed results • Cellular phone studies have shown no meaningful associations; however, newer studies are being conducted on effects of long-term use
Occupational exposure: synthetic rubber and polyvinyl chloride manufacturing, petroleum refining or production work, licensed pesticide application, agricultural work, and parental workplace exposures	• No definitive links have been made between occupational exposure and the risk of brain tumors • Many exposures show increased brain tumor mortality in certain industries, but these findings are not statistically significant • No evidence for increased risk from prenatal or postnatal exposure
Lifestyle factors: diet; tobacco and alcohol use	• *N*-nitroso compounds, especially those in cured foods, and decreased consumption of vitamin-rich fruits and vegetables increase the risk of brain tumors • Studies have been hampered by selection biases and difficulties in collecting information on food intake

(continued)

Table 1–2. *(continued)*   **Established and Potential Risk Factors for Primary Brain Tumors of the Neuroepithelium or Meninges**

Risk Factor	Summary of Current Findings
Lifestyle factors *(continued)*	• Studies on tobacco smoke have been inconclusive • Prenatal alcohol exposure is associated with no risk or low risk of brain tumors • Wine and beer are slightly protective against brain tumors in adults
Medical history and medication use: head trauma and seizures; medications	• Head trauma is suspected to increase the risk of meningiomas and acoustic neuromas • Assessment of seizure has been confounded by a lack of temporality • Headache, sleep, and pain medications may be protective against brain tumors • Diuretics and antihistamines may increase the risk for meningiomas • No other drug effects have been identified
Infectious agents or immunologic response: influenza, varicella-zoster, BK, and JC viruses; *Toxoplasma gondii*; allergies	• Increased risk of brain tumors is seen with some viruses • *Toxoplasma gondii* may increase the risk of meningiomas • Varicella-zoster virus and allergies may have a possible protective effect against brain tumors

Sources: Bondy et al, 1994; Berleur and Cordier, 1995; Wrensch et al, 1997, 2002; Minn et al, 2002.

An estimated 5% to 10% of brain tumors are due to genetic predisposition, but this range may be an underestimate. Patients with brain tumors do not routinely see clinical geneticists, and genetic syndromes may be hard to diagnose. The occurrence of brain tumors in individuals with hereditary syndromes such as tuberous sclerosis, neurofibromatosis types 1 and 2, nevoid basal cell carcinoma syndrome, and syndromes involving adenomatous polyps indicates a genetic predisposition to brain tumors (Bondy et al, 1994). With some cancer family syndromes such as the Li-Fraumeni syndrome, which is linked to alterations in the *p53* gene, individuals in affected families have an increased risk of developing a wide variety of cancers. With regard to brain tumors, germline *p53* mutations have been found to be more frequent in patients with gliomas, multifocal gliomas, or a family history of cancer. Further research is under way to determine the frequency of *p53* mutations and whether specific *p53* mutations correlate with certain environmental exposures. Studies of frequencies of alterations in other important cell cycle regulator genes such as *p16*, *RB*, and *MDM2* are also being conducted.

Although familial cancer aggregation suggests a genetic etiology, common exposure to environmental agents may also contribute to the induction of brain tumors in families. Significant familial aggregation of brain tumors and of brain tumors with other cancers has been reported in some studies but not others, and the relative risk of brain tumors has ranged from nearly 1 to 9 (Bondy et al, 1994; Wrensch et al, 1997). The fact that some studies have revealed a higher than expected frequency of siblings with brain tumors supports a genetic etiology; however, studies of twins have not supported this idea.

It seems likely that most familial brain tumors are associated with gene–environment interactions in which susceptible individuals develop cancer after exposure to endogenous or exogenous carcinogenic agents. The term "genetic susceptibility" is often used to refer to relatively common genetic alterations that influence metabolism, carcinogenesis, and DNA stability and repair; these alterations are distinguished from the highly penetrant genes, which are rare alterations that lead to genetic predisposition to a disease. The role of genetic polymorphisms (i.e., alternative states of genes established in the population) in modulating susceptibility to carcinogenic exposures has been explored in some detail for tobacco-related cancers but much less so for other cancer types, including gliomas. Recent advances in genetic technology have allowed the inclusion of potentially relevant polymorphisms in large-scale epidemiologic evaluations of brain tumors. In particular, studies of polymorphisms in cytochrome p450 (*CYP2D6*) and glutathione transferase θ (*GSTT1*) have started to reveal an increased risk for gliomas and a few other brain tumor types.

Because it is unlikely that any single polymorphism would predict risk for a substantial proportion of patients, researchers are developing panels of possibly relevant polymorphic genes to integrate with epidemiologic data. It is hoped that such an approach may help clarify the role of genetic polymorphisms in brain tumor risk.

Ionizing and Non-ionizing Radiation

Ionizing Radiation

Therapeutic ionizing radiation is the only established environmental risk factor for brain tumors. Relatively low doses (1.5 Gy) used to treat ringworm of the scalp (tinea capitis) and skin hemangioma in children and infants have been associated with an increased risk for nerve sheath tumors, meningiomas, and gliomas. An increased risk of adult-onset gliomas has been shown for people who had received radiotherapy for acute lymphoblastic leukemia as children. In addition, an elevated risk of subsequent primary or recurrent brain tumors has been observed after radiotherapy for childhood cancer other than leukemia. Results from preliminary studies have suggested that the ability to repair DNA and the predisposition to cancer are related to differences in sensitivity to γ-radiation. Clearly, much work remains to be done to establish the importance of sensitivity to radiation exposure to the risk of developing gliomas. However, it is conceivable that individuals sensitive to γ-radiation have an increased risk for developing brain tumors.

Other types of radiation exposure have been consistently suspected but not consistently implicated in brain tumor risk. For example, parental exposure to ionizing radiation before conception of the affected child has not been shown to be a risk factor for childhood brain tumors, and findings for *in utero* exposure have been mixed. Diagnostic radiation exposures (medical or dental) have not been shown to play any appreciable role in the development of gliomas but could be involved in the development of meningiomas. Working in nuclear facilities and materials production has been suspected to slightly increase the risk for brain tumors; however, no specific radiation or chemical exposures have been implicated. Inconsistent reports of increased mortality from brain tumors among airline pilots point to a potential role for cosmic radiation at high altitude in the formation of brain tumors.

Electromagnetic Fields

Widespread interest in the potential health effects of electromagnetic fields stems from residential studies that have shown an increased risk of brain tumors and leukemia in children living in homes with higher exposure to electromagnetic fields. Occupational studies of workers have also indicated higher brain tumor mortality and incidence among presumably exposed workers. Although a causal connection between electromagnetic fields and brain tumors has not been established, neither has the effect of electromagnetic fields on the risk of brain tumors been definitively disproven.

Cellular Telephones

Considerable concern over the health effects of using cellular telephones has prompted studies of whether the use of such phones influences the risk of developing brain tumors. Several recent studies were unable to detect any meaningful or significant association between the use of analog cell phones and the risk of brain tumor. Additional studies may be needed to determine whether any risks are possible from digital cell phone use. Previous studies could not consider the long-term effects of cell phone use nor the effects of long-term cell phone use, or whether some small proportion of users might be especially susceptible to developing brain tumors from cell phone use. The International Agency for

Research on Cancer is the lead institute in the European INTERPHONE Group that studies associations between cell phone use and brain tumors. A recent study from this group showed that regular use of a cell phone over 10 years was associated with a 4-fold increased risk of acoustic neuromas but not other types of brain tumors (Lonn et al, 2004). Most other study findings thus far have been negative, but cell phone use is still a public health concern because of its widespread and increasing usage.

Occupational Exposure

People can be exposed to a wide range of potentially carcinogenic chemical, physical, or biologic agents in their workplace. Despite the likelihood that brain tumors arise from specific workplace exposures, no definitive links have been made even with known or strongly suspected carcinogens. Although animal studies have suggested many likely candidates, pinpointing culprits in occupational studies is especially difficult because workers are rarely exposed to only a single hazardous substance and because agents might interact with each other to increase or decrease risk. Also, there are often only a few cases of brain tumors even in large occupational cohort studies. This limitation precludes the subgroup analyses that would be necessary to identify harmful chemicals, physical agents, work processes, or interactions. A limited understanding of the basic natural history and pathogenesis of brain tumors, such as the latency period between exposure and development of clinical disease, also hinders efforts to establish specific causes.

Because of these limitations and inconsistent findings from epidemiologic studies, controversy exists for occupations and industries that have shown a slightly positive or significantly positive association with the risk of brain tumors. Several industries associated with the use of potential and known carcinogenic compounds have not been consistently associated with an increased risk for brain tumors. The use of some pesticides and other agricultural chemicals has been associated with as much as a 3-fold increased risk among applicators but not among workers manufacturing these compounds. The reported increased risk of brain tumors for synthetic rubber production and processing workers and for polyvinyl chloride production workers has also varied depending on the study. Most studies have shown an increased risk of brain tumor mortality among petrochemical and oil refinery workers of 20% to 80%, but the increases have not been statistically significant. The absence of statistical significance could be due to small numbers of cases, and the positive findings in individual studies may simply be due to chance. Even so, the general consistency of findings (despite the low statistical power and likely nondifferential exposure misclassification, both of which would tend to conceal true associations) and the multiple, possibly carcinogenic exposures support arguments favoring a true causal connection.

Parental Occupational Exposure

Parental occupational exposures might increase the risk of cancer in children. Exposures may alter the father's DNA before conception, or prenatal maternal exposures might directly affect the developing fetus. However, no definitive evidence of the importance of fetal or postnatal infant exposure has emerged, and results from studies of prenatal and postnatal maternal exposures have been inconsistent. A risk of childhood brain tumors has been reported to be associated with paternal work with (or in industries of) oil or chemical refining; paper and pulp; solvents; painting, printing, or graphic arts; metallurgy; aerospace industry; farming in general; and pig farming, chicken farming, grain farming, horticulture, pesticides, or contact with horses. For farming exposures, postnatal exposures may be as relevant or more relevant than prenatal exposures because study results have been strongest for subjects who grew up on a farm and whose parents had farming exposures.

Lifestyle Factors

Epidemiologic studies of diet and of tobacco and alcohol use experience problems with obtaining accurate measurements of exposures to extremely common and widespread compounds. In addition, assessing each compound's individual effects is difficult because exposure to several compounds, especially in the diet, is unavoidable.

Diet

The potential mechanisms for the carcinogenic effects of N-nitroso compounds in the brain have been examined. Childhood brain tumors could be due to prenatal or postnatal exposures to these compounds. It also is possible that prenatal or early childhood exposures could increase the risk of adult-onset tumors, but very little is known about the latency of brain tumor development. About half of human exposures to N-nitroso compounds come from endogenous digestive processes; however, exogenous sources such as tobacco smoke, cosmetics, and auto interiors also contribute to these exposures. An added complication is that some sources, such as vegetables that are high in nitrites, also contain vitamins that may block the formation of N-nitroso compounds. Some study results of dietary N-nitroso compounds support their association with brain tumors in both children and adults. Greater consumption of cured foods and lower consumption of fruits and vegetables or vitamins that might block nitrosation have been observed among individuals with brain tumors (or their mothers) than among control subjects. However, these findings are also consistent with other hypotheses regarding oxidative burden and antioxidant protection. Selection bias favoring the participation of control subjects with "healthier" diets could falsely accentuate case-control differences. In addition, inherent difficulties in accurate dietary assessment often cause misclassification of exposures and tend to obscure any true differences between cases and controls.

Vitamin supplementation during pregnancy may be protective against PNETs, astroglial tumors, and other brain tumors. The observation that maternal dietary folate might protect against PNETs suggests the continuing need to develop and pursue fresh or understudied hypotheses about brain tumor etiology. To investigate the individual variation in response to environmental toxins, new studies are examining polymorphisms in genes involved in oxidative metabolism and carcinogen detoxification in addition to assessing environmental exposures.

Tobacco and Alcohol Use

Epidemiologic studies of cancer are often concerned with the use of tobacco and alcohol as potential carcinogenic agents. Although cigarette smoke is a major environmental source of carcinogens, including polycyclic hydrocarbons and N-nitroso compounds, studies of smoking and adulthood or childhood brain tumors have generally shown no evidence of an important association. However, some studies have suggested an increased risk of brain tumors from smoking unfiltered cigarettes. Maternal alcohol consumption, although perhaps associated with impaired cognitive development in offspring, seems to have little if any role in the offspring's risk of brain tumors. Few studies have shown an increased risk among children prenatally exposed to alcohol; only 1 study has produced significant results. On the other hand, results for adults have suggested a decreased risk for gliomas with consumption of wine. Much more research is needed on lifestyle factors that modulate the risk of developing brain tumors.

Medical History and Medication Use

Head Trauma and Seizure

Serious head trauma has been suspected as a cause of some types of brain tumors, especially meningiomas and acoustic neuromas, but not gliomas. An increased prevalence of birth trauma or other head injury has been reported for children with brain tumors compared with control children; however, differential recall of head injuries by individuals or mothers of these children and by mothers of control children lessens the confidence in a possible causal association. To minimize this source of bias, investigators are restricting their studies to severe, memorable injuries or are using control groups of subjects who are likely to recall events similar to the cases. An increased risk of brain tumors has been linked to a history of seizure in several studies involving persons with epilepsy. However, the determination of temporality for causation is problematic because it is difficult to determine whether the seizures were due to the tumor or whether the tumor was due to the seizures or the medications used to control them.

Medications

Little is known about the effects of most medications on the risk of brain tumors. Nonsignificant protective associations have been observed for headache, sleep, and pain medications. Diuretics and antihistamines have been associated with a nonsignificantly increased risk of meningiomas but have showed either the opposite or no effect for adulthood gliomas. Prenatal exposures to fertility drugs, oral contraceptives, sleeping pills or tranquilizers, barbiturates, pain medications, antihistamines, neuroactive drugs, and diuretics have been examined in relation to the risk of childhood brain tumors, but very few significant or consistent findings have been observed. One class of drugs that should be assessed for risk of brain tumors is nonsteroidal anti-inflammatory drugs, which are known to be protective against other tumor types.

Infectious Agents and Immunologic Response

Several types of viruses, including retroviruses, polyomaviruses, and adenoviruses, cause brain tumors in experimental animals, but with the exception of studies of HIV-related brain lymphomas, few epidemiologic studies have addressed the potential role of viruses in causing human brain malignancies (reviewed in Minn et al, 2002; Wrensch et al, 2002).

The possible roles of viruses and other infectious agents in causing human brain tumors have not been adequately investigated despite decades of calls for more research in this area. The paucity of studies in this area is likely due to the difficulties in designing meaningful studies and the limited availability of qualified investigators with sufficient cross training or experience to design and conduct such studies. Studies of the effects of SV40-contaminated polio vaccine on cancer incidence have found unconvincing results of an association with brain tumors. With regard to the varicella-zoster virus, the agent for chickenpox and shingles, 1 study found that more mothers of children with medulloblastomas than control mothers were exposed to chickenpox during pregnancy, while another study did not. Other research showed that adults with gliomas in the San Francisco Bay area were significantly less likely than control subjects to report having had either chickenpox or shingles. This observation was supported by serologic evidence indicating that case subjects were less likely than control subjects to have antibodies against the varicella-zoster virus.

Toxoplasma gondii is a parasitic agent that has been investigated with regard to human tumors, at least partly because it is capable of causing gliomas in experimentally exposed animals (reviewed in Wrensch 1993; Berleur 1995). Although 1 study convincingly linked astrocytomas with the presence of antibodies against *Toxoplasma gondii*, a more recent study found an association of this parasite with meningiomas but not with gliomas.

Other studies have shown that people with brain cancer are less likely than control subjects to report allergies and common infections. Therefore, further study of the role of common infections and allergies in preventing brain tumors may be warranted.

KEY PRACTICE POINTS

- Increasing trends in the incidence of brain tumors, especially among the elderly and children, seem largely due to advances in diagnostic technologies (i.e., computed tomography and magnetic resonance imaging).
- Sex differences exist for certain types of tumors. Neuroepithelial tumors are more prevalent in men, whereas meningiomas are more prevalent in women.
- For all brain tumor types, survival rates decrease dramatically with increasing age at diagnosis.
- Molecular, rather than traditional histologic, categorization of tumors may create more homogeneous groups of patients amenable to individualized treatment.
- Studies of genetic polymorphisms and brain tumor risk point to multiple genetic alterations enhanced by gene–environment interactions as factors that increase the risk of brain tumors.
- Exposure to ionizing radiation is the only established risk factor for brain tumors. Larger studies of other environmental factors are needed to clarify their roles in brain tumor development.
- The potential associations of common medications and infections with brain tumor development need to be further investigated.

SUGGESTED READINGS

Aldape KD, Okcu MF, Bondy ML, Wrensch M. Molecular epidemiology of glioblastoma. *Cancer J* 2003;9:99–106.

American Cancer Society. *Cancer Facts and Figures—2006*. Atlanta, GA: American Cancer Society; 2006.

Berleur MP, Cordier S. The role of chemical, physical, or viral exposures and health factors in neurocarcinogenesis: implications for epidemiologic studies of brain tumors. *Cancer Causes Control* 1995;6:240–256.

Bondy M, Wiencke J, Wrensch M, Kyritsis AP. Genetics of primary brain tumors: a review. *J Neurooncol* 1994;18:69–81.

Central Brain Tumor Registry of the United States. *Statistical Report: Primary Brain Tumors in the United States, 1998–2002*. Hinsdale, IL: CBTRUS; 2005. Available at: http://www.cbtrus.org/reports/reports.html.

Counsell CE, Grant R. Incidence studies of primary and secondary intracranial tumors: a systematic review of their methodology and results. *J Neurooncol* 1998;37:241–250.

Davis FG, McCarthy BJ. Epidemiology of brain tumors. *Curr Opin Neurol* 2000;13:635–640.

Davis FG, McCarthy BJ. Current epidemiological trends and surveillance issues in brain tumors. *Expert Rev Anticancer Ther* 2001;1:395–401.

Devesa SS, Grauman DG, Blot WJ, Pennello G, Hoover RN, Fraumeni JF Jr. *Atlas of Cancer Mortality in the United States, 1950–1994*. Washington, DC: National Institutes of Health, National Cancer Institute; 1999.

El-Zein R, Bondy M, Wrensch M. Epidemiology of brain tumors. In: Ali-Osman F, ed. *Contemporary Cancer Research: Brain Tumors*. Totowa, NJ: Humana Press; 2002:3–18.

Gurney JG, Kadan-Lottick N. Brain and other central nervous system tumors: rates, trends, and epidemiology. *Curr Opin Oncol* 2001;13:160–166.

Inskip PD, Linet MS, Heineman EF. Etiology of brain tumors in adults. *Epidemiol Rev* 1995;17:382–414.

Jemal A, Murray T, Ward E, et al. Cancer statistics, 2005. *CA Cancer J Clin* 2005;55:10–30.

Lonn S, Ahlbom A, Hall P, Feychting M. Mobile phone use and the risk of acoustic neuromas. *Epidemiology* 2004;15:653–659.

Lusis E, Gutmann DH. Meningioma: an update. *Curr Opin Neurol* 2004;17:687–692.

Minn Y, Wrensch M, Bondy ML. Epidemiology of primary brain tumors. In: Prados M, ed. *Atlas of Clinical Oncology: Brain Cancer*. Hamilton, Ontario: BC Decker; 2002:1–15.

Preston-Martin S, Mack W. Neoplasms of the nervous system. In: Schottenfeld D, Fraumeni JF, eds. *Cancer Epidemiology and Prevention*. 2nd ed. New York, NY: Oxford University Press; 1996:1231–1281.

Surawicz TS, McCarthy BJ, Kupelian V, Jukich PJ, Bruner JM, Davis FG. Descriptive epidemiology of primary brain and CNS tumors: results from the Central Brain Tumor Registry of the United States, 1990–1994. *Neurooncology* 1999;1:14–25.

Wrensch M, Bondy ML, Wiencke J, et al. Environmental risk factors for primary malignant brain tumors: a review. *J Neurooncol* 1993;17:47–64.

Wrensch M, Lee M, Miike R, et al. Familial and personal medical history of cancer and nervous system conditions among adults with glioma and controls. *Am J Epidemiol* 1997;145:581–593.

Wrensch M, Minn Y, Chew T, Bondy M, Berger MS. Epidemiology of primary brain tumors: current concepts and review of the literature. *Neurooncology* 2002;4:278–299.

2   NEUROPATHOLOGY AND MOLECULAR BIOLOGY OF INTRACRANIAL TUMORS

Gregory N. Fuller and Kenneth D. Aldape

Chapter Overview 23
Introduction 24
Cornerstones of Clinical Oncologic Neuropathology 24
    Knowledge of Normal Morphology 24
    Knowledge of Disease Morphology 25
    Knowledge of the Patient's Clinical Information 25
        Anatomic Location of the Lesion 25
        Neuroimaging Features 26
        Type and Duration of Clinical Signs and Symptoms 26
Handling of Biopsy Tissue During Intraoperative Consultation 26
    Preparation of Cytologic Specimens 26
    Preparation of Frozen Tissue Sections 27
    Preparation of Formalin-Fixed, Paraffin-Embedded Tissue Sections 28
    Preparation of Tissue for Ultrastructural Examination 28
Immunocytochemical Studies in Oncologic Neuropathology 28
    New Immunohistochemical Markers 28
    Proliferation Markers 29
New Tumor Entities 29
Molecular Biologic Studies in Oncologic Neuropathology 30
    Molecular Testing of Oligodendroglial Tumors for Deletion Status
    of Chromosome Arms 1p and 19q 30
    Molecular Testing of Glioblastomas for *MGMT* Promoter
    Methylation Status 31
    Molecular Testing of Glioblastomas for *EGFR* Alterations 31
Sources of Error in the Interpretation of Brain Tumor Histopathology 31
Conclusion 33
Key Practice Points 34
Suggested Readings 35

CHAPTER OVERVIEW

More than 120 types of primary brain tumor have been recognized and codified by the World Health Organization. As part of the patient's clinical team, the neuropathologist identifies the tumor type and grade. Contemporary oncologic neuropathology uses a broad array of morphologic, immunohistochemical, and molecular biologic techniques to accomplish this task. Knowledge of normal morphology, disease morphology, and the patient's clinical information (including age, relevant clinical history, location of the lesion, neuroimaging features of the lesion, and type and duration of the presenting symptoms) are prerequisites for competent histopathologic diagnosis of brain and spine tumors. The neuropathologist must stay abreast of developments in this dynamic field because new tumor types, diagnostic antibodies, and molecular tests are being introduced into the practice of surgical neuropathology with increasing frequency.

INTRODUCTION

At M. D. Anderson Cancer Center, the neuropathologist works closely with other members of the clinical team to deliver the best possible care for patients with brain tumors. The neuropathologist uses morphologic, immunohistochemical, and molecular biologic techniques to identify tumor types and grades. The increasing use of molecular genetic evaluation of tumors is rapidly changing the practice of clinical oncologic neuropathology.

CORNERSTONES OF CLINICAL ONCOLOGIC NEUROPATHOLOGY

The competent diagnosis of central nervous system (CNS) lesions relies on knowledge of normal morphology, knowledge of disease morphology, and knowledge of the patient's clinical information. Familiarity with these 3 cornerstones is critical not only for facilitating an accurate diagnosis but also for avoiding the common pitfalls and the subsequent adverse sequelae of misdiagnosis.

Knowledge of Normal Morphology

Accurate identification of the abnormal is predicated on a thorough knowledge of the normal. Normal microscopic morphology of the CNS includes not only the hematoxylin and eosin (H&E)-stained, immunocytochemical, and ultrastructural features of various cell types (Table 2–1) but also the specialized regional histology seen throughout the CNS. The most salient regions include the pituitary gland, pineal gland, choroid plexus, olfactory bulbs and tracts, optic nerves and their meningeal coverings, lumbar cistern and its contents, circumventricular organs, and cerebellopontine angle. Several reference works are available to those who seek to become more fully conversant in normal neurohistology (see Suggested Readings).

Table 2–1. Unique Cell Types of the CNS

Neuron	Choroid plexus cell
Microglial cell	Arachnoid cell
Astrocyte	Melanocyte
Ependymal cell	Pineocyte
Oligodendrocyte	Pituicyte

Knowledge of Disease Morphology

More than 120 types of primary tumor of the brain and meninges have been recognized by the World Health Organization. The neuropathologist must be familiar with the different entities and the broad range of morphologic variations that each tumor may assume. Many of these variants have not been formally classified by the World Health Organization, but the neuropathologist must be able to recognize them. An important example of such morphologic variation is seen in glioblastoma, for which there are at least 10 morphologic variants: giant cell, small cell, spindle cell, bland cell, myxoid, epithelioid, inflammatory, lipid rich, rhabdoid, and gliosarcoma.

Knowledge of the Patient's Clinical Information

It is critical that the neuropathologist be familiar with the patient's clinical information before rendering a diagnosis. Essential clinical information includes the anatomic location of the lesion, the neuroimaging characteristics of the lesion, and the type and duration of clinical signs and symptoms that lead to clinical presentation. The patient's age and relevant clinical history (e.g., history of CNS or systemic malignancy) must also be known. Each of these factors affects the neuropathologist's formulation of the differential diagnosis before surgery as well as the final diagnosis that follows the thorough evaluation of the histopathologic, immunophenotypic, and clinical features of the lesion.

Anatomic Location of the Lesion

Knowledge of the anatomic location of the lesion is very important. For example, a solitary mass located in the lumbar cistern is most likely a schwannoma, meningioma, myxopapillary ependymoma, or paraganglioma of the filum terminale. Similarly, specific tumors are the most likely possibilities for a mass located in the lateral ventricle, the cerebellopontine angle, and many other specific neuroanatomic regions. The anatomic relationship of the lesion to intracranial structural compartments can also provide useful diagnostic information. For example, the differential diagnosis for an extra-axial, dural-based mass may include specific mesenchymal and hematopoietic tumors as well as several nonneoplastic entities.

Neuroimaging Features

The neuropathologist is not expected to match the expertise of radiologists in interpretating neuroimaging studies. However, the neuropathologist must be aware of the major features of the patient's preoperative magnetic resonance (MR) images, computed tomographic images, and special imaging studies, which can be obtained from the radiologist's reports and, whenever possible, from direct examination of the imaging studies.

Type and Duration of Clinical Signs and Symptoms

For the neuropathologist's purposes, the type and duration of clinical signs and symptoms can often be simplified as acute (e.g., headache, nausea, vomiting, incoordination, visual disturbance, or paresis) or chronic (e.g., seizure). A long-standing history of chronic symptoms tends to indicate a more indolent lesion than acute-onset presentation does.

HANDLING OF BIOPSY TISSUE DURING INTRAOPERATIVE CONSULTATION

The intraoperative review of biopsy samples sent for frozen section is one of the most important tasks performed by the surgical pathologist. Proper tissue handling is particularly crucial at this stage of the patient's care. For almost all tumors, regardless of the sample size (e.g., obtained by stereotactic biopsy, partial resection, or lobectomy), 3 types of specimens are prepared: cytologic specimens, frozen tissue sections, and permanent formalin-fixed, paraffin-embedded tissue sections. In some instances, it is also prudent to place a small representative piece of tissue in glutaraldehyde for possible ultrastructural examination.

Preparation of Cytologic Specimens

Cytologic specimens prepared during intraoperative consultation can be very helpful. The cytologic preparation, which uses fixation in 95% ethanol, yields exquisite cytoplasmic and nuclear detail that is free of the distortion produced by freezing.

One of 4 cytologic preparation techniques can be used, depending on the type and consistency of the tumor (Table 2–2). For a suspected pituitary adenoma, the procedure of choice is always the touch (also called imprint) preparation. This procedure takes advantage of the differentially greater shedding by adenomas than by the normal adenohypophysis, the cells of which are tightly packaged by fibrovascular septa that adenomas lack. By taking advantage of the differential adhesion of various cell types of the tumor ex vivo, the squash (also called smear or crush) preparation can be very informative for the vast majority of intra-axial brain tumors,

Table 2–2.   Rapid Intraoperative Cytologic Techniques

Technique	Tumor Tissue Characteristics	Representative Tumors
Touch (imprint) preparation	Soft and discohesive	Pituitary adenoma, lymphoma, melanoma
Squash (smear, crush) preparation	Soft or friable	Glioma, metastatic carcinoma
Scrape preparation	Dense, hard, rubbery, or desmoplastic	Desmoplastic primary tumor, dural metastasis, some meningiomas
Drag preparation	Necrotic or cauterized	Extensively necrotic metastasis

including gliomas and metastases. Scrape preparations are used for densely desmoplastic or fibrous tumors, such as many dural metastases and paraspinal tumors, which do not squash or smear very well and tend to show mostly red blood cells on touch preparations. In the scrape procedure, a scalpel is used to repeatedly scrape the cut surface of the tissue, and the material thus collected on the scalpel blade is then smeared onto a glass slide. The drag preparation is useful for extensively necrotic tumors for which a single frozen section or squash preparation is likely to show only nonspecific necrosis. In this procedure, as large an area as possible of the resected tissue is sampled for the potential presence of small remaining clusters of viable tumor cells. Multiple necrotic tissue fragments, one after another, are rapidly dragged with forceps across the same glass slide. This technique maximizes the chance of detecting isolated viable tumor cell clusters in an otherwise overwhelmingly necrotic tissue sample while avoiding the time, labor, and expense of freezing an entire Petri dish of tissue fragments.

For the fixation and staining of cytologic preparations, the preferred approach is rapid fixation with no air-drying artifact in 95% ethanol, H&E staining, and coverslipping with permanent mounting medium. As an alternative or in addition, a 1-step DiffQuick stain with water coverslipping can be used for a quick "first look."

Preparation of Frozen Tissue Sections

Depending on the procedures in place at the neuropathologist's hospital and frozen section laboratory, some representative tumor tissue may be snap frozen in liquid nitrogen for archiving in the tissue bank. If diagnostic tissue is present in the frozen section block, this sample can be stored frozen in the tissue bank rather than processed into paraffin.

In contrast to cytologic preparations, which provide cytoplasmic and nuclear detail, frozen sections provide a snapshot of the architectural features of the tissue. Thus, the cytologic and frozen tissue section preparations reveal unique morphologic information and complement each other.

Preparation of Formalin-Fixed, Paraffin-Embedded Tissue Sections

This technique is standard in all U.S. pathology laboratories and typically involves immersion in 10% formalin for fixation and then automated enclosure in a paraffin block for long-term storage. Not all immunostains work on tissue processed in this way, and antibodies to new antigenic targets should always be validated by comparing their reactivity against frozen sections of similar tissue.

Preparation of Tissue for Ultrastructural Examination

It is sometimes prudent to place a representative piece of tissue in glutaraldehyde for possible ultrastructural examination (i.e., electron microscopy). If glutaraldehyde fixative is not available, the next best approach is to retain some tissue in formalin without processing it into paraffin; procedures are available for "postfixing" wet tissue in formalin for electron microscopy. Ultrastructural examination of tissue retrieved from paraffin blocks may also be warranted in some circumstances, but this procedure yields the poorest results.

One of the most common procedures for which tissue is placed "on hold" in glutaraldehyde is spinal cord biopsy. The 2 most common tumors of the spinal cord are diffuse astrocytoma and ependymoma. In very small biopsy samples (which spinal cord biopsy samples tend to be), it may be difficult to distinguish these 2 tumor types on H&E-stained tissue sections if the characteristic perivascular pseudorosettes of ependymoma are not seen in the limited amount of tissue available for examination. Immunohistochemical analysis conducted with currently available differentiation marker antibodies cannot resolve the issue because both tumor types are gliomas, which typically show immunoreactivity for the glial markers S-100 protein and glial fibrillary acidic protein. In contrast, the hallmark ultrastructural features of extensive intercellular junctional complexes and lumens filled with microvilli and cilia are characteristic of ependymoma but not astrocytoma.

IMMUNOCYTOCHEMICAL STUDIES IN
ONCOLOGIC NEUROPATHOLOGY

New Immunohistochemical Markers

New immunohistochemical markers of potential clinical utility are constantly being introduced. These markers can be loosely categorized as "homegrown" monoclonal and polyclonal antibodies generated by research laboratories, as commercially available antibodies that are not easy to use or have not been adequately independently validated, or as commercially available antibodies that perform well and have been independently verified by multiple experienced laboratories as markers that contribute useful

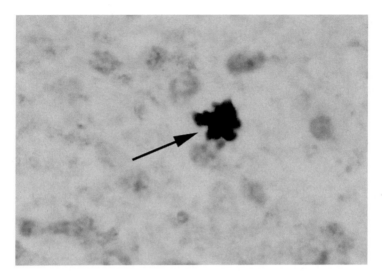

Figure 2–1. Commercially available antibody directed against pHH3 facilitates rapid identification and quantitation of mitotic figures (arrow) (pHH3 immunostain with hematoxylin counterstain, original magnification × 400).

diagnostic or prognostic information. Examples of the latter category of recently introduced markers relevant to oncologic neuropathology are the anti-INI1/hSNF5/SMARCB1/BAF47 antibody for atypical teratoid/ rhabdoid tumors and the anti-OCT4 antibody for germinoma.

Proliferation Markers

Currently, the most widely used proliferation marker is the Ki-67 antigen, for which there is a commercially available antibody (MIB-1) that works well in formalin-fixed, paraffin-embedded tissue. An increasingly popular class of proliferation markers, as typified by anti-phosphohistone H3 (pHH3) antibody, essentially functions as mitotic figure immunostains (Figure 2–1). Immunostaining for pHH3 has several advantages over traditional mitotic figure quantitation using H&E-stained tissue sections, including the unambiguous identification of mitoses based on the combination of chromogenic reaction product and morphologic features of mitotic figures and the greatly expedited microscopic review secondary to the ease of mitotic figure identification.

New Tumor Entities

Brain tumor classification is not a static field. In addition to the increasing contributions of molecular and genomic testing to the refinement of

Table 2–3.   Brain Tumor Types Newly Described In the Past 30 Years

Tumor Type	Year Described
Pleomorphic xanthoastrocytoma	1979
Central neurocytoma	1982
Dysembryoplastic neuroepithelial tumor	1988
Chordoid glioma	1988
Papillary glioneuronal tumor	1988–1989
Rosetted glioneuronal tumor	1988–1989
Pilomyxoid astrocytoma	1999
Rosette-forming glioneuronal tumor of the fourth ventricle	2002
Papillary tumor of the pineal region	2003
Monomorphous angiocentric bipolar glioma	2005

tumor stratification within long-standing brain tumor categories, new tumor entities are periodically identified. Ten types of brain tumor newly described in the past 30 years are listed in Table 2–3.

MOLECULAR BIOLOGIC STUDIES IN ONCOLOGIC NEUROPATHOLOGY

The 3 most common molecular or cytogenetic markers being studied as potential prognostic or diagnostic markers are chromosome arms 1p and 19q deletion status, O^6-methylguanine-DNA methyltransferase (*MGMT*) promoter methylation status, and epidermal growth factor receptor (*EGFR*) gene amplification or overexpression. Other potential markers are chromosome arms 9p and 10q deletion status and *EGFRvIII*, *PTEN*, *TP53*, and *P16^{INK4a}* amplification, overexpression, or mutation.

Molecular Testing of Oligodendroglial Tumors for Deletion Status of Chromosome Arms 1p and 19q

Over the past 7 years, studies have shown that the combined deletion of chromosome arms 1p and 19q predicts an increased response to chemotherapy and radiotherapy for both low-grade and high-grade oligodendrogliomas, thereby resulting in increased recurrence-free survival rates. Initial reports that this combined loss is predictive of response to chemotherapy in particular have been revised with additional experience. The current thinking is that this molecular signature is predictive of a more treatment-responsive tumor in general.

Several methods are available for testing the deletion status of a chromosome, including conventional loss of heterozygosity, fluorescence in situ hybridization, and quantitative microsatellite analysis. Additional details are provided in the resources listed in Suggested Readings. Because fluorescence in situ hybridization has several advantages, it is the preferred method of deletion testing at many institutions.

Molecular Testing of Glioblastomas for *MGMT* Promoter Methylation Status

Recent studies have demonstrated a correlation between gene silencing of *MGMT* through methylation of its promoter and response to temozolomide chemotherapy in patients with glioblastomas. As of this writing, this finding has not been independently confirmed, and *MGMT* promoter methylation testing as a means to determine therapy for the individual patient awaits validation.

Molecular Testing of Glioblastomas for *EGFR* Alterations

The recent finding that *EGFR* alterations are predictive of response to anti-EGFR therapies in patients with lung cancer has spurred interest in whether *EGFR* amplification in glioblastomas is predictive of response to those therapies. To date, there is no evidence that *EGFR* aberrations in gliomas are associated with response to targeted therapies; additional information is required for a definitive answer. Nevertheless, the fact that *EGFR* amplification is essentially restricted to glioblastoma has a diagnostic application. Occasional cases are encountered in which high-grade features (e.g., marked hypercellularity and prominent mitotic activity) are present but the requisite diagnostic criteria (i.e., microvascular proliferation and tumor necrosis) for glioblastoma are lacking in the tissue available for examination. In such cases, strong EGFR positivity suggests that the tumor will exhibit the clinical behavior typical of glioblastoma.

SOURCES OF ERROR IN THE INTERPRETATION OF BRAIN TUMOR HISTOPATHOLOGY

Almost all diagnostic mistakes made in surgical neuropathology fall under at least 1 of the 10 major categories of error (Table 2–4). There are many different examples of each type of error, and active awareness of the various sources of diagnostic error goes a long way toward preventing their occurrence.

A common source of serious diagnostic error that warrants specific mention is overgrading (i.e., misdiagnosing a circumscribed low-grade tumor as a high-grade tumor), which can lead to inappropriate therapy. Table 2–5 lists the most common circumscribed low-grade tumors of the CNS, which typically show little infiltration of the surrounding brain parenchyma and are often initially treated with surgical resection alone. The neuropathologist should be familiar with the clinicopathologic

Table 2–4. Categories of Diagnostic Error in Interpreting Brain Tumor Histopathology

Mistaking normal structures for pathologic processes
Mistaking nonneoplastic diseases for tumors
Mistaking one tumor type for another
Not recognizing common tumors arising in uncommon locations
Not being familiar with rare tumor types
Not being familiar with recently described tumor types
Being misled by sample preparation artifacts
Not recognizing inadequate or nonrepresentative biopsy samples
Not performing appropriate diagnostic procedures
Not formulating an appropriate differential diagnosis

Table 2–5. The Most Common Circumscribed Low-Grade Tumors of the CNS

Pilocytic astrocytoma
Pleomorphic xanthoastrocytoma
Subependymal giant cell astrocytoma
Desmoplastic cerebral astrocytoma of infancy
Chordoid glioma of the third ventricle
Circumscribed and dorsally exophytic brain stem gliomas
Myxopapillary ependymoma
Subependymoma
Dysplastic gangliocytoma of the cerebellum
Central neurocytoma
Cerebellar liponeurocytoma
Paraganglioma of the filum terminale
Ganglioglioma
Dysembryoplastic neuroepithelial tumor
Hemangioblastoma
Papillary tumor of the pineal region

features of each of these types of circumscribed tumor, the details of which are provided in the sources listed in Suggested Readings.

Another source of diagnostic error is mistaking a nonneoplastic disease for a tumor. Mass lesions such as demyelinating pseudotumors, abscesses, infarcts, and other rare lesions can mimic neoplasms on neuroimaging scans and tissue sections. The most deceptive of these is the demyelinating pseudotumor. The principal morphologic hallmark of demyelinating disease on H&E-stained tissue sections is the presence of macrophages. The identity of these cells may not always be readily apparent because infiltrating macrophages can mimic infiltrating glioma cells. A cytologic squash preparation performed at the time of intraoperative biopsy sample consultation will usually unmask the presence of macrophages. If doubt remains, one of several commercially available immunostains for macrophages, such as anti-CD68 or anti-HAM56 antibody, may be ordered.

A third common diagnostic pitfall is nonrepresentative biopsy sampling of a high-grade diffuse glioma. By definition, diffuse gliomas infiltrate brain parenchyma and exhibit a gradient of cellularity and key diagnostic features, such as necrosis and microvascular proliferation. The latter 2 features often present only in the densely cellular areas of the tumor and are absent in the peripheral areas of sparse glioma cell infiltration. Biopsy of the latter areas will give the misleading impression of a low-grade glioma. This pitfall may be avoided by simply checking the preoperative MR images for contrast enhancement, which excludes a diagnosis of diffuse low-grade glioma. In addition, low-grade gliomas are very unusual in patients aged 60 years or older. Histologic features of low-grade glioma in a biopsy sample of an older patient, particularly in the setting of a contrast-enhanced lesion on MR images, strongly suggest that the tumor was undersampled (i.e., that the biopsy was taken from an area of the lesion that was not fully representative).

A final frequently encountered clinical scenario is a new contrast-enhanced mass lesion seen in a patient who has had a high-grade brain tumor surgically resected and who has also undergone radiotherapy. The differential diagnosis in this situation may include recurrent tumor, radiation necrosis, textiloma (i.e., gossypiboma), and postoperative abscess. These principal entities are not mutually exclusive. Glioma and radiation necrosis of brain parenchyma may coexist, or one may be overwhelmingly predominant. Textiloma is a form of pseudotumor in which there is a marked inflammatory reaction to resorbable hemostatic agents. This reaction results in striking contrast enhancement on MR images and often in clinical symptoms secondary to inflammation-related edema; all of these features mimic recurrent glioma. In modern neurosurgical practice, postoperative abscess is uncommon.

Conclusion

The role of the neuropathologist has expanded as discoveries of new ways of classifying brain tumors, on both the molecular and microscopic levels, have multiplied. A brain tumor is best assigned a diagnosis by a specialized pathologist who is trained in neuropathology and is familiar with the nuances of such classification.

KEY PRACTICE POINTS

- Because brain tumor pathology is a rapidly evolving field—new tumor types, diagnostic antibodies, and molecular diagnostic tests are constantly emerging—frequent continuing medical education in this area is essential.
- The foundation of competent histopathologic tumor diagnosis rests on knowledge of normal morphology, disease morphology, and the patient's clinical information.
- The approach to brain tumor diagnosis begins with a review of the major aspects of the patient's clinical information, including anatomic location of the lesion, preoperative neuroimaging features of the lesion, type and duration of the presenting symptoms, patient age, and relevant medical history.
- During consultation of intraoperative biopsy samples, cytologic preparations (touch, squash, scrape, or drag) can provide morphologic information that complements that provided by frozen tissue sections.
- If possible, the entire tissue specimen should not be submitted for frozen section. Some representative tissue should be saved for permanent formalin-fixed sections, which will be free of freezing artifact.
- In certain clinical situations, such as small spinal cord biopsy samples (in which astrocytomas and ependymomas cannot be distinguished with certainty on H&E-stained tissue sections), glutaraldehyde fixation and ultrastructural evaluation by electron microscopy may be required. If glutaraldehyde fixation is not available, some tumor tissue can be saved in formalin for subsequent postfixing.
- Immunohistochemical analysis, electron microscopy, fluorescence in situ hybridization, and molecular biologic studies may be required to develop a definitive diagnosis.
- The presence of histologic features of low-grade glioma in a biopsy sample from a patient aged 60 years or older, particularly in the setting of a contrast-enhanced lesion on MR images, strongly suggests undersampling of the tumor.
- If a confident diagnosis cannot be reached, a board-certified oncologic neuropathologist should be consulted.
- When expert consultation on difficult cases is being solicited, if at all possible, a compact disc with the preoperative MR images (or at least the preoperative radiology report) and a representative paraffin block or 6 to 10 unstained slides should be sent. These measures will facilitate rapid review and mitigate potential delays in consultation.
- When a patient is referred to M. D. Anderson, the tissue section slides, surgical pathology report, and preoperative neuroimaging studies with reports should be forwarded by registered postal courier well in advance of the patient's appointment.

SUGGESTED READINGS

Burger PC, Scheithauer BW. *Tumors of the Central Nervous System. AFIP Atlas of Tumor Pathology.* Series IV. Washington, DC: American Registry of Pathology; in press.

Colman H, Giannini C, Huang L, et al. Assessment and prognostic significance of mitotic index using the mitosis marker phospho-histone H3 in low and intermediate-grade infiltrating astrocytomas. *Am J Surg Pathol* 2006;30:657–664.

Fuller GN. Molecular classifications. In: Barnett GH, ed. *High-Grade Gliomas: Diagnosis and Treatment.* Current Clinical Oncology series. Totawa, NJ: Humana Press; 2006.

Fuller GN, Burger PC. Central nervous system. In: Mills SE, ed. *Histology for Pathologists.* 3rd ed. New York, NY: Raven Press; 2006.

Fuller GN, Goodman JC. *Practical Review of Neuropathology.* Philadelphia, PA: Lippincott, Williams & Wilkins; 2001.

Fuller GN, Ribalta T. Metastases. In: McLendon R, Rosenblum M, Bigner DD, eds. *Russell and Rubinstein's Pathology of Tumors of the Nervous System.* 7th ed. London, UK: Hodder Arnold; 2006.

Hegi ME, Diserens AC, Gorlia T, et al. *MGMT* gene silencing and benefit from temozolomide in glioblastoma. *N Engl J Med* 2005;352:997–1003.

Louis DN, Ohgaki H, Wiestler OD, Cavenee W, Eds., *WHO Classification of Tumours of the Central Nervous System.* Lyon, France: IARC; 2007.

McDonald JM, Colman H, Perry A, Aldape K. Molecular and clinical aspects of 1p/19q loss in oligodendroglioma. In: Zhang W, Fuller GN, eds. *Genomic and Molecular Neuro-Oncology.* Boston, MA: Jones and Bartlett; 2004:17–30.

McDonald JM, See SJ, Tremont I, et al. Prognostic impact of histology and 1p/19q status in anaplastic oligodendroglial tumors. *Cancer* 2005;104:1468–1477.

McLendon R, Rosenblum M, Bigner DD, eds. *Russell and Rubinstein's Pathology of Tumors of the Nervous System,* 7th ed. London, UK: Hodder Arnold; 2006.

Mischel PS, Cloughesy TF, Nelson SF. DNA-microarray analysis of brain cancer: molecular classification for therapy. *Nat Rev Neurosci* 2004;5:782–792.

Nigro JM, Misra A, Zhang L, et al. Integrated array-comparative genomic hybridization and expression array profiles identify clinically relevant molecular subtypes of glioblastoma. *Cancer Res* 2005;65:1678–1686.

Prayson RA. *Neuropathology.* Philadelphia, PA: Elsevier; 2005.

Ribalta T, McCutcheon IE, Aldape KD, Bruner JM, Fuller GN. The mitosis-specific antibody anti-phosphohistone-H3 (PHH3) facilitates rapid reliable grading of meningiomas according to WHO 2000 criteria. *Am J Surg Pathol* 2004;28: 1532–1536.

Ribalta T, McCutcheon IE, Neto AG, et al. Textiloma (gossypiboma) mimicking recurrent intracranial tumor. *Arch Pathol Lab Med* 2004;128:749–758.

3 RADIOLOGY OF BRAIN TUMORS: STRUCTURE AND PHYSIOLOGY

J. Matthew Debnam, Leena Ketonen,
Leena M. Hamberg, and George J. Hunter

Chapter Overview 37
Introduction 38
Computed Tomography 38
    Computed Tomography Angiography and Venography 38
    Computed Tomography Perfusion 40
Magnetic Resonance Imaging 41
    Magnetic Resonance Angiography and Venography 42
    Magnetic Resonance Spectroscopy 44
    Magnetic Resonance Perfusion Imaging 47
    Functional Magnetic Resonance Imaging 47
Positron Emission Tomography 48
Catheter Angiography 50
Key Practice Points 51
Suggested Readings 51

CHAPTER OVERVIEW

This chapter provides the practicing oncologist with a basic understanding of the current and rapidly evolving technologies used at M. D. Anderson Cancer Center to evaluate patients with cerebral neoplasms. The radiologic assessment of these intracranial neoplasms depends primarily on the features seen with magnetic resonance imaging. Other modalities, such as computed tomography and catheter angiography, also aid in the diagnostic workup, although to a lesser degree. New and developing technologies such as computed tomography and magnetic resonance angiography and venography, magnetic resonance spectroscopy, computed tomography perfusion or magnetic resonance perfusion imaging, and positron emission tomography add significant information to the evaluation of patients with cerebral neoplasms. Functional magnetic resonance imaging complements intraoperative cortical mapping in locating the eloquent cortex before surgical resection of an intracranial neoplasm. Catheter angiography is expanding into the realm of treatment for several of these intracranial lesions, including selective embolization and administration of chemotherapy.

INTRODUCTION

In neuro-oncologic imaging of the brain, several basic modalities may be used to assess brain lesions and form a differential diagnosis. These methods include computed tomography (CT), magnetic resonance imaging (MRI), and catheter angiography. Although they continue to evolve rapidly, advanced imaging techniques are used in clinical practice today, such as CT and MR angiography and venography, MR spectroscopy (MRS), diffusion-weighted MRI, CT perfusion and MR perfusion imaging, functional MRI, and positron emission tomography (PET). The use of catheter angiography is also expanding, and newer applications go beyond that of the routine diagnostic cerebral angiogram. Plain film radiography has been relegated to relatively little, if any, use in the modern era. In this chapter, we discuss the basic neuroimaging techniques, CT and MRI, and provide an introductory discussion on the more advanced techniques to give the reader insight into what we feel will soon become standard practice. The reader is referred to the list of suggested readings at the end of the chapter for more detailed discussion of these advanced techniques.

COMPUTED TOMOGRAPHY

CT has played a vital role in neuro-oncologic imaging. It is most commonly used as a screening tool in patients referred to us from the M. D. Anderson Emergency Center to assess for brain metastases and their sequelae (e.g., mass effect and herniation) and to exclude hemorrhage and other common presentations (e.g., acute stroke). CT can also be used to search for metastases in patients who are unable to undergo MRI, such as patients with pacemakers or other indwelling metallic devices. Newer techniques using CT include CT angiography, CT venography, and CT perfusion.

Computed Tomography Angiography and Venography

CT angiography and venography are quickly replacing catheter angiography in the contrast evaluation of the more proximal arterial vessels and the larger venous structures of the head and neck. The use of CT angiography and venography in this situation involves venous injection of a bolus of contrast material and thin-section imaging of the neck and brain while the contrast material fills the vascular structures. Common indications of CT angiography for oncologic patients are to exclude a proximal arterial thrombus in patients with stroke-like symptoms, to assess the arterial supply and venous drainage of the tumors (Figure 3–1), to further define the arterial anatomy in relation to the tumors (Figure 3–2), and to assess the proximal

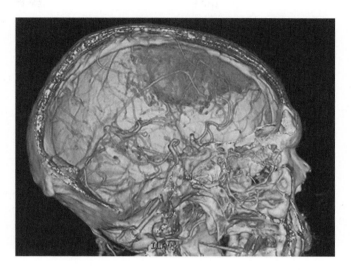

Figure 3–1. A CT angiogram (surface-shaded reconstructed image) demonstrating the vascularity of a large, left frontal meningioma.

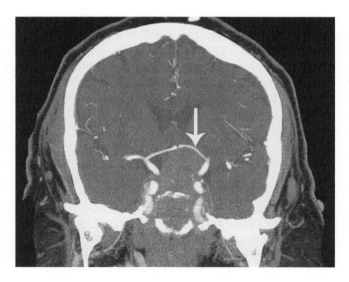

Figure 3–2. A CT angiogram (coronal plane) showing a pituitary macroadenoma with superior extension and upward displacement of the left greater than right A1 segments of the anterior cerebral artery (arrow).

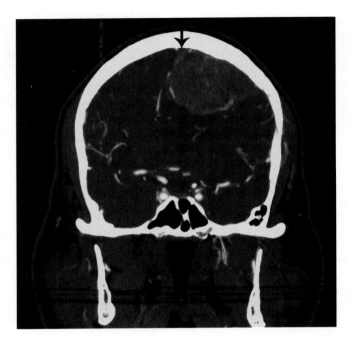

Figure 3–3. A CT venogram (coronal plane) illustrating a large meningioma invading and occluding the superior sagittal sinus, which is characterized by a lack of enhancement (arrow).

vessels in patients with entities such as vasculitis or vasospasm. In the venous system, CT venography can be used to assess the anatomy of venous structures in relation to adjacent tumors, such as a meningioma (Figure 3–3), or to exclude venous sinus thrombosis. CT angiography and venography have a major advantage over catheter angiography in that they are not invasive procedures and hence are not associated with complications such as dissection, stroke, and groin hematoma. However, CT angiography and venography are more limited in their ability to evaluate the distal arterial vessels and smaller venous structures, and therefore catheter angiography would be necessary for a complete evaluation.

Computed Tomography Perfusion

CT perfusion involves the rapid venous injection of a contrast agent through a focused volume of tissue with CT, starting before the arrival of the agent in the vessels and continuing during its initial and subsequent passages through the brain. This procedure permits calculation of physiologic parameters such as cerebral blood volume, tissue transit time, cerebral blood flow, and—of most interest to oncologists—tissue permeability, as exemplified by parameters reflecting leakage of contrast out of the vascular tree into the tumor (K1) or leakage of contrast out of the tumoral tissue back

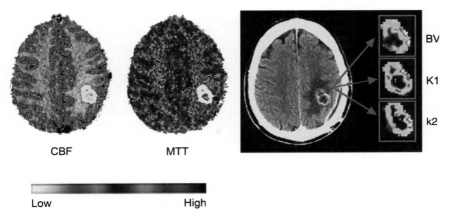

CBF   MTT

Low   High

Figure 3–4. CT perfusion images of a brain of a patient with a recurrent glioblastoma multiforme in the left parietal lobe. Normal brain has no leakage of contrast out of the blood vessels because of an intact blood-brain barrier. The tumor has leakage of contrast, and the parameters of blood volume (BV) and constants related to permeability (K1 and k2) are shown in the insets. There is measurable variability in these parameters around the tumor periphery. This recurrent lesion had central necrosis. Abbreviations: CBF, cerebral blood flow; MTT, mean transit time. Low–High scale indicates level of contrast.

into the vascular tree (k2). This technique can be used to evaluate benign and malignant intracranial and skull base tumors and to investigate the vascular pathologic features coincidentally occurring in patients with primary intracranial malignancies (Figure 3–4).

MAGNETIC RESONANCE IMAGING

MRI is the most powerful tool in neuro-oncologic radiologic practice. MR involves using a radiofrequency pulse to excite hydrogen protons within a magnetic field to elevate the protons to a higher-energy state. When the protons return to their resting, lower-energy state, they release electromagnetic energy. This energy is received by a coil, or antenna, and converted into an image. The time that it takes the hydrogen protons to return to their resting state is called the relaxation time. The relaxation time depends on the chemical composition of the tissues subjected to the pulse.

A standard MR study of the brain uses T1-weighted, fast spin-echo T2-weighted, fluid-attenuated inversion recovery (FLAIR), and diffusion-weighted imaging sequences. The T1-weighted sequence best demonstrates normal anatomy and can be performed with the intravenous contrast agent gadolinium. Gadolinium accumulates where the blood-brain barrier breaks down, which occurs in many cerebral neoplasms. The fast spin-echo T2-weighted sequence highlights tissues with a high concentration of water as a bright signal or hyperintensity. On the FLAIR sequence, the cerebrospinal fluid signal is suppressed, thereby improving lesion conspicuity, especially along the ventricular system. With the diffusion-weighted imaging sequence, the movement of protons through tissues or spaces, such as the extracellular space, is decreased and there is signal hyperintensity. Common causes of signal hyperintensity on this sequence include acute cerebral infarction and, in certain tumors such as lymphoma, dense cell packing. Decreased diffusion is also present in cerebral abscesses, which distinguishes them from centrally necrotic tumors, which do not demonstrate decreased diffusion. T1-weighted post-gadolinium sequences in 3 orthogonal directions (axial, coronal, and sagittal) are used to identify the enhancement characteristics of normal and abnormal intracranial tissue. With this sequence, tumors tend to be enhanced substantially more than normal brain does. A fifth series that we often acquire at M. D. Anderson is a gradient echo sequence, which demonstrates signal hypointensity in cases of hemorrhage, melanin, or calcification. This sequence is particularly useful in the evaluation of lesions such as hemorrhagic metastases or melanomas.

Magnetic Resonance Angiography and Venography

When assessment of the cerebral vasculature is necessary, an MR angiogram or venogram may be performed. MR angiography uses techniques that make vessels with flowing blood appear brighter than adjacent, stationary tissue. MR venography is performed using a 2-dimensional time-of-flight sequence, which samples tissues in multiple thin imaging slices. MR arteriography uses a 3-dimensional time-of-flight sequence, in which a volume of tissue is sampled to obtain the necessary data. The data from MR angiography or venography are then reconstructed into 3-dimensional images of the arterial or venous structures (Figure 3–5), similar to a conventional angiogram or venogram, by using techniques called maximum intensity projection and volume rendering. These images may be rotated to allow evaluation of the vessels from different angles. Similar to CT angiography, MR angiography and venography can assess the arterial supply and venous drainage of tumors and further define the vascular anatomy in relation to a tumor (Figure 3–6).

The major advantage that MR assessment of the cerebral arterial and venous systems has over CT angiography, especially in patients with renal failure, is that it does not require the use of radiation or iodinated contrast material. However, we prefer CT angiography and venography over MR angiography and venography because the former offer superior resolution of the vasculature and result in fewer artifacts in situations of slow flow, turbulent flow, or vessel motion.

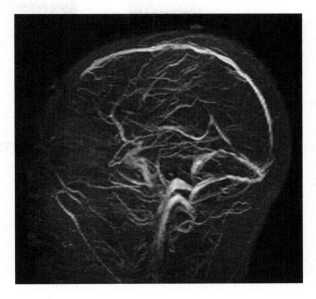

Figure 3–5. An MR venogram of normal superficial cerebral venous structures.

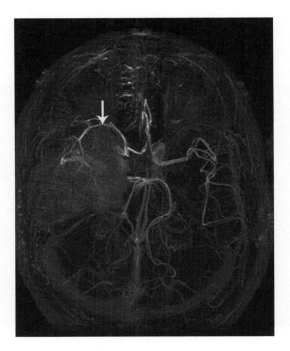

Figure 3–6. An MR angiogram showing a hemangiopericytoma in the right temporal lobe anteriorly displacing the right middle cerebral artery (arrow).

Magnetic Resonance Spectroscopy

Proton MRS is becoming a common clinical tool because it can add an important functional aspect to conventional anatomic brain imaging. MRS can distinguish normal brain tissue from abnormal tissue by analyzing certain metabolites in the brain and calculating their ratios. The most notable metabolites are N-acetylaspartate (NAA), choline, and creatine (Figure 3–7). Because the MRS metabolite pattern of the normal brain at a given age is known and predictable, deviation from the normal pattern can provide additional information about the tumor composition, the grade of a malignancy, and any change over time. Successful application of MRS to pediatric patients requires knowledge and understanding of the differences between a young child's and an adult's level of metabolic activity in the brain.

In MRS studies, the highest peak is that of NAA, which is a marker of mature neuronal density and viability and is therefore decreased in tumor tissue because malignant cells in a tumor replace healthy neurons. The choline peak is one of the most important for analyzing brain tumors because it reflects the metabolism of cellular membrane turnover. This peak is increased in all primary and secondary brain tumors. The level of choline activity is usually compared with the level of creatine activity: an elevated ratio of choline to creatine suggests the presence of a tumor. An elevated choline level is also seen in young, developing brains and with remyelination in demyelinating disorders (e.g., multiple sclerosis and

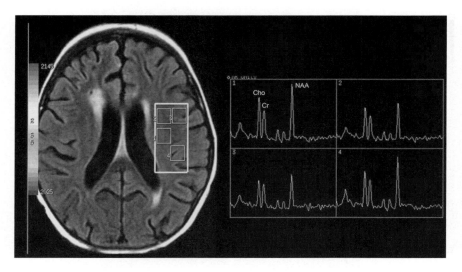

Figure 3–7. MR spectroscopy illustrating the normal choline (Cho), creatine (Cr), and NAA peaks. The insets at right correspond to the numbered sections at left.

acute disseminated encephalomyelitis). The typical pattern of a high-grade malignancy demonstrates a spectrum with an elevated choline-to-creatine ratio and a depressed NAA peak (Figure 3–8). Another metabolite that is useful in evaluating intracranial malignancy is lactate. The presence of lactate indicates that the normal metabolic respiration of tissue has been altered. This situation occurs in highly active and cellular lesions that outgrow their blood supply and enter an anaerobic metabolic state. Tumors that are necrotic or areas of treatment-induced necrosis exhibit lipid metabolites, which can also be identified with MRS. In an untreated tumor, the presence of lipids is usually an indicator of high-grade malignancy.

MRS analyzes metabolites by using a single-voxel or multivoxel technique. A voxel is the prescribed volume in which tissues are assessed. With a multivoxel approach, spectra are simultaneously generated from a large number of volume elements within a slab of tissue, which allows large parts of the brain to be evaluated at the same time (Figure 3–8). The reliability of MRS findings is dependent on voxel position (Figure 3–9). The ideal location of a single sample volume is at the enhanced edge of the tumor. This position yields a spectrum that more accurately reflects the lesion pathology than a spectrum obtained from the lesion center does. In contrast, multivoxel MRS covers a large volume, and even heterogeneous lesions are more likely to be properly sampled. However, other technical factors such as complex shimming, long acquisition time, complicated postprocessing, and artifacts related to the bone and air spaces may make multivoxel MRS less useful in inexperienced hands.

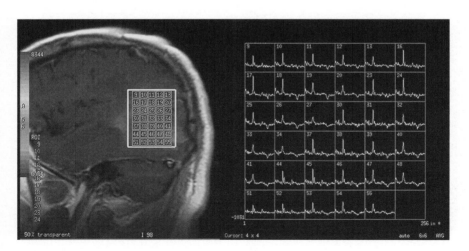

Figure 3–8. Multivoxel MR spectroscopy of a grade III anaplastic astrocytoma showing significant elevation of the choline-to-creatine ratio and depression of the NAA peak. This pattern is consistent with a high-grade neoplasm. The insets at right correspond to the numbered sections at left.

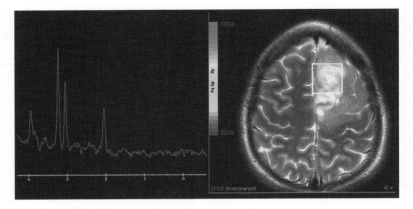

Figure 3–9. Single-voxel MR spectroscopy of a grade II oligodendroglioma showing mild elevation of the choline-to-creatine ratio and depression of the NAA peak. This pattern is not consistent with a high-grade malignancy. The chart at left corresponds to the boxed section at right.

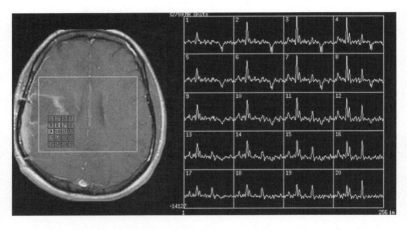

Figure 3–10. Multivoxel MR spectroscopy illustrating significant elevation of the choline-to-creatine ratio and depression of the NAA peak (voxels 6 and 10) in the area of enhancement surrounding a resection cavity. This pattern is consistent with a recurrent tumor. The insets at right correspond to the numbered sections at left. Same patient as in Figure 3–13.

MRS can facilitate the differential diagnosis of various brain lesions and provide information about a tumor's biologic characteristics and response to treatment. The change in the biologic degree of malignancy may also be seen with MRS. This imaging technique may also be used to determine whether a tumor has recurred (Figure 3–10) or treatment has induced tissue injury. MRS is not limited to tumor diagnosis: it can easily be performed at the same time as conventional MRI and is helpful in distinguishing abscesses from other ring-enhancing lesions such as necrotic tumors.

Magnetic Resonance Perfusion Imaging

MR perfusion imaging involves the rapid venous injection of the contrast agent gadolinium through a focused volume of tissue with imaging, starting before the arrival of the gadolinium and continuing during its passage through the volume of interest. There are 2 main approaches to MR perfusion imaging. The first-pass (susceptibility) approach uses T2- or T2*-weighted images acquired rapidly for 60 seconds or so, whereas the dynamic approach uses T1-weighted images acquired over several minutes to visualize the extravascular phase of contrast enhancement that may not be apparent with a first-pass paradigm. Both approaches permit calculation of physiologic parameters such as cerebral blood volume, tissue transit time, cerebral blood flow, and tissue permeability. However, the first-pass technique more accurately measures transit times and cerebral blood volume, whereas the dynamic technique is more sensitive to changes in tumor permeability. Both techniques are used to evaluate benign and malignant intracranial and skull base tumors. MR perfusion imaging methods, particularly permeability variations, are sensitive to tumoral angiogenesis and may be useful in grading primary brain neoplasias and in monitoring the effects of therapy on neovascular proliferation. Another use for MR perfusion imaging is to assist the surgeon in identifying the most active part of a tumor so that optimal biopsy locations can be chosen.

Voxel-by-voxel analysis of MR perfusion imaging studies allows mapping of the distribution of cerebral blood volume, cerebral blood flow, mean tissue transit time, and tissue permeability (Figure 3–11). These maps are interpreted at the same time as conventional anatomic imaging and spectroscopic data.

Functional Magnetic Resonance Imaging

Functional MRI involves the detection of eloquent cortex, which should be avoided during tumor resection, and is a useful adjuvant to neurosurgical cortical mapping. Functional MRI operates on the premise that areas of the brain that are activated during certain activities will have increased blood flow due to the higher oxygen demand of that tissue. This increase in blood flow brings more oxygen into the local environment. The higher oxygen concentration changes the signal that is produced during an MR examination. This change in signal is measured by the blood oxygen level–dependent functional MRI technique whereby both language activity and motor activity are assessed. During this study, the patient is placed in an MRI unit and is asked to perform multiple tasks designed to cause increased, measurable blood flow to eloquent language and motor cortices (Figure 3–12).

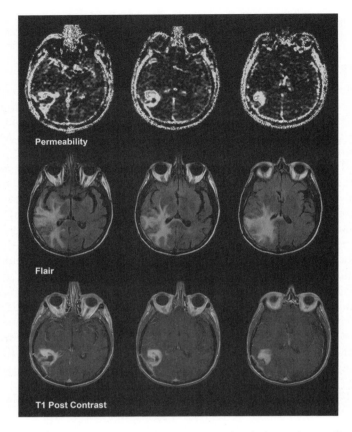

Figure 3–11. MR perfusion images using a T1-weighted, dynamic paradigm. There is a recurrent glioblastoma multiforme in the right parietal lobe with surrounding edema. (*Top*) The permeability map shows details of permeability changes due to tumoral angiogenesis. Note the variability of this process within the tumor. Areas of higher permeability (white) are considered to be sites of more active vascular prolif-eration than are those with low permeability (black) and therefore are considered to be more malignant. Central necrosis is evidenced by a lack of both blood volume and permeability. Normal brain lacks permeability but has normal blood volume. (*Middle*) The FLAIR preconstrast images show the extent of edema or gliosis around the tumor. (*Bottom*) Conventional T1-weighted postcontrast images show enhance-ment in the periphery.

POSITRON EMISSION TOMOGRAPHY

Currently, the most common use of PET involves the administration of cyclotron-produced fluoride 18-labeled fluorodeoxyglucose (FDG), which competes with serum glucose for cellular uptake within the body. Tumors within the body, including those within the brain, use more glucose than

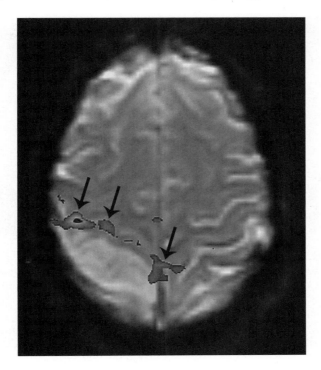

Figure 3–12. A map of the motor cortex anterior to a right parietal oligodendroglioma (arrows) as determined by functional MRI using a finger tapping paradigm.

normal tissue does because they have higher metabolic demands. When FDG is taken up by the cells of a tumor, it becomes phosphorylated by the enzyme hexokinase, which slows the degradation of FDG by the glycolytic cycle and reduces the diffusibility of FDG out of the cell. In addition to their increased use of glucose, tumors have increased amounts of transport proteins and the hexokinase enzyme, which leads to even greater accumulation of FDG.

FDG decays and emits 2 photons, which are detectable by a coincidence scanner. The images that are then produced reflect the concentration of FDG within the tumor and adjacent normal brain parenchyma. The main use of FDG PET imaging in the brain is to determine whether an area of enhancement around a tumor resection cavity is recurrent tumor, which has higher metabolic activity and glucose uptake (Figure 3–13), or radiation necrosis, which has lower metabolic activity and glucose uptake. The reported sensitivity of FDG PET in detecting tumor versus radiation necrosis is 80% to 90%, and the specificity is 50% to 90%. Experimental PET imaging using labeled amino acids, such as tyrosine or methionine, as well as choline may prove to be more accurate in the future, although these techniques are expensive and not yet proven.

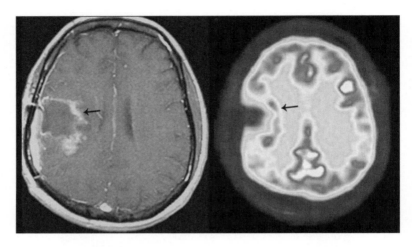

Figure 3–13. An FDG PET study demonstrating hypermetabolic activity in a similar location as the thick enhancement around a resection cavity (arrows). This pattern is consistent with a tumor recurrence. Same patient as in Figure 3–10.

CATHETER ANGIOGRAPHY

Cerebral angiography is the injection of contrast material into the major blood vessels in the neck while dynamic fluoroscopic imaging of the brain is being performed. This technique has long been the standard method for evaluating the intracranial vasculature. However, the evaluation of the proximal arterial and larger venous structures is quickly being replaced by the less invasive techniques of MR and CT angiography.

Rapidly evolving techniques in cerebral angiography involve the placement of microcatheters into the intracerebral vasculature by a specially trained neuro-interventionalist. This procedure is now common practice in many centers for thrombolysis of an occluded proximal artery in patients with acute cerebral infarctions. For patients with cancer, the microcatheters can be navigated through the cerebral vasculature to a feeding vessel that lies just proximal to a cerebral neoplasm. The vessel can then be closed off by using liquid glue, coils, or agents such as polyvinyl alcohol. This embolization technique is particularly beneficial for neoplasms such as hemangioblastomas, meningiomas, and certain hemorrhagic metastases; it can also be used for head and neck cancers (e.g., juvenile nasal angiofibromas and paragangliomas) and neoplasms of the spine. Embolization can significantly reduce the amount of blood loss that occurs during the subsequent resection of these hemorrhagic lesions. The microcatheter technique can also be used to selectively administer chemotherapeutic agents into a tumor.

KEY PRACTICE POINTS

- CT is most commonly used as a screening tool for patients referred from the M. D. Anderson Emergency Center to assess for the sequelae of intracranial lesions (e.g., mass effect and herniation) and to exclude hemorrhage and acute stroke.

- CT angiography and venography are quickly replacing catheter angiography in the contrast evaluation of the more proximal arterial vessels and the larger venous structures of the head and neck and the brain.

- Breakdown of the blood-brain barrier, which occurs in most cerebral neoplasms, leads to the accumulation of an intravenously administered contrast agent and appears as an area of enhancement on CT scans and on the T1-weighted postcontrast MRI sequence.

- Common causes of signal hyperintensity on the diffusion-weighted MRI sequence include acute cerebral infarction and, in certain tumors such as lymphoma, dense cell packing. Signal hyperintensity (an indicator of decreased diffusion) is also present in cerebral abscesses, which distinguishes them from centrally necrotic tumors, which do not demonstrate decreased diffusion.

- The typical pattern of a high-grade malignancy on MRS is a spectrum with an elevated choline-to-creatine ratio and a depressed NAA peak.

- MR perfusion imaging methods are sensitive to tumoral angiogenesis and may be useful in grading primary brain neoplasms, in monitoring the effects of therapy on neovascular proliferation, and in assisting the surgeon in identifying the most active part of a tumor so that optimal biopsy locations can be chosen.

- Functional MRI involves the detection of eloquent cortex, which should be avoided during tumor resection, and is a useful adjuvant to neurosurgical cortical mapping.

- The main use of FDG PET imaging in the brain is to determine whether an area of enhancement around a tumor resection cavity is recurrent tumor, which has higher metabolic activity and glucose uptake, or radiation necrosis, which has lower metabolic activity and glucose uptake.

- A neuro-interventionalist may navigate microcatheters just proximal to a cerebral neoplasm for vascular embolization and for administration of chemotherapeutic agents to a tumor.

Suggested Readings

Dowling C, Bollen AW, Noworolski SM, et al. Preoperative proton MR spectroscopic imaging of brain tumors: correlation with histopathologic analysis of resection specimens. *AJNR Am J Neuroradiol* 2001;22:604–612.

Hamberg LM, Rhea JT, Hunter GJ, Thrall JH. Multi-detector row CT: radiation dose characteristics. *Radiology* 2003;226:762–772.

Hirai T, Korogi Y, Ono K, Uemura S, Yamashita Y. Preoperative embolization for meningeal tumors: evaluation of vascular supply with angio-CT. *AJNR Am J Neuroradiol* 2004;25:74–76.

Hoeffner EG, Case I, Jainet R, et al. Cerebral perfusion CT: technique and clinical applications. *Radiology* 2004;231:632–644.

Langleben D, Segall GM. PET in differentiation of recurrent brain tumor from radiation injury. *J Nucl Med* 2000;41:1861–1867.

Law M, Yang S, Wang H, et al. Glioma grading: sensitivity, specificity, and predictive values of perfusion MR imaging and proton MR spectroscopic imaging compared with conventional MR imaging. *AJNR Am J Neuroradiol* 2003;24: 1989–1998.

Majós C, Julià-Sapé M, Alonso J, et al. Brain tumor classification by proton MR spectroscopy: comparison of diagnostic accuracy at short and long TE. *AJNR Am J Neuroradiol* 2004;25:1696–1704.

Smirniotopoulos JG. The new WHO classification of brain tumors. [Review] *Neuroimaging Clin N Am* 1999;9:595–613.

Wetzel SG, Kirsch E, Stock KW, Kolbe M, Kaim A, Radue EW. Cerebral veins: comparative study of CT venography with intraarterial digital subtraction angiography. *AJNR Am J Neuroradiol* 1999;20:249–255.

Yetkin FZ, Mueller WM, Morris GL, et al. Functional MR activation correlated with intraoperative cortical mapping. *AJNR Am J Neuroradiol* 1997;18: 1311–1315.

4   SURGICALLY CURABLE BRAIN TUMORS OF ADULTS

Franco DeMonte

Chapter Overview 54
Meningiomas 54
   Epidemiology 55
   Etiology 55
      Trauma 55
      Irradiation 56
      Genetics and Molecular Biology 56
      Gonadal Steroid Hormones and Receptors 57
      Other Receptors and Growth Factors 57
   Clinical Presentation 58
   Diagnostic Imaging 59
   Pathologic Subtypes 61
      Grade I Meningiomas 61
      Grade II Meningiomas 61
      Grade III Meningiomas 62
   Management 62
      Surgical Approach 63
      Adjuvant Radiotherapy 63
      Adjuvant Chemotherapy 66
   Recurrence 66
Schwannomas 67
   Vestibular Schwannomas (Acoustic Neuromas) 67
      Epidemiology 67
      Etiology and Genetics 68
      Clinical Presentation 68
      Diagnostic Imaging 68
      Management 71
         Observation 71
         Surgery 71
         Radiosurgery and Stereotactic Radiotherapy 71
   Other Cranial Nerve Schwannomas 73
      Trigeminal Schwannomas 73
      Facial Nerve Schwannomas 74
      Jugular Foramen Schwannomas 75
      Schwannomas of the 3rd, 4th, 6th, and 12th Cranial Nerves 77
Craniopharyngiomas 77
   Epidemiology 77

Etiology 77
Clinical Presentation 78
Diagnostic Imaging 79
Pathology 80
Management 80
Epidermoid and Dermoid Cysts 81
Epidemiology 81
Etiology and Pathogenesis 82
Clinical Presentation 82
Diagnostic Imaging 83
Management 84
Choroid Plexus Papillomas 84
Epidemiology 84
Etiology 84
Clinical Presentation 84
Diagnostic Imaging 85
Management 86
Hemangioblastomas 86
Epidemiology and Genetics 86
Clinical Presentation 87
Diagnostic Imaging 87
Management 87
Key Practice Points 89
Suggested Readings 90

CHAPTER OVERVIEW

Although more than half of the tumors of the central nervous system are high-grade neuroglial tumors with generally poor median patient survival times, there is a substantial subset of tumors for which surgery alone has curative potential. With the use of modern microsurgical techniques and technologies such as imaging guidance, intraoperative ultrasonography, and magnetic resonance imaging, surgical morbidity and mortality have decreased significantly. Although some incompletely resected or recurrent benign tumors may require adjuvant treatment after surgery or may be treated with nonsurgical options, surgery is generally considered essential for cure. This chapter discusses non-glial central nervous system tumors in adults only. For information on surgically curable astroglial tumors, please see chapter 5.

MENINGIOMAS

Meningiomas are usually benign growths that originate from the leptomeninges. Of all intracranial meningiomas, 85% are located supratentorially, one third to one half of which are located along the

Table 4–1. Common Sites and Relative Incidence of Intracranial
             Meningiomas in Adults

Site	Relative Incidence (%)
Parasagittal or falcine	25
Convexity	19
Sphenoid ridge	17
Tuberculum sella	9
Posterior fossa	8
Olfactory groove	8
Middle fossa or Meckel's cave	4
Tentorial region	3
Peritorcular region	3
Lateral ventricle	1–2
Foramen magnum	1–2
Orbital or optic nerve sheath	1–2

Based on data from Cushing H, Eisenhardt L. *Meningiomas: Their Classification, Regional Behavior, Life History, and Surgical End Results.* Springfield, IL: Charles C. Thomas; 1938. Gautier-Smith C, Lamouche M. *Parasagittal and Falx Meningiomas.* London, UK: Butterworths, 1970. Quest D. Meningiomas: an update. *Neurosurgery* 1978;3:219–225. MacCarty C, Taylor W. Intracranial meningiomas: experiences at the Mayo Clinic. *Neurol Med Chir (Tokyo)* 1979;19:569–574. Rohinger M, Sutherland G, Louw D, Sima A. Incidence and clinicopathological features of meningioma. *J Neurosurg* 1989;71:665–672.

base of the anterior and middle fossae. Table 4–1 lists the most common sites of occurrence and their relative incidence.

Epidemiology

The incidence of meningiomas among primary intracranial neoplasms is approximately 20%, and the reported incidence per 100,000 population varies from less than 1% to more than 6%. The male-to-female incidence ranges from 1:1.4 to 1:2.8 (Drummond et al, 2004). The average incidence is higher for African Americans than for Caucasian Americans. The incidence of intracranial meningiomas rises with increasing age and has been reported to be 3.5 times higher in patients older than 70 years of age than in younger patients, regardless of sex (Kuratsu and Ushio, 1997). The tumor growth rate, however, seems to be lower in the elderly. Meningiomas are multiple in 5% to 40% of patients, especially when they are associated with neurofibromatosis type 2 (NF2).

Etiology

Trauma

Although numerous case-control studies have reported an increased association between a history of head trauma (vs no head trauma) and the development of meningiomas, Annegers et al (1979) found no significant increase in the number of any intracranial tumors in a prospective study of

2,953 patients with head injuries over 29,859 person-years. Similarly, a population-based cohort study conducted in Denmark with 228,055 patients who were hospitalized with head injuries between 1977 and 1992 found no significant increase in the subsequent incidence of meningiomas (Inskip et al, 1998).

Irradiation

Exposure to ionizing radiation is a known etiologic factor in the development of meningiomas (see also chapter 1). An increased rate of meningioma formation has been seen in patients after irradiation for tinea capitis, in patients after treatment for primary head and neck malignancies, and in survivors of radiation exposure from the atomic bomb explosions in Hiroshima and Nagasaki. The latency period from radiation exposure to tumor detection varies inversely with the radiation dose. Compared with non–radiation-induced meningiomas, radiation-induced meningiomas are more biologically aggressive, possess more atypical histology, are more likely to recur, are more likely to occur in multiple locations, have different cytogenetic characteristics, and do not exhibit tumor behavior that correlates with their proliferation index.

Genetics and Molecular Biology

Thirty to eighty percent of sporadic meningiomas and nearly all neurofibromatosis-related meningiomas have mutations in the *NF2* gene (located in chromosome band 22q12) that result in mutations in the protein MERLIN. Chromosomal mapping techniques have identified chromosome subband 22q12.3-qter, which is near the *NF2* gene but is believed to represent a separate and distinct locus in meningioma formation. Loss of expression of another tumor suppressor gene, *DAL-1*, which is located in 18p11.3, has been found in 30% to 70% of meningiomas and is thought to play a role in both early tumorigenesis and meningioma evolution. Other tumor suppressor genes implicated in the development or progression of meningiomas are *SMARCB2* (22q11.2), *p53* (17p), and *CDKN2B* (9p21). The fact that malignant and atypical meningiomas tend to have more chromosomal aberrations than benign tumors do suggests progressive loss of tumor suppressors and potential activation of oncogenes. Some of the genes implicated in meningioma oncogenesis are c-*sis*, C-*myc*, Ha-*ras*, K-*ras*, c-*fos*, c-*erbB*, and *S6k*. A variety of other chromosomal aberrations have been implicated in the formation and progression of meningiomas, including losses on 1p, 2p, 6q, 10, and 14q and gains on 1q, 9q, 12q, 15q, 7q, and 20. Alterations on chromosomes 1, 10, and 14 and reactivation of the telomerase subunit hTERT seem to be particularly important in the progression of more biologically aggressive meningiomas. Radiation-induced meningiomas have been shown to express genetic aberrations that are different than those of sporadic meningiomas. In particular, there are fewer losses of genetic material on chromosome 22 and more losses on chromosomes 1p, 6q, 9q, 18q, and 19q.

Gonadal Steroid Hormones and Receptors

Estrogen receptors have been reported in 0% to 94% of meningiomas and progesterone receptors in 40% to 100%. Recent studies using modern experimental and laboratory techniques have revealed minimal amounts of functional estrogen receptor. This finding is supported by the generally disappointing results of antiestrogen agents (i.e., tamoxifen and mepitiostane) in treating meningiomas. Most investigators have identified high levels of progesterone receptors in meningiomas, and the presence of these receptors has correlated with less aggressive tumor biology, more favorable prognosis, and a lower incidence of recurrence. Antiprogesterone agents used to treat meningiomas have yielded varied results; the most recent phase III double-blind, randomized, placebo-controlled trial of mifepristone reported no significant benefit (Grunberg et al, 2001). Androgen receptors are found in meningiomas with about the same frequency as progesterone receptors and are expressed in 69% of males and 31% of females (Carroll et al, 1993). Testosterone stimulates in vitro meningioma cell growth, and it has been speculated that androgen receptors may help modulate progesterone receptor activity.

Other Receptors and Growth Factors

Using polymerase chain reaction analysis, Carrol et al (1996) detected D_1 receptor mRNA in meningiomas, particularly in females, as well as D_2 receptor mRNA and prolactin receptor mRNA, but the functional importance of these findings is unclear. Somatostatin receptors, particularly type 2a (hsst2a) receptors, have also been reported at high levels in meningiomas. There have been a few reports of success using somatostatin analogs to treat meningiomas, but the role of somatostatin receptors in tumor progression or growth is still unclear. Growth hormone receptor mRNA is ubiquitously expressed in meningiomas. Growth hormone receptor blockade by pegvisomant has been shown to result in decreased growth rates of primary meningioma cell cultures and reduced tumor growth and regression in an in vivo animal model.

Westphal and Hermann (1986) discovered functionally intact epidermal growth factor (EGF) receptors, a product of the oncogene c-*erb*, and reported increased DNA synthesis after EGF treatment of meningioma cell cultures. Weisman et al (1986) noted a modulatory effect on this receptor by platelet-derived growth factor (PDGF) and revealed near maximal levels of DNA synthesis in meningioma cell cultures when PDGF and EGF were added together. Subsequent studies using Northern blot analysis and polymerase chain reaction revealed that activated forms of EGF receptor, ErbB2, and ErbB4 mRNA are present in meningiomas, that EGF receptors in meningiomas are capable of inducing *ras* signaling pathways, and that ErbB2 expression levels decrease with increasing World Health Organization (WHO) tumor grade.

The finding of c-erb/EGF receptor expression in meningiomas prompted searches for other oncogene receptor–mitogen systems. Using Northern blot analysis, Maxwell et al (1990) demonstrated that meningiomas express both the c-*sis*/PDGF-2 proto-oncogene and the PDGF receptor (PDGFR) gene. In situ hybridization localized the c-*sis*/PDGF-2 and PDGFR mRNAs and their protein products in the tumor cells of the meningiomas but not in normal tissue. Further studies revealed that PDGFR-β is expressed in meningiomas, that PDGF-BB increases c-*fos* expression in meningioma cell cultures, and that overexpression of PDGFR-β and PDGF-BB is associated with higher grade and proliferative activity in meningiomas. These results support the concept of PDGFR activation by an autocrine-paracrine loop and the idea that PDGFR activation contributes to tumor cell proliferation or malignant transformation. Autocrine loops of leukemia inhibitory factor, interleukin-6, and oncostatin M have also been identified in meningiomas, although the exact function of these loops is unknown. Oncostatin M expression has been shown to be associated with decreased meningioma cellular proliferation in vitro. Vascular endothelial growth factor (VEGF) levels are associated with increased angiogenesis, edema, and frequency of recurrence in meningiomas. The hematopoietic growth factors granulocyte colony-stimulating factor and granulocyte-macrophage colony-stimulating factor have been identified in meningioma samples, and their expression has correlated with angiogenesis, tumor proliferation, and meningioma grade. Fibroblast growth factor and insulin-like growth factor 1 have also been identified in meningiomas and implicated in tumor progression.

Many of the growth factor receptors (e.g., PDGFR, EGF receptor, and VEGF receptor) are protein tyrosine kinase receptors that activate *ras* and associated intracellular cascades, which mediate cellular proliferation, differentiation, and transformation. Shu et al (1999) reported that indirect *ras* inhibition via dominant-negative Ha-*ras* gene transfer to meningioma cells in culture and direct inhibition of *ras* by microinjecting inhibitory antibodies inhibited meningioma cell proliferation in vitro.

Clinical Presentation

There is no single symptom or sign that identifies patients who harbor intracranial meningiomas. A variety of presenting features depend primarily on the tumor's size and location; these features include headache, paresis, seizure, personality change or confusion, and visual impairment. Headache and paresis are the most common symptom and sign; each occurs in a third of patients. Meningiomas in particular locations may produce a consistent set of signs and symptoms. Tumors of the olfactory

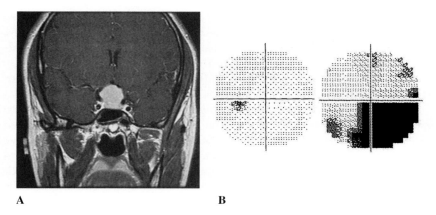

A   B

Figure 4–1. (A) T1-weighted, postcontrast coronal MR image reveals the typical appearance of a tuberculum sellae meningioma. (B) Visual field maps for the same patient. (Courtesy of The University of Texas M. D. Anderson Cancer Center, Department of Neurosurgery, Houston, Texas)

groove have been associated with the Foster–Kennedy syndrome (anosmia, ipsilateral optic atrophy, and contralateral papilledema); tuberculum sellae meningiomas may cause significant and early visual loss (typically a "chiasmal syndrome" with ipsilateral optic atrophy and an incongruent bitemporal hemianopia) (Figure 4–1); cavernous sinus meningiomas may result in proptosis, diplopia, or primary aberrant oculomotor regeneration; and foramen magnum tumors often have associated nuchal and suboccipital pain with stepwise appendicular sensory and motor deficits.

Diagnostic Imaging

Computed tomography (CT) with contrast can detect most meningiomas. CT can optimally identify bone involvement, including both hyperostosis and bone erosion or remodeling. On nonenhanced CT scans, meningiomas are generally homogeneously isodense or slightly hyperdense compared with normal brain. Because small meningiomas can be missed, contrast-enhanced studies are indicated. Calcification may range from tiny punctate areas to dense calcification of the entire lesion. With intravenous contrast, meningiomas are typically enhanced homogeneously and often demonstrate morphologic features such as sharp demarcation and a broad base against bone or free dural margins (Figure 4–1). Approximately 15% of benign meningiomas have an unusual appearance on CT images. Areas of hyperdensity, hypodensity, or nonuniform enhancement may be seen. These areas may represent hemorrhage, cystic degeneration, or necrosis, respectively.

The magnetic resonance imaging (MRI) characteristics of meningiomas are generally consistent. On T1-weighted images, 60% to 90% of meningiomas are isointense and the remainder are mildly hypointense compared with gray matter (Figure 4–2A). On T2-weighted images, 30% to 45% of meningiomas have increased signal intensity and approximately 50% are isointense compared with gray matter (Figure 4–2C). Their typical extraparenchymal location heightens the neuroradiologist's ability to diagnose these tumors.

There is increased interest in using MRI characteristics to subtype meningioma tissue before surgery. The results of these studies have been variable: some have reported 75% to 96% accuracy, whereas others have found no correlation. The MRI characteristics that allowed accurate preoperative identification of meningioma subtypes were confined to findings on T2-weighted images. Specifically, meningothelial and angioblastic

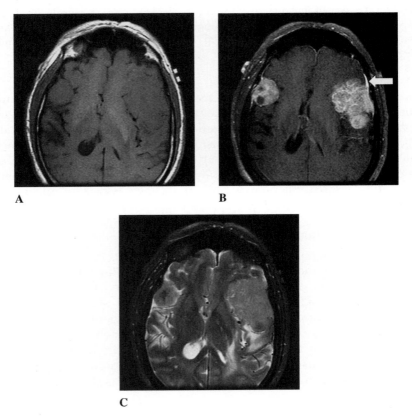

A   B

C

Figure 4–2. T1-weighted, precontrast (A), T1-weighted, postcontrast (B), and T2-weighted (C) axial MR images of a patient with multiple meningiomas. Note the presence of areas of cystic degeneration and the typical dural tail associated with meningioma (arrow in B). (Courtesy of The University of Texas M. D. Anderson Cancer Center, Department of Neurosurgery, Houston, Texas)

variants had a higher signal intensity on T2-weighted sequences than fibroblastic and transitional meningiomas did. The amount of cerebral edema associated with the meningiomas was also found to be greater in meningothelial or angioblastic variants. Finally, a high signal intensity on T2-weighted images has been correlated with microscopic hypervascularity and soft tumor consistency.

Contrast-enhanced MRI provides the most sensitive and specific means of detecting meningiomas. Most meningiomas are enhanced intensely and homogeneously with intravenous contrast material, and in 10% of cases, small additional meningiomas are encountered that are missed on unenhanced MR images. Contrast enhancement of the dura mater extending away from the margins of the mass is typical of meningiomas, although this pattern can be seen with other dural-based lesions. This "dural tail" (Figure 4–2B) can represent either tumor extension or reactive change, and its resection is important to reduce the risk of recurrence. Postoperative enhanced MRI has also been found to be sensitive and specific in detecting residual or recurrent meningiomas. Thick and nodular enhancement has a high correlation with recurrent or residual neoplasm.

In vivo MR spectroscopy is an evolving area of study (see chapter 3). Compared with the MR spectra of normal brain, the typical MR spectra for meningiomas reveal a markedly increased choline peak and reduced N-acetylaspartate and phosphocreatine/creatine peaks. An additional peak present in some meningiomas at 1.47 ppm has been attributed to alanine.

Pathologic Subtypes

Microscopically, meningiomas have a varied but characteristic histopathologic appearance. This diversity forms the basis for their pathologic classification (Table 4–2). The current system is based on the 2000 WHO classification system, which associates histopathology with information on recurrence and aggressiveness. There are 3 grades of meningiomas: grade I meningiomas are associated with a low risk of recurrence and aggressive growth, whereas grade II and III meningiomas have a greater likelihood of one or both of these characteristics.

Grade I Meningiomas

Of the 9 subtypes of grade I meningiomas, the 3 most common are meningothelial, fibrous, and transitional. Although it is important that these and the other subtypes are recognized, the prognostic significance of each one is unclear but they are currently considered equivalent.

Grade II Meningiomas

Apart from brain invasion and metastatic spread, which define malignancy, certain features of grade II meningiomas that may be seen by light microscopy suggest increased tumor aggressiveness and an increased

Table 4–2. WHO Classification of Tumors of the Meninges

Grade	Classification
I	Meningothelial
	Fibrous (fibroblastic)
	Transitional (mixed)
	Psammomatous
	Angiomatous
	Microcystic
	Secretory
	Lymphoplasmacyte rich
	Metaplastic (xanthomatous, myxoid, osseous, cartilagenous, etc.)
II	Atypical
	Clear cell
	Choroid
III	Anaplastic (malignant)
	Papillary
	Rhabdoid

Adapted from Kleihues P, Cavenee WK, eds. *World Health Organization Classification of Tumours: Pathology and Genetics of Tumours of the Nervous System.* Lyon, France: IARC Press; 2000 with permission.

recurrence rate. Among these atypical features are loss of architectural pattern, high cellularity, increased number of mitotic figures (more than 4 mitoses per 20 high-powered fields), necrosis, prominent nucleoli, and nuclear pleomorphism. The 3 subtypes of grade II meningiomas are atypical, choroid, and clear cell.

Grade III Meningiomas

The diagnosis of a grade III (i.e., malignant) meningioma traditionally requires histologic evidence of brain invasion or distant metastasis, which in most cases is accompanied by further evidence of biologic aggressiveness such as cellular sheeting, nuclear pleomorphism, increased cellularity and mitoses (more than 20 mitoses per 20 high-powered fields), and necrosis. When dissemination occurs, the most common locations for metastases are the lungs and pleura, abdominal viscera (especially the liver), lymph nodes, and bones. Patients with meningiomas associated with frank malignancy are reported to have only a 2-year median survival duration. The 3 subtypes of grade III meningiomas are anaplastic (malignant), papillary, and rhabdoid.

Management

The treatment of a meningioma depends primarily on the size and location of the tumor, the age of the patient, and associated symptoms and neurologic deficits. The mainstay of treatment is surgical resection, although small, asymptomatic, incidental meningiomas can typically be managed with observation and serial imaging. After surgery, re-imaging is typically performed at 6-month intervals initially, which may be extended to longer intervals if there are no radiographic signs of tumor growth and the patient remains asymptomatic. Treatment should be initiated when symptoms arise or tumor growth is documented. Critical parameters that affect the ease of surgical removal include the tumor's location, size, and consistency; vascular and neural involvement; and in the case of recurrence, prior surgery or radiotherapy. New and innovative approaches have been devised to reach and widely expose meningiomas in any location. Furthermore, a greater appreciation of risk factors for and patterns of tumor recurrence has changed surgical planning and goals. The surgical goal now is to decrease the incidence of recurrence by resecting all of the neoplasm and all involved dura mater, soft tissue, and bone. However, the tumor size and location and the involvement of adjacent structures may not allow all meningiomas to be completely resected in this manner.

Surgical Approach

In the operating room, the patient should be positioned to maximize the accessibility of the tumor, the chances of unimpeded venous drainage, the beneficial effects of gravity, the surgeon's comfort, and above all the patient's safety. In any position that places the patient's head above heart level, monitoring for air embolism should be used, particularly because many meningiomas are located close to the venous sinuses and their large tributaries.

To the surgeon's advantage, a layer of arachnoid usually separates meningiomas from the brain, cranial nerves, and blood vessels. By accessing and staying within this surgical plane, the surgeon can minimize the chances of neural or vascular injury (Figure 4–3). Early extensive tumor debulking allows the tumor capsule to collapse inward, thus facilitating the definition of the arachnoid plane. The method used to debulk the tumor—which may be suction, coagulation, sharp excision, ultrasonic aspiration, or laser vaporization—depends on the tumor's consistency, vascularity, and location. Once the tumor mass has been resected, careful attention must be given to the resection of the involved dura mater and bone. The involved dura mater is resected as widely as possible and then repaired with autologous pericranium, fascia lata, or temporalis fascia or a dural graft from cadaveric dura mater, synthetic collagen matrix, or bovine pericardium. Vascularized pericranium, temporalis muscle, or free tissue transfer is used to separate intracranial contents from the paranasal sinuses, aerodigestive tract, and middle ear. Cranioplasty is performed as required to reconstruct calvarial defects.

Adjuvant Radiotherapy

Although there have been no randomized, controlled, or prospective studies with long-term follow-up conducted to evaluate the efficacy of

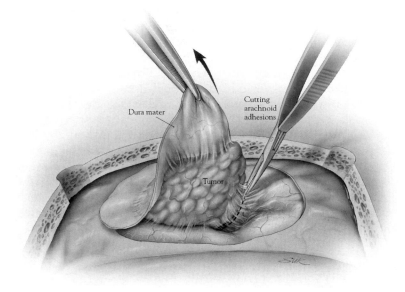

Figure 4–3. Artist's representation of the technique of removal of a convexity meningioma. Careful, sharp dissection divides arachnoid adhesions and allows separation of the tumor from the brain. Reprinted from Conrad CA, Pro B, Prabhu SS, McCutcheon IE, DeMonte F. Primary brain tumors. In: Markman M, ed. *Atlas of Cancer.* Philadelphia, PA: Lippincott, Williams, and Wilkins; 2003:561–593 with permission.

radiotherapy in treating meningiomas, the use of external-beam irradiation has become an important part of the management of these tumors, particularly as adjuvant treatment for patients after subtotal tumor resection. In a retrospective analysis of 140 patients with benign meningiomas who were treated by subtotal resection plus adjuvant radiotherapy over 23 years, Goldsmith et al (1994) reported 5- and 10-year progression-free survival rates of 89% and 77%, respectively. In patients treated using CT planning (after 1980), the 5-year progression-free survival rate was 98%. Recently, Soyuer et al (2004) compared 92 patients with WHO grade I benign cerebral meningiomas who underwent gross total resection, subtotal resection plus adjuvant radiotherapy, or subtotal resection plus delayed radiotherapy. At a median follow-up of 7.7 years, the 5-year progression-free survival rates were 77%, 91%, and 38%, respectively. The overall 5- and 10-year survival rates were not statistically different among the 3 groups or from the age-adjusted expected survival rate. Thus, delaying radiotherapy until tumor recurrence without compromising overall patient survival is possible and may spare the patient from the potential toxicity of radiation. The data do not permit determination of which strategy is optimal. For meningiomas that are considered inoperable because of their location, poor patient health, or patient refusal of surgery, external-beam radiotherapy would seem beneficial for aggressive (e.g., atypical or anaplastic) tumors, but very little information exists to support this theory.

Stereotactic irradiation in the form of radiosurgery or conformal, fractionated, or intensity-modulated radiotherapy has increasingly been used to treat meningiomas with improved efficacy and diminishing untoward effects. Stereotactic irradiation uses various forms of energy, the most common of which are photons from cobalt 60 γ-ray sources (e.g., the Gamma Knife) or linear accelerators (LINAC) and heavy particles (e.g., protons) from cyclotrons. Radiosurgery provides effective tumor control of small meningiomas. Kondziolka et al (1999) observed a 93% tumor control rate in patients whose meningiomas were treated by Gamma Knife radiosurgery and a 61% incidence of tumor shrinkage in 99 patients who were followed for 5 to 10 years. The incidence of new neurologic deficits in this group of patients was 5%. In a recent retrospective study, Pollock et al (2003) reported that Gamma Knife radiosurgery of small- or medium-sized benign meningiomas provided progression-free survival rates equivalent to that of complete surgical resection after a mean follow-up of 64 months. Gamma Knife radiosurgery has also been shown to be an effective treatment for difficult-to-resect cavernous sinus meningiomas. Lee et al (2002) reported an actuarial tumor control rate of 93% at 5 years for benign cavernous sinus meningiomas; adverse effects of radiation were experienced by 6.7% of patients.

LINAC-based radiosurgery also offers effective control of small meningiomas. A recent study of 43 patients who underwent LINAC-based radiosurgery for skull base meningiomas reported a 7-year local control rate of 89.7% (Chuang et al, 2004). This value correlated with the 5-year control rate of 89% and a complication rate of 5% in a previous study of 127 patients (Hakim et al, 1998). Spiegelmann et al (2002) reported that both the 3- and 7-year actuarial tumor growth control rates were 97% for cavernous sinus meningiomas treated by LINAC-based radiosurgery. They also reported a low incidence of long-term cranial neuropathies.

Despite the promising results of stereotactic irradiation, there are some limitations and uncertainties with this modality. The targeted tumor is limited to 35 to 40 mm because this is the size at which the tumor can receive a single dose of appropriate strength with a 1% risk of radiation necrosis. However, the increased availability and use of fractionated delivery of stereotactic irradiation have overcome this size limitation. Alheit et al (1999) reported a 1-year progression-free survival rate of 100% in 24 patients who underwent fractionated stereotactically guided conformal radiotherapy for meningiomas. Seven of the 15 patients who had neurologic deficits before treatment improved, and 2 patients experienced early side effects (1 facial palsy and 1 addisonian state). Other recent studies have reported benefit from stereotactic conformal radiotherapy for atypical and malignant meningiomas and for large cavernous sinus meningiomas.

Intensity-modulated radiotherapy delivers fractionated, conformal radiotherapy more effectively than traditional techniques to tumors with complex shapes. Initial reports have shown that this method is effective in treating meningiomas and controlling tumor growth and carries a low risk of side effects.

Adjuvant Chemotherapy

Little information is available regarding the efficacy of traditional anti-neoplastic agents against benign or malignant meningiomas. Adjuvant chemotherapy (intravenous or intra-arterial *cis*-platinum, or dacarbazine and doxorubicin) for malignant meningiomas and for recurrent benign or atypical meningiomas has been administered to a small number of patients but has generally been unsuccessful despite its effectiveness against other soft tissue tumors. Hydroxyurea has been shown to arrest meningioma cell growth in the S phase of the cell cycle and to induce apoptosis in vitro. Although a similar beneficial effect has been seen in a small subgroup of patients with recurrent and unresectable meningiomas, subsequent studies have shown little, if any, benefit. Interferon-α has been reported to be effective in prolonging the time to recurrence in a small group of patients with aggressive meningiomas and to have lower toxic-ity than traditional chemotherapeutic agents. The Southwest Oncology Group used tamoxifen to treat 19 patients with unresectable or refractory meningiomas and observed tumor progression in 10 patients, temporary stabilization of the disease process in 6 patients, and a partial or minor response in 3 patients (Goodwin et al, 1993). A recent phase III, double-blind, randomized study of mifepristone did not show any benefit (Grunberg et al, 2001).

Recurrence

The completeness of the tumor resection is the primary factor influencing the meningioma recurrence rate. Stafford et al (1998) found a 25% recur-rence rate at 10 years in patients who had undergone a gross total tumor resection and a 61% recurrence rate in those who had undergone partial resection. Jääskeläinen (1986) found an overall recurrence rate at 20 years of 19% (lifetable analysis). Multivariate analysis showed that strong risk factors for recurrence included no coagulation of dural origin, invasion of bone, and soft consistency of the tumor. The recurrence rate at 20 years was 11% for patients with none of these risk factors, 15% to 24% for 1 risk fac-tor, and 34% to 56% for 2 risk factors. In a second study from the same group, the diagnosis of atypical or anaplastic meningioma carried an increased risk of recurrence of 38% and 78% at 5 years, respectively (Jääskeläinen et al, 1986). The fact that the cumulative relative survival rates (i.e., the observed-to-expected survival rates) at 1, 5, 10, and 15 years were 83%, 79%, 74%, and 71%, respectively, indicated increased mortality in patients with meningiomas. Using multivariate analysis, Stafford et al (1998) found that age younger than 40 years, male sex, incomplete surgical resection, optic nerve involvement, and 4 or more mitotic figures per 10 high-powered fields were associated with a decreased progression-free survival rate. Other factors that have been implicated in the recurrence of meningiomas include mitoses, focal necrosis, brain invasion, syncytial tumors, hypervascularity, hemosiderin deposition, sheets of tumor cells, prominent nucleoli, nuclear pleomorphism, and elevated proliferation index.

The use of Ki-67 labeling to develop a "proliferation index" is a common immunocytochemical technique for predicting a tumor's biologic aggressiveness and potential for recurrence (see chapter 2). Labeling indices averaging 1%, 5.5%, and 12% have been identified for benign, atypical, and anaplastic meningiomas, respectively (Abramovich and Prayson, 1998). Other markers of proliferation currently being investigated are progesterone receptors, topoisomerase IIα, telomerase, transforming growth factors, mitosin, survivin, and other apoptosis-related proteins. Positron emission tomography studies of glucose utilization have also been used to assess a tumor's biologic aggressiveness and potential for recurrence.

SCHWANNOMAS

Intracranial nerve sheath tumors constitute 4% to 8% of all intracranial neoplasms. The most common are the vestibular schwannomas, which are followed distantly by trigeminal nerve sheath tumors. These neoplasms can arise, although infrequently, from other cranial nerves both intracranially and extracranially. All schwannomas may develop as an isolated disease process (spontaneous mutation), but most intracranial nonvestibular tumors and 5% of vestibular schwannomas are associated with NF2.

Vestibular Schwannomas (Acoustic Neuromas)

The solitary benign vestibular schwannoma is the most common tumor of the cranial nerves. Improved diagnostic modalities have resulted in the ability to diagnose, follow, and treat smaller and even asymptomatic vestibular schwannomas. Early interventions using improved microsurgical and navigational techniques as well as adjuvant and primary nonsurgical alternatives such as radiosurgery and radiotherapy have resulted in a marked reduction in the morbidity and mortality of therapy for these tumors.

Epidemiology

Vestibular schwannomas account for 80% to 90% of tumors found in the cerebellopontine angle (CPA). Overall, they account for 6% to 8% of all intracranial tumors and have a yearly incidence of about 1 per 100,000 population. In the United States, 2,000 to 3,000 new cases are diagnosed each year. Race and sex do not appear to be contributing factors in the development of these tumors.

Etiology and Genetics

Vestibular schwannomas occur in sporadic and hereditary forms. Unilateral sporadic tumors account for 95% of cases. Approximately 5% of vestibular schwannomas are associated with neurofibromatosis, mainly NF2. Only 2% of patients with NF1 present with unilateral vestibular schwannomas, and bilateral vestibular schwannomas in the presence of NF1 are exceedingly rare. NF2 affects 1 in every 50,000 individuals and represents 10% of all cases of neurofibromatosis. Patients with NF2 present with bilateral vestibular schwannomas in more than 90% of cases. Using polymorphic DNA markers, Seizinger et al (1986) showed loss of heterozygosity for genes on chromosome 22 in 50% of tumor specimens analyzed from patients with NF2 and in 44% of specimens from patients with sporadic vestibular schwannomas. The product of the *NF2* gene, the protein MERLIN, is one of several cytoskeletal proteins that link the cell membrane to the cytoskeleton. The difference between sporadic and hereditary forms of the disease is that in the latter, the defect in bilateral vestibular schwannomas is present in the germ cell line. Comparative genomic hybridization analysis has identified 2 additional areas that may be involved in vestibular schwannoma formation: a gain in chromosome band 9q34 in 10% of tumors, and a gain in chromosome arm 17q in 5% of tumors (Lanser et al, 1992).

Clinical Presentation

Compression of the cochlear division of the vestibulocochlear nerve results in slowly progressive unilateral sensorineural hearing loss, which is by far the most common symptom of vestibular schwannomas. Other symptoms may include tinnitus, headache, dysequilibrium, and vertigo. As the tumor grows into the CPA, trigeminal nerve compression may occur with resulting facial hypoesthesia or, more commonly, diminution of the corneal reflex. Other abnormalities on physical examination may include nystagmus, papilledema, and ataxia. Despite the intimate relationship of this tumor with the seventh cranial nerve, patients rarely present with facial weakness. Formal hearing evaluation will usually disclose a pattern consistent with sensorineural hearing loss. Speech discrimination is usually decreased, whereas the speech reception threshold is increased (Figure 4-4).

Diagnostic Imaging

Schwannomas are generally isodense or very slightly hyperdense to adjacent brain on CT images. These tumors are intensely enhanced by contrast. Larger lesions may have a heterogeneous pattern of enhancement secondary

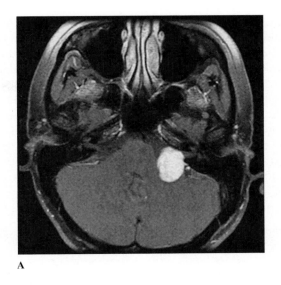

A

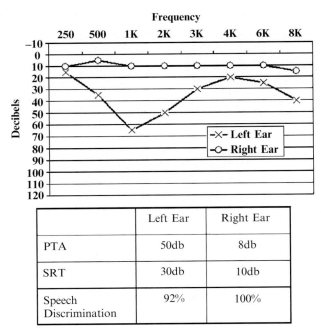

	Left Ear	Right Ear
PTA	50db	8db
SRT	30db	10db
Speech Discrimination	92%	100%

B

Figure 4-4. (A) T1-weighted, postcontrast axial MR image reveals the typical appearance of a left vestibular schwannoma. (B) Audiogram for the same patient reveals asymmetrical hearing loss with an elevated speech reception threshold (30 db) and decreased speech discrimination (92%). (Courtesy of The University of Texas M. D. Anderson Cancer Center, Department of Neurosurgery, Houston, Texas)

to cystic degeneration and xanthomatous change. High-resolution, thin-cut CT images allow assessment of mastoid aeration, assessment of the position of the jugular bulb, and measurement of the distance from the posterior lip of the internal auditory meatus to the posterior semicircular canal; these parameters are important influences on the choice of surgical approach.

MRI with gadolinium enhancement is the most sensitive and specific study with which to evaluate for the presence of a vestibular schwannoma. T1-weighted images reveal an extra-axial lesion at the level of the internal auditory meatus. The tumor is usually isointense or hypointense relative to brain. It is brightly enhanced with gadolinium, and the intracanalicular portion of the tumor is well visualized. On T2-weighted images, schwannomas tend to exhibit increased signal intensity (Figure 4–5).

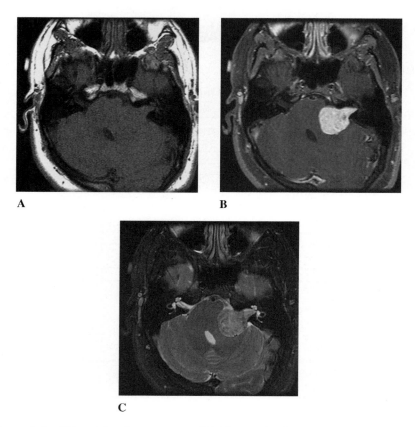

A   B

C

Figure 4–5. T1-weighted, precontrast (A), T1-weighted, postcontrast (B), and T2-weighted (C) axial MR images for a patient with a left vestibular schwannoma. Note the expansion of the internal auditory canal and increased signal intensity of the tumor on the T2-weighted scan. (Courtesy of The University of Texas M. D. Anderson Cancer Center, Department of Neurosurgery, Houston, Texas)

Management

The treatment options for patients with vestibular schwannomas include observation, microsurgical removal, radiosurgery, and stereotactic radiotherapy. The approach chosen must take into account the patient's age and medical condition, the quality of the patient's hearing, the tumor size, and the experience of the surgical and radiosurgical team.

Observation.   Not all patients with vestibular schwannomas require treatment. Patients older than 65 years with ipsilateral hearing loss without evidence of brainstem compression or hydrocephalus may simply be followed clinically and radiographically with serial CT or MRI performed at regular intervals. Progression of symptoms and signs or tumor growth require intervention.

Surgery.   The ideal treatment for symptomatic patients with vestibular schwannomas is complete microsurgical excision of the tumor. Concomitant goals include the preservation of facial nerve function, low morbidity and mortality, and when possible, preservation of hearing.

The choice of surgical approach should take into account the size and degree of tumor extension into the internal auditory canal, the quality of the patient's hearing, and the experience of the surgical team. Every attempt should be made to preserve useful hearing, although it must be realized that when the tumor is larger than 2 cm or fills the fundus of the internal auditory canal, this goal is far less frequently realized. With all surgical approaches, the rate of anatomic preservation of the facial nerve is higher than 95%. Functional facial nerve preservation for tumors larger than 3 cm is also higher than 75%, regardless of the approach used, which highlights the importance of surgical technique and experience. Facial nerve monitoring has improved preservation of facial nerve function and should be used. Hearing preservation depends on the tumor size, the degree of preoperative hearing, and the experience of the operating surgeon. Hearing preservation rates have been reported to be 35% to 80% in selected patients. Long-term hearing preservation is significantly increased when functional hearing is preserved in the immediate postoperative period. Total tumor removal can be accomplished in most cases with a mortality rate of less than 1%. Tumor recurrence rates of less than 3% have been reported after complete tumor excision.

Radiosurgery and Stereotactic Radiotherapy.   Radiosurgery is the principal alternative to microsurgical resection of vestibular schwannomas. The goals of radiosurgery are the prevention of tumor growth, the maintenance of neurologic function, and the prevention of new neurologic deficits.

In reviewing their 15 years of experience with 829 cases of vestibular schwannoma treated by Gamma Knife radiosurgery, Lunsford et al (2005) reported a tumor control rate of 97% at 10 years, preservation of hearing in 50% to 77% of patients, facial neuropathy in less than 1%, and trigeminal dysfunction in less than 3%. Other recent trials have reported tumor control rates of 87% to 97%, preservation of functional hearing in 37% to 83% of patients, and facial and trigeminal neuropathies in 0% to 11% of patients. Fractionated stereotactic radiotherapy has also been found to be effective in treating vestibular schwannomas: tumor control rates of 90% to 100% at 3 to 5 years, preservation of functional hearing in 60% to 93% of patients, and facial and trigeminal neuropathies in 2% to 18% of patients have been reported.

Radiosurgical and stereotactic radiotherapeutic modalities have not been directly compared in prospective randomized trials. Gamma Knife radiosurgery has traditionally been limited to tumors smaller than 3 cm, and stereotactic radiotherapy has been reserved for larger, nonsurgically treated tumors as well as incompletely resected tumors. Retrospective comparisons show similar tumor control rates for the 2 modalities. In addition, the rate of facial and trigeminal nerve injuries is similar between stereotactic radiotherapy and low-dose radiosurgery and higher for high-dose radiosurgery. Should radiosurgery or radiotherapy be unsuccessful, subsequent surgical resection may be necessary. These salvage surgeries are more technically challenging operations, require longer operative times, have higher rates of incomplete tumor resection, and are associated with a worse prognosis for postoperative cranial nerve function, especially facial nerve function.

A useful management algorithm is presented in Figure 4–6. In elderly patients, tumors 2.5 cm in diameter or smaller without brainstem compression are best managed by close clinical observation and monitoring by MRI. Younger patients with tumors 2.5 cm or smaller are candidates for microsurgical excision or radiosurgery. Accurate data regarding

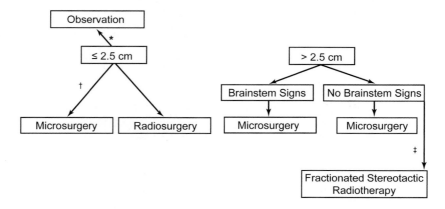

Figure 4–6. Management algorithm for vestibular schwannomas. *For elderly patients. † Preferable for patients less than 40 years of age. ‡ For elderly patients, infirm patients, or patients who refuse surgery. (Courtesy of The University of Texas M. D. Anderson Cancer Center, Department of Neurosurgery, Houston, Texas)

the surgeon's or radiosurgeon's personal outcome data should be shared with the patient so that the patient can make an informed decision. A bias exists toward surgery for patients under 40 years of age. Tumors larger than 2.5 cm associated with signs of brainstem compression are best managed by surgical excision. For tumors of this size without signs of brainstem compression, surgical excision is typically also recommended, but fractionated stereotactic radiotherapy can be used for elderly or infirm patients or for patients who refuse surgery.

Other Cranial Nerve Schwannomas

Trigeminal Schwannomas

Schwannomas of the trigeminal nerve account for less than 0.5% of intracranial tumors and up to 8% of intracranial Schwann cell tumors (Figure 4–7). Half are located in the middle fossa arising from the ganglionic segment of the trigeminal nerve. Trigeminal schwannomas of the ganglionic segment result in facial numbness or pain and corneal hypoesthesia in 80% to 90% of patients. These are the initial complaints in about 60% of patients, although in 10% to 20% of patients, trigeminal dysfunction never develops. Tumors of the ganglionic segment are more frequently associated with facial pain than are those of the trigeminal root.

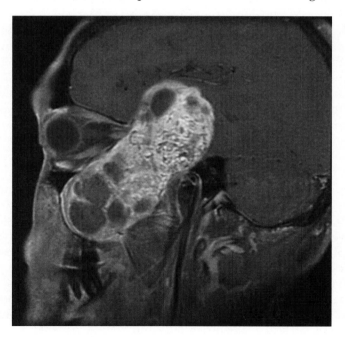

Figure 4–7. T1-weighted, postcontrast sagittal MR image of a giant trigeminal schwannoma arising from the second division of the nerve. Areas of cystic degeneration in tumors of this size are common. (Courtesy of The University of Texas M. D. Anderson Cancer Center, Department of Neurosurgery, Houston, Texas)

Diplopia, usually on the basis of an abducens palsy, is the initial symptom in 15% of patients but is present in 50% by the time of diagnosis. Facial weakness and hearing loss are rare symptoms of this lesion. When they occur, the presumptive mechanism is involvement of the greater superficial petrosal nerve, the facial nerve, and the eustachian tube or cochlea in the temporal bone. Impairment of lower cranial nerve function and long tract signs are noted at diagnosis in 30% to 50% of patients.

As for vestibular schwannomas, complete excision of trigeminal schwannomas nearly always results in cure and is the goal of any surgical procedure. Tumors of the trigeminal root are generally approached through a retrosigmoid craniectomy, while a variety of approaches are available for middle fossa or dumbbell-shaped tumors. Trigeminal nerve deficits are the most common morbidity of surgery, although improvements in trigeminal nerve function have been noted. Al-Mefty et al (2002) reported a series of 25 patients who had trigeminal schwannomas that were totally resected. After a mean follow-up of 33 months, there was improvement in trigeminal deficits in 44% of patients, decreased facial pain in 73%, and improvement in trigeminal motor deficits in 63%. Twelve percent of the patients experienced a persistent, new, or worse cranial nerve function after surgery, and tumors recurred in 3 patients after an average of 22.3 months. Sarma et al (2002) reported on 26 patients who underwent gross total resection of trigeminal nerve schwannomas. Improvement in trigeminal nerve function was seen in 44.4% and improvement in facial nerve function was seen in 75% of patients with preoperative dysfunction. There were no recurrences, 38.4% of the patients experienced new cranial nerve deficits (the most common of which was a cranial nerve IV deficit), and 0.4% reported worsening of trigeminal function postoperatively. Finally, in a study of Gamma Knife radiosurgical treatment of 56 patients who had trigeminal schwannomas, a tumor control rate of 93% was achieved (Pan et al, 2005). Trigeminal nerve dysfunction was reported in 13 of the patients.

Facial Nerve Schwannomas

Slowly progressive facial weakness is the typical clinical presentation of a facial nerve schwannoma. Sudden facial weakness, however, occurs in about 10% of cases, and a full third of patients with facial nerve schwannomas never manifest facial weakness. Facial spasm has been reported in up to 17% of patients. Conductive, sensorineural, or mixed hearing loss occurs in 50% of patients. Tinnitus and vertigo occur in 13% and 10% of patients, respectively. External manifestations of the tumor, such as a mass, pain, or otorrhea, occur in 30% or more of patients. Facial nerve schwannomas are rare and account for only 1.5% of CPA tumors. These tumors involve the tympanic or vertical segments in 60% and 50% of patients, respectively. Multiple segments are almost always affected (Figure 4–8). If the tumor is small, it may be separable from the nerve, but in most cases resection and facial nerve grafting are required. Complete excision is curative.

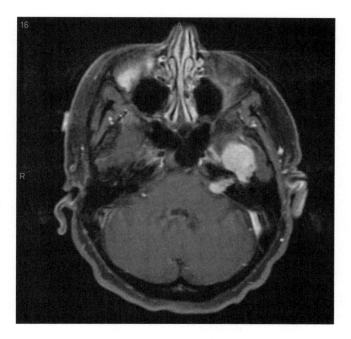

Figure 4–8. T1-weighted, postcontrast axial MR image of a patient with left facial weakness reveals a schwannoma of the facial nerve with involvement of the internal auditory canal and middle fossa along the course of the greater superficial petrosal nerve. (Courtesy of The University of Texas M. D. Anderson Cancer Center, Department of Neurosurgery, Houston, Texas)

Jugular Foramen Schwannomas

Jugular foramen tumors comprise up to 4.0% of intracranial schwannomas. Although it is difficult, if not impossible, to identify the specific nerve of origin, the clinical presentation and the surgical management of a jugular foramen schwannoma are more a function of anatomic location than of specific nerve origin. These tumors are typically classified as type A, B, or C based on their location (Kaye et al, 1984). Type A tumors are primarily intracranial masses with only minor extension into the foramen. Tumors within the bony foramen, with or without an intracranial component, are classed as type B. Type C tumors are primarily extracranial and have only minor extension into the foramen or the posterior fossa. A fourth category, type D, has been suggested for tumors that have both intracranial and extracranial extensions with a saddlebag or dumbbell-shaped appearance on images (Figure 4–9). Patients with type B and C tumors present with various forms of the jugular foramen syndrome (Table 4–3), although hoarseness is usually the initial symptom. Type A tumors may be clinically indistinguishable from vestibular schwannomas.

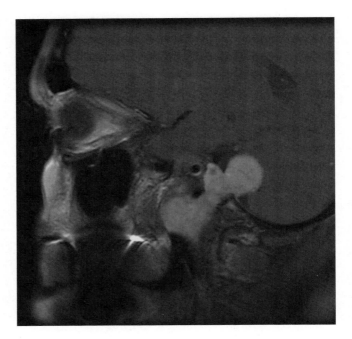

Figure 4–9. T1-weighted, postcontrast sagittal MR image of a schwannoma of the left jugular foramen. Note the dumbbell shape of this intracranial and extracranial tumor. (Courtesy of The University of Texas M. D. Anderson Cancer Center, Department of Neurosurgery, Houston, Texas)

Table 4–3.   Jugular Foramen Syndromes

Signs	Syndrome
Palsies of cranial nerves IX, X, and XI	Vernet's
Palsies of cranial nerves IX, X, XI, and XII	Collet-Sicard
Palsies of cranial nerves IX, X, XI, and XII and the sympathetic nerves	Villaret's

Total resection of jugular foramen schwannomas is essentially curative, although postoperative cranial nerve morbidity rates of up to 38% have been reported. A recent study of 6 patients with dumbbell-shaped jugular foramen tumors operated on by Kadri and Al-Mefty (2004) reported no additional postoperative cranial nerve deficits, improvement in 9th and 10th cranial nerve function in 2 patients, and no recurrence during a mean follow-up of 32.8 months.

Radiosurgery is a good alternative for small jugular foramen schwannomas. Tumor control was achieved in 16 of 17 patients treated by Muthukumar et al (1999) at a mean follow-up of 3.5 years. They concluded that radiosurgery is best reserved for small tumors, patients without lower cranial nerve deficits, and patients with residual or recurrent tumor.

The management of lower cranial nerve dysfunction is by far the most important aspect of patients' care. If extensive jugular foramen dissection is necessary, early tracheostomy may be warranted to avoid aspiration pneumonitis. Patients must not be allowed to eat or drink until definite objective evidence of an adequate swallowing mechanism without aspiration is obtained. A modified barium swallow, consultation with speech pathology, and laryngoscopy should be obtained. Pooling of secretions, a dysfunctional swallowing mechanism, or aspiration identifies patients who require further rehabilitation.

Schwannomas of the 3rd, 4th, 6th, and 12th Cranial Nerves

Schwannomas of the cranial nerves subserving extraocular muscle function are extremely rare. The clinical presentation usually involves diplopia due to dysfunction of the tumor's nerve of origin. Other symptoms may include decreased visual acuity, hemiparesis, ataxia of gait, paresthesia, and symptoms of intracranial hypertension. Treatment is surgical resection, which may occasionally be associated with functionally normal eye movements.

When they occur, hypoglossal schwannomas are usually located entirely within the intracranial compartment. Less commonly, they are shaped like dumbbells and have both intracranial and extracranial components. Purely extracranial tumors can also occur. Unilateral lingual atrophy, deviation, and fibrillation are nearly universal findings. Intracranial hypertension, long tract signs, ataxia, and dysfunction of the other lower cranial nerves may occur.

CRANIOPHARYNGIOMAS

Epidemiology

Craniopharyngiomas account for up to 4% of all intracranial tumors. They have a bimodal age distribution with peaks at 5 to 14 years and 50 to 60 years. The overall incidence of this tumor is 0.5 to 2.5 per 1,000,000 population. There is no apparent sex or racial variance. No definite genetic relationships have been identified, and familial cases are rare. The most common location of craniopharyngiomas is the suprasellar region. These tumors account for 13% of all suprasellar tumors and 56% of suprasellar tumors in children, in whom they represent 5% to 10% of all intracranial tumors.

Etiology

Two hypotheses have been advanced to explain the origin of craniopharyngiomas. The embryogenetic theory relates to the development of the adenohypophysis and transformation of the remnant cells of the craniopharyngeal duct and Rathke's pouch. During the fourth week of gestation, the infundibulum, which is a downward evagination of the diencephalon, comes into contact with Rathke's pouch, an invagination of the primitive oral cavity (stomodeum). The neck of the pouch is the craniopharyngeal duct, which eventually narrows, closes, and separates from the stomodeum by the end of the second month of gestation. This newly formed vesicle then flattens and surrounds the infundibulum, and its walls form the structures of the hypophysis. The vesicle itself involutes into a cleft or may disappear completely. It is from the cells of the embryologic craniopharyngeal duct or Rathke's pouch that, according to this theory, craniopharyngiomas arise. In contrast, the metaplastic theory advances the possibility that craniopharyngiomas arise from squamous metaplasia of residual epithelial cells derived from the primitive stomodeum and normally contained within the adenohypophysis. Both theories are likely operative, thus explaining the histopathologic spectra of craniopharyngiomas. The adamantinomatous variety, which is most prevalent in childhood, is likely derived from embryologic remnants, whereas the squamous-papillary form of the tumor, which is the predominant type found in adults, may be attributed to metaplasia of cellular foci derived from mature cells of the anterior hypophysis.

Clinical Presentation

The clinical presentation of craniopharyngiomas is typically insidious. An interval of 1 to 2 years between the onset of symptoms and diagnosis is common. The most common presenting symptoms are headache, endocrine dysfunction, and visual disturbance. Headache, which is reported by 55% to 86% of patients, is dull but progressively severe, continuous, and at times positional. The etiology of the headache may be increased intracranial pressure secondary to hydrocephalus or compression of the sellar dura mater or sellar diaphragm. On presentation, 66% to 90% of patients have some degree of endocrine dysfunction. The most common manifestation is hypothyroidism, which occurs in 40% of patients. Almost a fourth of patients have associated signs of adrenal insufficiency, and 20% have diabetes insipidus. Eighty percent of adults complain of decreased libido. Impotence and amenorrhea are common. Visual disturbance, which is due to compression of the optic nerves, chiasm, or tracts, occur in 40% to 70% of patients.

Three distinct clinical syndromes have been described which relate to the anatomic localization of the tumor. A prechiasmal localization typically results in progressive decline of visual acuity and constriction of visual fields with the associated finding of optic atrophy. Hydrocephalus and signs of increased intracranial pressure are most commonly associated with retrochiasmal craniopharyngiomas. Intrasellar craniopharyngiomas usually manifest as headache and endocrinopathy.

Diagnostic Imaging

The radiologic hallmark of a craniopharyngioma is the appearance of a suprasellar calcified cyst. Not all craniopharyngiomas, however, are calcified or cystic. CT is the most sensitive method for demonstrating calcification, which is present in 85% of craniopharyngiomas. Calcification is more common in children (90%) than in adults (50%). CT is also useful for defining the cystic portion of the tumor. Up to 75% of craniopharyngiomas are cystic. The cyst contents usually have the same density as cerebrospinal fluid (CSF), and administration of contrast enhances the cyst capsule. With its multiplanar imaging capacity, MRI is essential for defining the local anatomy and is the most important imaging modality used for surgical planning and patient follow-up (Figure 4–10). But because MRI does not identify calcifications well, CT is used to complement it. Cysts are typically hyperintense on T1-weighted images, whereas the solid components are isointense and become hyperintense on administration of intravenous paramagnetic contrast agents.

Other important investigations necessary for all patients with presumed craniopharyngiomas are complete endocrinologic and neuro-ophthalmologic evaluations and neuropsychologic assessments. Differential diagnostic possibilities include pituitary adenoma, hypothalamic-optic pathway glioma, epidermoid or dermoid tumor, meningioma, hypothalamic hamartoma, germ cell tumor, metastasis, inflammatory processes such as sarcoidosis, histiocytosis X, and carotid or basilar aneurysm.

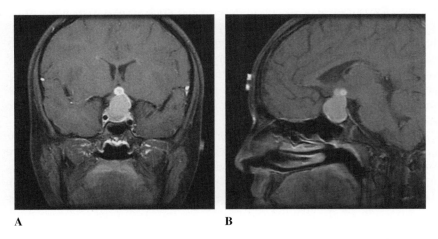

A   B

Figure 4–10. T1-weighted, postcontrast coronal (A) and sagittal (B) MR images of a patient with decreased vision and endocrinopathy reveal a cystic sellar and suprasellar craniopharyngioma. (Courtesy of The University of Texas M. D. Anderson Cancer Center, Department of Neurosurgery, Houston, Texas)

Pathology

Cystic craniopharyngiomas usually consist of a single large cyst or multiple cysts filled with turbid, brownish-yellow proteinaceous material. This material has been compared with crankcase machinery oil and may sparkle or glitter because of the high content of cholesterol crystals floating in the emulsion. The tumor most frequently arises on the pituitary stalk and projects into the hypothalamus. It may extend anteriorly into the prechiasmatic space and subfrontal region; posteriorly into the prepontine, interpeduncular, or cerebellopontine cisterns; superiorly into the third ventricle; or laterally into the middle fossa. Purely intraventricular craniopharyngiomas have been described. Metastatic craniopharyngiomas are extremely rare.

Three histopathologic variants of craniopharyngiomas have been described. Adamantinomatous craniopharyngiomas consist of reticular epithelial masses resembling the enamel pulp of developing teeth. Squamous-papillary craniopharyngiomas are composed of islands of simple squamous epithelium and fibrovascular islands of connective tissue. The third variant is a mixed tumor evidencing features of the first 2 variants.

Management

The management of craniopharyngiomas requires a multidisciplinary approach involving specialists in neurosurgery, endocrinology, neuroophthalmology, neuropsychology, and radiation oncology. A full endocrinologic assessment is necessary. Particular attention must be paid to the presence of hypothyroidism, adrenal insufficiency, and diabetes insipidus because the presence of any or all of these has been shown to increase intraoperative and postoperative morbidity. Potential adrenal insufficiency needs to be addressed (by steroid replacement) before the hypothyroidism is treated, as the initiation of thyroid replacement before steroid replacement can precipitate acute adrenal insufficiency. Symptomatic acute hydrocephalus needs to be treated by prompt external ventricular drainage. The presence of untreated preoperative hydrocephalus negatively affects patient outcome.

Consensus has not been reached on the surgical treatment of choice for craniopharyngiomas. Gross total resection would seem the most intuitive treatment, but it can be associated with morbidity and mortality rates as high as 20% and 12%, respectively (this rate excludes endocrinopathies). The recurrence rate may also be as high as 20%. The surgical approaches for resection of a craniopharyngioma include pterional, orbitocranial, subfrontal, transsphenoidal, and transcallosal. At times, a combination of approaches is required. Some authors have proposed limited surgery with the goals of pathologic confirmation of the tumor and surgical decompression of the optic nerves, chiasm, and tracts. Surgery would then be followed by external-beam radiotherapy at a dose of 54 to 55 Gy delivered at 1.8 Gy per fraction. The incidence of tumor progression after planned limited surgery and radiotherapy ranges from 12% to 25% and is similar to that seen with failed gross total resection and radiotherapy. Thus, the optimal surgical approach should strive for *safe* gross total resection, with the fact kept in mind that hypothalamic injury correlates directly with the degree of psychosocial impairment and ultimate outcome. External-beam radiotherapy should follow failed gross total resection or limited resections, since tumor progression occurs in more than half of these cases. Radiotherapy at the time of tumor progression is associated with a posttreatment progression rate of 29%. Early studies have shown that stereotactic radiosurgery may be beneficial, particularly for patients with small solid tumors.

Potential morbidity associated with treatment of craniopharyngiomas includes seizure, worsening of visual deficit, hypothalamic injury, stroke, and CSF leakage. Endocrinopathy is very common. Permanent diabetes insipidus occurs in 65% to 75% of adults. Replacement of 2 or more of the anterior pituitary hormones is necessary in 80% to 90% of patients, and obesity occurs in 50%.

Another treatment that may be useful in managing craniopharyngiomas, especially at recurrence, is intermittent cyst aspiration by stereotactic puncture or Ommaya reservoir placement. In addition, intracystic injection of bleomycin or radioisotopes can be tried. Such injection is rarely done, however, because of the possibility of leakage of the therapeutic agent with subsequent arachnoiditis and damage to the brain or cranial nerves. Overall, the 5- and 10-year survival rates for patients with craniopharyngiomas are 91% and 90%, respectively (Yasargil et al, 1990).

EPIDERMOID AND DERMOID CYSTS

Epidermoid and dermoid cysts have a similar appearance, derivation, pathogenesis, and clinical outcome. Both are thought to be congenital lesions that increase in size secondary to desquamation of keratin, cholesterol, and cellular debris. Epidermoid cysts typically expand and conform to subarachnoid spaces, but dermoid cysts do not. The tumors may be further differentiated by patient age at clinical onset, rate of progression, preferential location, and frequency of associated lesions.

Epidemiology

Intracranial epidermoid cysts have an incidence of less than 2% and represent less than 2% of all intracranial tumors. The ratio of epidermoid to dermoid cysts is approximately 10 to 1.5. Recent studies suggest a mild female predominance for both tumors. Epidermoid cysts are most commonly diagnosed in the third to fifth decades of life, whereas dermoid cysts typically become symptomatic in the first and second decades.

Epidermoid cysts have an affinity for the subarachnoid cisterns at the base of the brain and are most commonly found in the parachiasmal suprasellar cistern and the CPA. The CPA is the most common site, and epidermoid cysts account for 7% of all CPA tumors. Epidermoid cysts may be present in other areas such as in the third ventricle, lateral ventricles, and temporal horns; beneath the frontal lobe in the anterior fossa; and at the temporal tip of the middle fossa. The fourth ventricle is not an uncommon location for either epidermoid or dermoid cysts. Dermoid cysts tend to occur in the midline.

Etiology and Pathogenesis

Both epidermoid and dermoid cysts are produced by the inward displacement of cutaneous epithelial tissue (ectoderm) during embryonic development. The tissue may be displaced into bone or into the soft tissue of an interspace such as a fontanelle or deeper tissues. During the third to fourth weeks of embryogenesis, the neural plate invaginates in the dorsal midline to form the neural groove. As the neural folds approach the midline to form the neural tube, ectopic epithelium may be deposited at sites between the neural canal and skin if the sequence of development is altered or incomplete. This theory is supported by identification of epithelial rests in tracts leading to deeply placed lesions. Secondary vesicles formed during development (otic and optic) may also result in epithelial misplacements, accounting for laterally placed squamous-lined cysts.

Clinical Presentation

Epidermoid cysts grow more slowly than dermoid cysts do by desquamation of epithelium and accumulation of cellular debris. As in stratified squamous epithelia elsewhere, the single basal layer of germinative cells gives rise to the other strata. Epithelial cells rest on a basement membrane anchored in a capsule of fibrous connective tissue. Enlargement of the tumors produces a lytic effect on the bone, resulting in a delicate, scalloped margin. Symptoms are due to compression of surrounding neurovascular structures.

The natural history of these lesions is one of slow, relentless progression of symptoms. Signs and symptoms generally depend on the cyst's location. Seizure is not uncommon with supratentorial tumors, whereas the presence of hydrocephalus is relatively rare even with tumors filling the aqueduct. Cranial nerve symptoms are typically irritative rather than dysfunctional. Epidermoid cysts of the CPA are strongly associated with facial pain. Rupture of a cyst's contents may trigger chemical meningitis and symptoms of meningeal irritation (i.e., Mollaret's meningitis, which is also occasionally seen with craniopharyngiomas).

If present, distinguishing features of dermoid cysts are dermal sinuses with external tufts of hair and focal areas of skin pigmentation. Some patients with dermoid cysts may have spina bifida occulta or vertebral segment anomalies. Dermal sinuses provide a potential portal of entry for organisms.

Diagnostic Imaging

Both epidermoid and dermoid cysts are of low attenuation (i.e., hypo-dense) on CT images. Dermoid cysts are more likely to contain calcification and have a greater range of attenuation. MRI is the imaging of choice for these tumors. Epidermoid and dermoid cysts are well defined, and on T2-weighted images they have an increased signal intensity. Fast fluid-attenuated inversion recovery (FLAIR) and diffusion-weighted images can be useful in revealing the subarachnoid extent of the tumor and narrowing the differential diagnosis, as these sequences are able to distinguish tumor from the surrounding CSF (Figure 4–11). These tumors are rarely enhanced by contrast. Cyst contents such as hair and sebum give

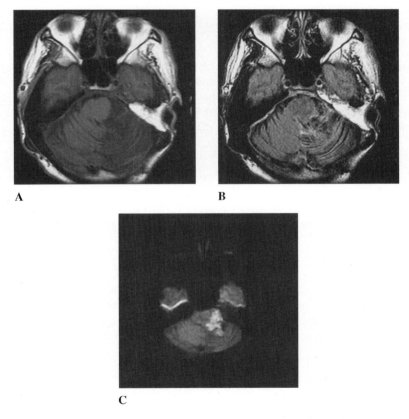

Figure 4–11. Axial T1-weighted (A), FLAIR (B), and diffusion-weighted MR (C) images of a patient with a recurrent left CPA epidermoid cyst. The lesion is indistinguishable from CSF on the T1-weighted image but shows internal structure on the FLAIR image and the restricted diffusion image (i.e., it is bright on the diffusion images). (Courtesy of The University of Texas M. D. Anderson Cancer Center, Department of Neurosurgery, Houston, Texas)

dermoid cysts a heterogeneous MRI signal, while the abundant lipid produces a high signal intensity on TI-weighted images.

Management

The treatment of choice is total resection of the contents of the cyst and its lining, but this is possible only in certain areas. These lesions tend to encircle or adhere to cranial nerves, blood vessels, and vital neurologic structures, thereby preventing complete resection in some circumstances. Small fragments of the cyst capsule left on the brainstem, basal vessels, or cranial nerves appear to have a benign course and low recurrence rates. Yasargil et al (1989) noted no cases of clinical or radiologic recurrence in their review of patients followed up for up to 20 years.

CHOROID PLEXUS PAPILLOMAS

Unlike choroid plexus papillomas of childhood, which generally present in the lateral ventricle, choroid plexus papillomas of adulthood generally present in the fourth ventricle or the CPA. These tumors may bulge into the CPA through the foramen of Luschka. Few surgical studies have evaluated outcomes for adult patients afflicted with this tumor.

Epidemiology

Choroid plexus papillomas are uncommon benign (WHO grade I) tumors in adults. The incidence of this tumor is approximately 0.5%. Males appear to have a higher incidence rate of 3:2 (McGirr et al, 1988). Ten percent of these tumors may undergo malignant transformation to choroid plexus carcinomas.

Etiology

Transgenic mice infected with SV-40 virus have DNA sequences similar to those of SV-40 virus found in choroid plexus tumors. This observation suggests the oncogenic properties of this polyomavirus. Malignant transformation of these tumors might also be the result of *TP53* germline mutations.

Clinical Presentation

Increased intracranial pressure secondary to obstructive hydrocephalus is the most common clinical presentation of choroid plexus papillomas. The obstruction of CSF flow out of the fourth ventricle is generally considered the main cause of the hydrocephalus. However, many patients continue to have hydrocephalus after tumor resection and often require ventriculoperitoneal shunting. Although the presiding consensus is that increased CSF production causes hydrocephalus in many patients, decreased CSF absorption secondary to occlusion of the arachnoid villi due to microdissemination of the tumor has also been implicated

Diagnostic Imaging

Choroid plexus papillomas are highly vascular neoplasms. They have a prominent vascular supply with enlarged choroidal arteries and early draining veins. On CT images, these tumors are isodense or hyperdense to surrounding brain in approximately 75% of cases. Calcification is not uncommon in adults. The tumors often have frond-like surfaces. Contrast enhancement is generally intense.

On MR images, choroid plexus papillomas are well circumscribed and usually compress (rather than invade) surrounding structures. They are generally isointense to surrounding brain on T1-weighted images and CSF is trapped between the papillae, which often gives these tumors a mottled appearance. On T2-weighted images, these tumors are generally isotense or hyperintense to brain. Contrast enhancement is intense. Hydrocephalus is often seen (Figure 4–12), and the presence of diffuse leptomeningeal metastases is not uncommon even in patients with histologically benign choroid plexus papillomas.

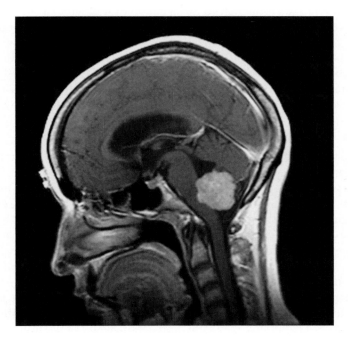

Figure 4–12. T1-weighted, postcontrast sagittal MR image of a patient with headache. This tumor was pathologically proven to be a choroid plexus papilloma. Note the presence of hydrocephalus. (Courtesy of The University of Texas M. D. Anderson Cancer Center, Department of Neurosurgery, Houston, Texas)

Management

Since choroid plexus papillomas are benign, surgical treatment alone should be curative and prevent recurrence. In a surgical series by McGirr et al (1988), only 1 of 14 patients with a gross total removal had a recurrence 11 years later. This study suggested that adjuvant radiation was not beneficial after subtotal resection. In a meta-analysis of studies of choroid plexus tumors, Wolff et al (2002) identified gross total resection as the most important factor affecting outcome and concluded that adjuvant treatment does not affect patient survival even for those who have subtotally resected tumors and evidence of recurrence. Radiotherapy may be used in patients with recurrent unresectable disease. The irradiation should be focal, and the recommended dose is 50 to 55 Gy.

HEMANGIOBLASTOMAS

Hemangioblastomas are benign vascular neoplasms of the central nervous system that typically present in the posterior fossa or upper cervical cord. Hemangioblastomas are the most common primary tumors of the posterior fossa in adults. A supratentorial presentation of this tumor is unusual. This tumor is often associated with von Hippel-Lindau disease (VHL). von Hippel was the first to describe the presence of a hemangioblastoma of the retina in 1904. It was Lindau who, in 1926, associated the coincidence of retinal, cerebellar, and visceral hemangioblastomas with a clinical entity or syndrome now referred to as VHL. Solitary hemangioblastomas of the posterior fossa in patients without the clinical criteria of VHL are called "Lindau tumors."

Epidemiology and Genetics

Approximately 75% of hemangioblastomas are sporadic. The remaining cases are associated with VHL, which is an autosomal dominant phakomatosis with a high degree of penetrance that results from a germline mutation in the *VHL* gene (on chromosome band 3p25-26). Cerebellar hemangioblastomas are present in 60% to 80% of patients with VHL. Patients with VHL typically have multiple tumors of the posterior fossa and the upper cervical cord. The *VHL* gene encodes the VHL protein (pVHL), which acts as a tumor suppressor. pVHL forms a complex with other proteins and proteolytically degrades the cellular components with which it binds. Hypoxia-inducible factor-1 (HIF-1) is regulated by pVHL. In the presence of normal oxygen levels, pVHL binds and degrades HIF-1. HIF-1 regulates growth factors and mitogens such as PDGFβ, VEGF, tumor growth factor α, and erythropoietin under the regulation of pVHL and oxygen levels. The absence or dysfunction of pVHL results in increased levels of HIF-1 and a pseudohypoxic state, both of which may contribute to hemangioblastoma formation and progression. PDGFβ and VEGF are known stimulators of angiogenesis; VEGF also causes vascular permeability, which could be associated with the common finding of peritumoral edema or cysts; and tumor growth factor α is a known mitogen, which also up-regulates growth factor receptors and may create an autocrine loop. pVHL also affects other targets not related to the HIF pathway, such as cell matrix-associated molecules, which may also be associated with tumorigenesis and progression. The vast majority of patients with VHL present in the first or second decades of life, and the mean age of onset of symptoms is approximately 33 years. Half of these patients have multiple lesions. Patients with sporadic (i.e., nonsyndromic) hemangioblastomas present in the fifth to sixth decades of life and classically have a single lesion in the cerebellum.

Clinical Presentation

Patients with hemangioblastomas usually have mild symptoms for approximately 1 year before diagnosis. With the advent of modern neuroimaging and the greater awareness of the importance of imaging family members of patients with VHL, tumors are now being identified earlier. The most common presentation includes occipital headache and associated cerebellar signs. Cranial nerve abnormalities are not uncommon in patients presenting with brainstem lesions. In patients with larger midline posterior fossa lesions, hydrocephalus may result. A distinguishing feature in up to 30% of patients with hemangioblastomas is polycythemia, which has been attributed to an erythropoietin-like substance secreted by these tumors.

Diagnostic Imaging

On CT scans, a hemangioblastoma appears as a low-density cyst with an enhanced vascular nodule or as a solid vascular mass. The solid portion of the tumor may at times be missed with contrast-enhanced CT imaging. MRI, however, clearly allows for visualization of the nodule (Figure 4–13). On T1-weighted images, the tumor is generally hypointense, and the mural nodule is enhanced with contrast. The tumor is classically associated with only a single cyst but may have multiple cysts. Angiography has been used to define the tumor by demonstrating its vascular pedicle and nodule. Angiography may be also used if preoperative embolization is to be considered.

Management

The treatment of a solitary hemangioblastoma is microsurgical resection. Preoperative embolization to decrease the vascularity of the tumor is warranted in some cases. Surgery involves resection of the mural nodule. The cyst does not need to be removed, as it disappears after tumor removal. Entry into the tumor during surgery can result in significant and at times torrential bleeding. The lesion should be removed en bloc and each feeding vessel near the tumor coagulated. Recurrence is unusual in cases when the mural nodule has been successfully resected.

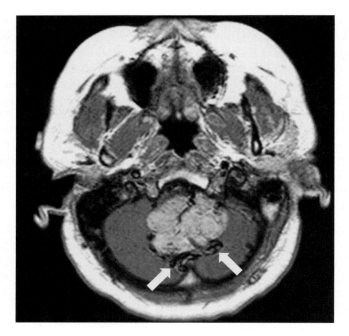

Figure 4–13. T1-weighted, postcontrast sagittal MR image reveals a giant poste-rior fossa hemangioblastoma. Note the marked vascularity of the lesion denoted by the large flow voids (arrows). (Courtesy of The University of Texas M. D. Anderson Cancer Center, Department of Neurosurgery, Houston, Texas)

Problems arise in the surgical management of hemangioblastomas when multiple tumors exist (often associated with VHL) or the tumors are located within functionally vital tissue. Although complete surgical resec-tion is still the treatment of choice in these cases, surgical resection with adjuvant radiotherapy or radiosurgery alone may be considered.

Radiosurgery in patients with hemangioblastomas theoretically should have effects similar to those observed for patients with arteriovenous mal-formations treated with radiosurgery. Wang et al (2005) treated 35 patients with hemangioblastomas with Gamma Knife irradiation of 17.2 Gy at the tumor margin (12 to 13 Gy at the brainstem) and followed the patients for a mean duration of 66 months. The 1- and 5-year actuarial tumor control rates were 94% and 71%, respectively. At the most recent follow-up, 6 patients had died, satisfactory tumor control was attained for 29, and stable or improved neurologic function was reported for 21. Ultimately, 8 of the 35 patients underwent surgical resection secondary to tumor-associated cyst enlarge-ment or the development of new tumors after radiosurgery, and 7 patients developed new hemangioblastomas; of the latter, 5 required additional radiosurgery. These findings are similar to those reported in other Gamma Knife and LINAC studies.

Wanebo et al (2003) recently reported on the natural history of hemangioblastomas among 160 patients with VHL treated at the National Institutes of Health. They noted that hemangioblastomas that have an associated cyst are more likely to become symptomatic than those that do not and that the rate of enlargement is far greater for the cysts than for the hemangioblastomas. Hemangioblastoma growth was typically phasic with sequential growth and quiescent phases, and over a median of 32 months, 44% of hemangioblastomas and 67% of their associated cysts grew. This phasic behavior may explain the relatively low response of hemangioblastomas to radiation. In that study, the presence of a tumor-associated cyst with a hemangioblastoma was considered a contraindication to radiosurgery.

KEY PRACTICE POINTS

- The incidence of intracranial meningiomas rises with increasing age, although the tumor growth rate decreases in the elderly.

- Compared with non–radiation-induced meningiomas, radiation-induced meningiomas are biologically more aggressive, possess more atypical histology, are more likely to recur, are more likely to occur in multiple locations, have different cytogenetic characteristics, and do not exhibit behavior that correlates with their proliferative index.

- Contrast-enhanced MRI provides the most sensitive and specific means of detecting meningiomas.

- Small, asymptomatic, incidentally identified meningiomas, particularly in elderly patients, can be managed with observation and serial imaging.

- Delaying radiotherapy until meningioma recurrence or progression of residual disease is possible without compromising overall patient survival.

- All patients with vestibular schwannomas 2.5 cm in diameter or smaller are candidates for microsurgical excision or radiosurgery and should be fully informed of the risks, benefits, and outcomes of both therapies in order to reach an informed decision.

- The assessment, identification, and management of lower cranial neuropathy are by far the most important aspects of care for patients with jugular foramen tumors.

- Optimal management of craniopharyngiomas strives for a safe gross total resection, since hypothalamic injury correlates directly with the degree of psychosocial impairment and the patient's ultimate outcome.

- Distinguishing features of intracranial dermoid cysts are dermal sinuses with external tufts of hair and focal areas of skin pigmentation.

- Piecemeal removal of hemangioblastomas may result in significant and at times torrential bleeding. The tumor should be removed en bloc and each nutrient vessel near the tumor coagulated.

90 — F. DeMonte

SUGGESTED READINGS

Abramovich C, Prayson R. MIB-1 labeling indices in benign, aggressive, and malignant meningiomas: a study of 90 tumors. *Hum Pathol* 1998;29:1420–1427.

Alheit H, Saran F, Warrington A, et al. Stereotactically guided conformal radiotherapy for meningioma. *Radiother Oncol* 1999; 50:145–150.

Al-Mefty O, Ayoubi S, Gaber E. Trigeminal schwannomas: removal of dumbbell-shaped tumors through the expanded Meckel cave and outcomes of cranial nerve function. *J Neurosurg* 2002;96:453–463.

Al-Mefty O, Topsakal C, Pravdenkova S, Sawyer JR, Harrison MJ. Radiation-induced meningiomas: clinical, pathological, cytokinetic, and cytogenetic characteristics. *J Neurosurg* 2004;100:1002–1013.

Annegers JF, Laws ER Jr, Kurland LT, Grabow JD. Head trauma and subsequent brain tumors. *Neurosurgery* 1979;4:203–206.

Betchen SA, Walsh J, Post KD. Long-term hearing preservation after surgery for vestibular schwannoma. *J Neurosurg* 2005;102:6–9.

Briggs RJ, Fabinyi G, Kaye AH. Current management of acoustic neuromas: a review of surgical approaches and outcomes. *J Clin Neurosci* 2000;7: 521–526.

Carroll R, Glowacka D, Dashner K, Black P. Progesterone and glucocorticoid receptor activation in meningiomas. *Cancer Res* 1993;53:1312–1316.

Carroll RS, Schrell UM, Zhang J, et al. Dopamine D_1, dopamine D_2, and prolactin receptor messenger ribonucleic acid expression by the polymerase chain reaction in human meningiomas. *Neurosurgery* 1996;38:367–375.

Chuang CC, Chang CN, Tsang NM, et al. Linear accelerator-based radiosurgery in the management of skull base meningiomas. *J Neurooncol* 2004;66:241–249.

Drummond KJ, Zhu JJ, Black PM. Meningiomas: updating basic science, management, and outcome. *Neurologist* 2004;10:113–130.

Dumanski J, Carlbom E, Collins V, Nordenskjöld M. Deletion mapping of a locus on human chromosome 22 involved in the oncogenesis of meningioma. *Proc Natl Acad Sci U S A* 1987;84:9275–9279.

Goldsmith BJ, Wara WM, Wilson CB, Larson DA. Postoperative irradiation for subtotally resected meningiomas: a retrospective analysis of 140 patients treated from 1967 to 1990. *J Neurosurg* 1994;80:195–201.

Goodwin JW, Crowley J, Eyre HJ, Stafford B, Jaeckle KA, Townsend JJ. A phase II evaluation of tamoxifen in unresectable or refractory meningiomas: a Southwest Oncology Group study. *J Neurooncol* 1993;15:75–77.

Gormley WB, Tomecek FJ, Qureshi N, Malik GM. Craniocerebral epidermoid and dermoid tumors: a review of 32 cases. *Acta Neurochir (Wien)* 1994;128:115–121.

Grunberg S, Rankin C, Townsend J, et al. Phase III double-blind randomized placebo-controlled study of mifepristone for the treatment of unresectable meningioma. [Abstract] *Proc Am Soc Clin Oncol* 2001;20.

Hakim R, Alexander E 3rd, Loeffler JS, et al. Results of linear accelerator-based radiosurgery for intracranial meningiomas. *Neurosurgery* 1998;43:446–453.

Inskip PD, Mellemkjaer L, Gridley G, Olsen JH. Incidence of intracranial tumors following hospitalization for head injury (Denmark). *Cancer Causes Control* 1998;9:106–116.

Jääskeläinen J. Seemingly complete removal of histologically benign intracranial meningioma: late recurrence rate and factors predicting recurrence in 657 patients. *Surg Neurol* 1986;25:461–469.

Jääskeläinen J, Haltia M, Servo A. Atypical and anaplastic meningiomas: radiology, surgery, radiotherapy and outcome. *Surg Neurol* 1986;25:233–242.

Kaba S, DeMonte F, Bruner J, et al. The treatment of recurrent unresectable and malignant meningiomas with interferon α-2B. *Neurosurgery* 1997;40:271–275.

Kadri PA, Al-Mefty O. Surgical treatment of dumbbell-shaped jugular foramen schwannomas. *Neurosurg Focus* 2004;17:56–61.

Kartush J, Lundy L. Facial nerve outcome in acoustic neuroma surgery. *Otolaryngol Clin North Am* 1992; 25:623–647.

Kaye AH, Hahn JF, Kinney SE, Hardy RW Jr, Bay JW. Jugular foramen schwannomas. *J Neurosurg* 1984;60:1045–1053.

Kondziolka D, Levy E, Niranjan A, Flickinger J, Lunsford L. Long-term outcomes after meningioma radiosurgery: physician and patient perspectives. *J Neurosurg* 1999;91:44–50.

Kuratsu J, Ushio Y. Epidemiological study of primary intracranial tumors in elderly people. *J Neurol Neurosurg Psychiatry* 1997;63:116–118.

Lanser M, Sussman S, Frazer K. Epidemiology, pathogenesis, and genetics of acoustic tumors. *Otolaryngol Clin North Am* 1992;25:499–520.

Lee JY, Niranjan A, McInerney J, Kondziolka D, Flickinger JC, Lunsford LD. Stereotactic radiosurgery providing long-term tumor control of cavernous sinus meningiomas. *J Neurosurg* 2002;97:65–72.

Limb CJ, Long DM, Niparko JK. Acoustic neuromas after failed radiation therapy: challenges of surgical salvage. *Laryngoscope* 2005;115:93–98.

Lonser RR, Glenn GM, Walther M, et al. von Hippel-Lindau disease. *Lancet* 2003;361:2059–2067.

Lunsford LD, Niranjan A, Flickinger JC, Maitz A, Kondziolka D. Radiosurgery of vestibular schwannomas: summary of experience in 829 cases. *J Neurosurg* 2005;102 Suppl:195–199.

Maxwell M, Galanopoulos T, Hedley-Whyte ET, Black PM, Antoniades HN. *Int J Cancer* 1990;46:16–21.

McCutcheon IE, Flyvbjerg A, Hill H, et al. Antitumor activity of the growth hormone receptor antagonist pegvisomant against human meningiomas in nude mice. *J Neurosurg* 2001;94:487–492.

McGirr S, Ebersold M, Scheithauer B, Quast LM, Shaw EG. Choroid plexus papillomas: long-term follow-up results in a surgically treated series. *J Neurosurg* 1988;69:843–849.

Muthukumar N, Kondziolka D, Lunsford LD, Flickinger JC. Stereotactic radiosurgery for jugular foramen schwannomas. *Surg Neurol* 1999;52:172–179.

Nakamura M, Roser F, Michel J, Jacobs C, Samii M. The natural history of incidental meningiomas. *Neurosurgery* 2003;53:62–70.

Pan L, Wang EM, Zhang N, et al. Long-term results of Leksell gamma knife surgery for trigeminal schwannomas. *J Neurosurg* 2005;102 Suppl:220–224.

Pollock BE, Stafford SL, Utter A, Giannini C, Schreiner SA. Stereotactic radiosurgery provides equivalent tumor control to Simpson Grade 1 resection for patients with small- to medium-size meningiomas. *Int J Radiat Oncol Biol Phys* 2003;55:1000–1005.

Samii M, Babu R, Tatagiba M, Sepehrina A. Surgical treatment of jugular foramen schwannomas. *J Neurosurg* 1995;82:924–932.

Samii M, Migliori M, Tatagiba M, Babu R. Surgical treatment of trigeminal schwannomas. *J Neurosurg* 1995;82:711–718.

Sarma S, Sekhar LN, Schessel D. Nonvestibular schwannomas of the brain: a 7-year experience. *Neurosurgery* 2002;50:437–448.

Seizinger B, Martuiza R, Gusella J. Loss of genes on chromosome 22 in tumorigenesis of human acoustic neuroma. *Nature* 1986;322:644–647.

Shu J, Lee JH, Harwalkar JA, Oh-Siskovic S, Stacey DW, Golubic M. Adenovirus-mediated gene transfer of dominant negative Ha-Ras inhibits proliferation of primary meningioma cells. *Neurosurgery* 1999;44:579–587.

Soyuer S, Chang EL, Selek U, Shi W, Maor MH, DeMonte F. Radiotherapy after surgery for benign cerebral meningioma. *Radiother Oncol* 2004;71:85–90.

Spiegelmann R, Nissim O, Menhel J, Alezra D, Pfeffer MR. Linear accelerator radiosurgery for meningiomas in and around the cavernous sinus. *Neurosurgery* 2002;51:1373–1380.

Stafford S, Perry A, Suman V, et al. Primary resected meningiomas: outcome and prognostic factors in 581 Mayo Clinic patients, 1978–1988. *Mayo Clin Proc* 1998;73:936–942.

Wanebo JE, Lonser RR, Glenn GM, Oldfield EH. The natural history of hemangioblastomas of the central nervous system in patients with von Hippel-Lindau disease. *J Neurosurg* 2003;98:82–94.

Wang EM, Pan L, Wang BJ, et al. The long-term results of Gamma Knife radiosurgery for hemangioblastomas of the brain. *J Neurosurg* 2005;102 Suppl: 225–229.

Weisman A, Villemure J, Kelly P. Regulation of DNA synthesis and growth of cells derived from primary human meningiomas. *Cancer Res* 1986;46:2545–2550.

Westphal M, Hermann H. Epidermal growth factor receptors on cultured meningioma cells. *Acta Neurochir (Wein)* 1986;83:62–66.

Wolff JEA, Sajedi M, Brant R, Coppes MJ, Egeler RM. Choroid plexus tumours. *Br J Cancer* 2002;87:1086–1091.

Yasargil M, Abernathy C, Sarioglu A. Microsurgical treatment of intracranial dermoid and epidermoid tumors. *Neurosurgery* 1989;24:561–567.

Yasargil MG, Curcic M, Kis M, Siegenthaler G, Teddy PJ, Roth P. Total removal of craniopharyngiomas. Approaches and long-term results in 144 patients. *J Neurosurg* 1990;73:3–11.

Yonehara S, Brenner AV, Kishikawa M, et al. Clinical and epidemiologic characteristics of first primary tumors of the central nervous system and related organs among atomic bomb survivors in Hiroshima and Nagasaki, 1958–1995. *Cancer* 2004;101:1644–1654.

5   LOW-GRADE GLIOMAS: EVIDENCE-BASED TREATMENT OPTIONS

Frederick F. Lang

Chapter Overview 93
Introduction 94
Diffusely Infiltrating Low-Grade Gliomas 95
   Clinical Features 95
   Neuroimaging Features 96
   Histopathologic Characteristics 96
   Molecular Profiles 98
   Clinical Prognostic Factors 99
   Therapeutic Options 100
      Surgery 100
         Timing of Surgery 100
         Extent of Resection 101
      Radiotherapy 104
         Radiation Dose 104
         Timing of Radiotherapy 104
      Chemotherapy 106
Circumscribed Low-Grade Gliomas: "Astroglial Variants" 108
   Clinical Features 109
   Neuroimaging Features 111
   Histopathologic Characteristics 112
   Therapeutic Options 114
      Surgery 114
      Radiotherapy 115
      Chemotherapy 116
Conclusion 116
Key Practice Points 117
Suggested Readings 118

CHAPTER OVERVIEW

Low-grade gliomas consist of the diffusely infiltrating low-grade gliomas (astrocytomas, oligodendrogliomas, and mixed gliomas) and the more circumscribed "astroglial variants" (pilocytic astrocytomas, gangliogliomas, pleomorphic xanthoastrocytomas, and subependymal giant cell astrocytomas). Diffusely infiltrating low-grade gliomas spread widely throughout the brain and typically progress to higher-grade tumors, whereas the astroglial variants are less invasive and only rarely transform to more aggressive forms. Because of these distinctions, astroglial variants can be effectively treated in most cases by surgical resection, even when the lesions are located in eloquent brain areas such as the brainstem or suprasellar region. In contrast, diffusely infiltrating low-grade gliomas must invariably be treated with multiple modalities. Surgery is usually undertaken to achieve as complete a resection as possible while preserving neurologic function. Radiotherapy is an important part of the management of these lesions, but the timing of its administration is controversial; recent prospective clinical trials support both early administration and application at the time of recurrence. Chemotherapy has become an increasingly attractive option, especially for oligodendrogliomas that demonstrate a specific molecular signature, namely loss of chromosomes 1p and 19q. Clinical trials remain critical to the continued progress of managing low-grade gliomas.

INTRODUCTION

Low-grade gliomas are primary brain tumors in adults and children that are histologically classified as grade I or II according to the World Health Organization (WHO) grading system. Because of differences in their growth pattern, neuroimaging characteristics, and prognosis, it is clinically practical to divide low-grade gliomas into 2 groups (Table 5–1).

Table 5–1. Classification and Characterization of Low-Grade Gliomas

Characteristic	Diffuse LGGs	Astroglial Variants
	Classification	
Histologic type	Fibrillary astrocytoma, oligodendroglioma, and mixed glioma	Pilocytic astrocytoma, ganglioglioma, PXA, and SEGA
WHO grade	II	I or II
Growth pattern	Infiltrative into normal brain parenchyma	Minimally invasive into normal brain; more circumscribed
Neuroimaging features	Nonenhanced; hypointense on T1-weighted MR images; hyperintense on T2-weighted MR images	Enhanced on T1-weighted MR images; often with cyst
Prognosis	Progression to anaplastic glioma or glioblastoma almost inevitable	Generally good; potentially curable with surgery only

The diffusely infiltrating low-grade gliomas (diffuse LGGs), which include astrocytomas, oligodendrogliomas, and mixed gliomas, appear as nonenhanced lesions on magnetic resonance (MR) images. Although patients with these tumors may survive for relatively long periods, diffuse LGGs usually progress to lethal, higher-grade glial tumors. More circumscribed gliomas, the "astroglial variants," include pilocytic astrocytomas, gangliogliomas, pleomorphic xanthoastrocytomas (PXAs), and subependymal giant cell astrocytomas (SEGAs). These variants are usually less invasive than diffuse LGGs and appear as enhanced and typically cystic lesions on MR images. Treatment of astroglial variants is typically associated with long-term survival and often cure, regardless of the fact that the lesions can arise in highly eloquent brain regions.

This chapter considers the management of diffuse LGGs and astroglial variants separately to provide perspective on current controversies surrounding each group. Evidence-based treatment approaches from current clinical trials are emphasized.

DIFFUSELY INFILTRATING LOW-GRADE GLIOMAS

Diffuse LGGs are not a single biologic disease; rather, they comprise 3 distinct histologic tumor types: astrocytomas, oligodendrogliomas, and mixed gliomas. These tumors are classified as grade II by the WHO grading system (Kleihues and Cavenee, 2000). Because they typically progress to higher-grade tumors (i.e., anaplastic astrocytoma [WHO grade III], anaplastic oligodendroglioma [WHO grade III], or glioblastoma multiforme [WHO grade IV]), which are invariably fatal to the patient, reference to these lesions as "benign gliomas" should be abandoned. Instead, these lesions should be considered early-grade malignancies that grow by invading the normal brain parenchyma and can spread widely throughout the brain.

Clinical Features

Diffuse LGGs typically present in the fourth and fifth decades of life. The most common presenting symptom is seizure, which occurs in one half to two thirds of patients. Approximately 50% of patients present with headache. Fewer patients present with symptoms referable to the location of the lesion. Focal signs and symptoms may be caused by direct invasion of tumor cells into functional brain regions or by local pressure. Larger tumors may produce signs of raised intracranial pressure. In the modern era, the routine use of magnetic resonance imaging (MRI) has resulted in an increasing trend to identify diffuse LGGs in patients with few or no symptoms and with normal neurologic function. This trend has increased the complexity of treating these patients.

Neuroimaging Features

On computed tomography scans, diffuse LGGs usually appear as low-density lesions. Compared with MRI, computed tomography has the advantage of more readily detecting calcification, which is present in 60% to 90% of oligodendrogliomas. However, MRI is more sensitive and provides multiplanar imaging, which improves localization. With MRI, diffuse LGGs are hypointense on T1-weighted images (Figures 5–1 and 5–2) and hyperintense on T2-weighted images. The absence of enhancement after gadolinium administration is a *sine qua non* of diffuse LGGs, but it should be remembered that nearly 30% of nonenhanced lesions are higher-grade tumors.

Histopathologic Characteristics

Macroscopically, low-grade gliomas are poorly defined lesions that tend to expand and distort involved structures. Microscopically, a unifying histologic feature of these tumors is the diffuse infiltration of the tumor cells into the surrounding brain parenchyma. Specifically, in most diffuse LGGs, the tumor cells are dispersed within normal brain parenchyma and disrupt the normal arrangement of potentially functional neurons.

The relationship between tumor cell infiltration and neuroimaging was elegantly analyzed by Daumas-Duport and colleagues (1987), who reported histologic correlates of serial biopsy specimens through MRI-defined areas

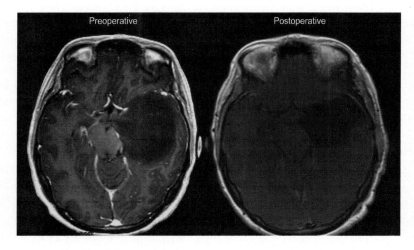

Figure 5–1. Preoperative and postoperative T1-weighted axial MR images show a nonenhanced tumor in the left temporal lobe of a 28-year-old woman who presented with a grand mal seizure. A total resection of the tumor was performed. The pathologic diagnosis was oligodendroglioma with LOH 1p/19q. Because of the patient's young age, the presence of small residual disease (posterior), and the LOH 1p/19q, the patient was subsequently treated with temozolomide.

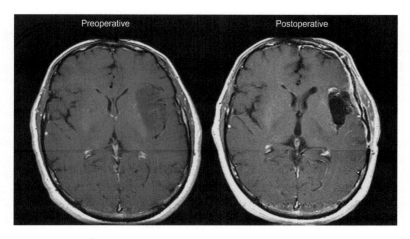

Figure 5–2. Preoperative and postoperative T1-weighted axial MR images of a nonenhanced tumor of the insular lobe in the left hemisphere of a 43-year-old man who presented with focal seizure. Tumors in this location are difficult to resect, but total resection was achieved. The pathologic diagnosis was grade II astrocytoma. The patient is being followed up until signs of recurrence, at which time radiotherapy is planned.

of glial tumors. In these specimens, contrast-enhanced regions on MRI corresponded to tumor tissue proper (i.e., tumor cells abutting each other without intervening brain), whereas areas of hypointensity on T1-weighted MR images and hyperintensity on T2-weighted images corresponded to isolated tumor cells infiltrating between essentially normal parenchymal structures. The density of infiltrating tumor cells may vary in these MRI-defined hypointense areas, from nearly all tumor cells with few neurons to rare scattered tumor cells with a predominance of neurons and edema. The density of tumor cells and the location of the tumor within, near, or away from eloquent brain areas are critical factors in making treatment decisions because the major challenge of all therapies is to eradicate the tumor cells without injuring the infiltrated normal brain.

Although all diffuse LGGs display an infiltrative pattern, it is also clear that 3 distinct histologic tumors are included under this rubric. Most common are the fibrillary astrocytomas, which are composed of cells resembling fibrillary astrocytes and whose astrocytic processes usually stain positive for glial fibrillary acidic protein (GFAP). Next frequent are the oligodendrogliomas, which resemble oligodendrocytes. Classic examples demonstrate uniform round nuclei and perinuclear halos, producing the so-called fried egg cytologic appearance, which is the diagnostically helpful artifact of delayed formalin fixation. The third and most controversial category is the mixed gliomas, which are composed of mixtures of neoplastic astrocytic cells and oligodendroglial cells. These may arise as biphasic variants in which the 2 cellular elements are distinct and juxtaposed, or as intermingled variants in which both components are intermixed and reactive astrocytes and neoplastic astrocytes are difficult to distinguish, or as cases in which the neoplastic cells appear to have intermediate features. These last variants are the most difficult to diagnose.

All diffuse LGGs are considered grade II in the WHO classification system because of their mild to moderate nuclear pleomorphism without evidence of mitotic activity, vascular hyperplasia, or necrosis. The progression of low-grade astrocytomas, oligodendrogliomas, or mixed gliomas to anaplastic astrocytomas, anaplastic oligodendrogliomas, or glioblastoma multiforme is common. Thus, low-grade gliomas are considered to be the least malignant stage of the continuous spectrum of infiltrating glial tumors.

In prior decades, astrocytoma and infiltrating glioma were common diagnoses. In the past decade, however, oligodendroglioma and mixed oligoastrocytoma have been increasingly diagnosed. This trend has correlated with an increasing recognition that the histologic subtype is a critical determinant of patient survival. A diagnosis of oligodendroglioma, and to a lesser extent mixed glioma, portends a better prognosis than does a diagnosis of pure astrocytoma. For example, the 5-year survival rate is approximately 70% for patients with oligodendrogliomas and 56% for patients with mixed gliomas, but 37% for patients with astrocytomas (Central Brain Tumor Registry of the United States, 2005). The differences between oligodendrogliomas and astrocytomas have raised important issues regarding patient inclusion criteria for clinical trials and treatment algorithms that group together all low-grade gliomas. Moreover, the trend toward loosening the diagnostic criteria for oligodendroglioma over the past few years has resulted in groups of "oligodendrogliomas" that lack histologic features of classic oligodendrogliomas, which in turn has led to an increased desire to identify features that distinguish oligodendrogliomas from astrocytomas.

Molecular Profiles

Recent work has identified important molecular markers in diffuse LGGs that may help identify histologic subsets of tumors, predict the responsiveness of the tumors to therapy, and define specific tumor types independent of histology.

For oligodendrogliomas, the most frequently reported molecular alteration is the loss of heterozygosity of chromosomes 1p and 19q (LOH 1p/19q). Loss of these chromosomes identifies a genetically favorable subset of oligodendrogliomas. In their seminal paper, Cairncross et al (1998) demonstrated that LOH 1p/19q in anaplastic oligodendrogliomas was statistically significantly associated with greater chemosensitivity and longer recurrence-free survival duration. Most recently, 2 randomized phase III trials validated that LOH 1p/19q is associated with improved survival in patients with anaplastic oligodendrogliomas (Cairncross et al, 1998; Jaeckle et al, 2006; van den Bent et al, 2006). However, because all patients in these trials received radiotherapy with or without chemotherapy, it is unclear whether anaplastic oligodendrogliomas with LOH 1p/19q are simply less aggressive or are more responsive to radiotherapy or chemotherapy (or both) compared with anaplastic oligodendrogliomas without LOH 1p/19q. Although both trials showed that adding chemotherapy before or after radiotherapy was of little benefit in tumors with LOH 1p/19q, they did not address whether tumors with LOH 1p/19q responded to chemotherapy alone. Nevertheless, these trials provide unequivocal evidence that LOH 1p/19q identifies a subgroup of anaplastic oligodendroglial tumors with a favorable prognosis.

Recent work has demonstrated that the findings just described for anaplastic (WHO grade III) oligodendrogliomas may also be true for low-grade (WHO grade II) oligodendrogliomas, which also frequently show LOH 1p/19q. As in anaplastic oligodendrogliomas, LOH 1p/19q in low-grade oligodendrogliomas may define a group with improved outcomes compared with tumors without LOH 1p/19q (Lang and Gilbert, 2006). LOH 1p/19q appears to be an early event in the genesis of oligodendrogliomas, and oligodendrogliomas with a classic appearance (i.e., perinuclear halos) are more likely to be associated with LOH 1p/19q than are oligodendrogliomas with an atypical appearance. Some studies have suggested that LOH 1p/19q in low-grade oligodendrogliomas is a marker of chemosensitivity, whereas others have not. Testing for LOH 1p/19q should be considered standard for all patients with histologically diagnosed oligodendrogliomas. Whether this molecular marker will replace histologic criteria for the diagnosis of a "true" oligodendroglioma remains to be seen. Clearly, LOH 1p/19q predicts a better prognosis for low-grade oligodendrogliomas, but well-designed phase III trials are needed to ultimately determine its role as a predictor of chemosensitivity.

Compared with oligodendrogliomas, LOH 1p/19q is rare in low-grade astrocytomas, and all studies have demonstrated a negative correlation between LOH 1p/19q and histologic characteristics of astrocytomas. The most common molecular alterations in astrocytomas are mutations in the *p53* tumor suppressor gene, which is located on chromosome 17p. Loss of *p53* is rare in oligodendrogliomas. Unfortunately, the identification of *p53* mutations in astrocytomas is not associated with tumor response to therapy, and it does not reliably predict prognosis. Immunohistochemical staining for the p53 protein (positive staining indicates mutated or abnormally regulated p53 protein) can be used to distinguish neoplastic astrocytes from reactive astrocytes on biopsy specimens and thus confirm the presence of astrocytic tumor cells in tumors with very low cellularity.

Clinical Prognostic Factors

Multiple studies have attempted to define clinical characteristics that may improve the survival of patients with diffuse LGGs. The European

Organization for Research and Treatment of Cancer (EORTC) reported one of the most comprehensive analyses. These investigators used the patient data sets from 2 large phase III trials of diffuse LGGs and found that in addition to tumors with histologic features of astrocytoma, 4 clinical factors negatively affected survival: patient age of 40 years or older, tumor size of 6 cm or larger in maximal diameter, tumor crossing the midline, and neurologic deficit before surgery (Pignatti et al, 2002). The investigators constructed a prognostic score based on the number of negative factors present. Patients with 0 to 2 factors were considered at low risk of dying of their disease (median survival time, 7.7 years), whereas patients with 3 to 5 factors were considered at high risk (median survival time, 3.2 years). A noteworthy caveat of this analysis is that the imaging data were based on computed tomography rather than on MRI, which is more sensitive to tumor size and determination of midline crossing. Hence, the prognostic importance of these variables may need further exploration.

Therapeutic Options

There is little consensus about the optimal treatment strategy for diffuse LGGs, and the clinical management of these tumors is one of the most controversial areas in neuro-oncology. The routine use of MRI, which has resulted in the early detection of diffuse LGGs in patients with few or no symptoms and with normal neurologic function, has increased the imperative to formulate treatment guidelines for patients with diffuse LGGs. The slow growth and low histologic grade of these tumors suggest that early intervention for cure may be possible, and many physicians recommend aggressive treatment, including extirpative surgery and radiotherapy, once diffuse LGGs are detected. In contrast, other physicians advocate a more conservative strategy and defer treatment until tumor progression, citing the potential morbidity associated with surgery and radiotherapy as well as the controversy surrounding the actual measurable benefits of these treatments. Adding to the complexity is recent evidence that patients whose tumors demonstrate LOH 1p/19q may benefit from chemotherapy, the use of which heretofore has been considered of little value. Although few studies have provided definitive evidence for one treatment strategy over another, the results of several recent randomized trials are beginning to provide answers.

Surgery

Although surgery is a critical part of the management of diffuse LGGs, there remains much debate about the effect of the timing of surgery and the extent of the surgery on the outcome of patients with diffuse LGGs.

Timing of Surgery. There is no phase III trial supporting early surgical intervention (i.e., at the time of detection of a nonenhanced tumor on

MR images) versus delayed surgical intervention (i.e., when the lesion increases in size or causes symptoms). However, for several reasons, at M. D. Anderson Cancer Center, we typically obtain surgical specimens for histologic diagnosis soon after a nonenhanced lesion is identified on MR images rather than waiting for tumor progression. First, although modern MRI is very effective in identifying nonenhanced lesions within the brain, the distinction between diffuse LGGs and nonneoplastic lesions (e.g., demyelination, inflammation, or infection) cannot be made with absolute certainty from radiographic studies alone, even when more advanced techniques such as MR spectroscopy and diffusion-weighted imaging are used as adjuncts. Second, imaging is currently not able to distinguish between histologic types of tumors, specifically astrocytomas versus oligodendrogliomas or mixed gliomas. These distinctions are critical for prognosis and subsequent intervention. Third and probably most important, radiographic studies cannot definitively determine the grade of a nonenhanced tumor. For example, 1 study showed that nearly a third of nonenhanced tumors were anaplastic gliomas at the time of detection rather than low-grade gliomas (Bernstein and Guha, 1994). This distinction is critical because the prognosis and treatment of anaplastic astrocytomas or anaplastic oligodendrogliomas (WHO grade III tumors) is decisively different from that of diffuse LGGs (WHO grade II tumors). Finally, an increasingly important reason is that radiographic studies cannot identify genetic alterations (e.g., LOH 1p/19q) in diffuse LGGs that predict patient survival and tumor response to treatment. Thus, despite the lack of phase III trials to support obtaining tissue early, the urgency of identifying the genetic makeup of tumors that may respond to therapy and of verifying that nonenhanced tumors do not have anaplastic features has led us to obtain tissue for histologic and molecular diagnosis soon after the identification of a nonenhanced lesion on MR images.

Extent of Resection.   Far more controversial than the timing of surgery is the nature of the surgical procedure that should be undertaken. The choice of aggressively removing diffuse LGGs to achieve a gross total resection, rather than performing a stereotactic biopsy or subtotal resection, has been one of the most controversial debates among neurosurgical oncologists. In other areas of oncology, surgery aims at complete tumor removal with a wide margin of normal tissue; however, the invasive nature of diffuse LGGs and their frequent juxtaposition to or within critically eloquent brain regions often preclude complete tumor removal and certainly prevent resection of a margin. Because even aggressive resections may leave tumor cells behind, many neurosurgeons opt against any intervention beyond a biopsy, but other neurosurgeons advocate as complete a removal as possible to minimize the tumor burden. To date, phase III clinical trials addressing this issue have not been completed, and recent attempts indicate that such a study is unlikely to be achieved; only retrospective reports are available to assist with decision making.

Nevertheless, at M. D. Anderson in the past decade, we have advocated and performed increasingly more complete resections rather than biopsies. Several reasons account for this trend. First, the technology that allows for achieving such resections has improved to the point that safe and maximal resection is feasible. Preoperative anatomic and functional MRI now provides precise localization of the tumor relative to critical motor, sensory, visual, and speech areas within the brain. This information provides accurate information about the potential for completely removing the lesion without causing neurologic deficit. More important, this information can be imported into the operating room using computer-assisted stereotactic surgical technology that allows the neurosurgeon to navigate through the brain, thereby identifying the borders of the tumor. This technology can be augmented by intraoperative ultrasonography, which provides real-time imaging of a lesion during resection, and by intraoperative functional mapping usually performed with the patient awake, which permits precise localization of brain regions subserving motor, sensory, and speech functions. M. D. Anderson is also now equipped with intraoperative MRI units that permit serial imaging during surgery (Figure 5–3). Taken together, these technologic advances have increased the feasibility of complete resection, and with this feasibility has come an increasing trend to resect nonenhanced lesions that historically

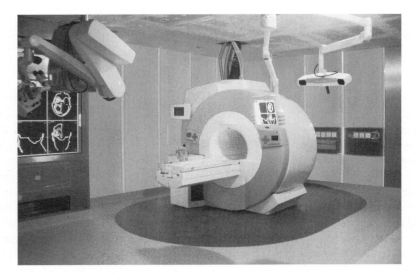

Figure 5–3. The use of intraoperative MRI, such as the setup at M. D. Anderson pictured here, helps the surgeon maximize the degree of safe tumor resection.

were difficult to define during surgery. Recent studies have indicated that these technologies have decreased surgical morbidity and mortality.

Second, more complete tumor removal may increase the accuracy of diagnoses. In a recent study from M. D. Anderson (Jackson et al, 2001), it was shown that even with expert neuropathologic review, there was a discrepancy in 38% of cases between diagnoses made from small biopsy specimens and those made from resected specimens. The incorrect diagnoses made from the small biopsy specimens affected the therapeutic regimens in 26% of cases and the prognostication in 38% of cases. Consequently, histologic assessment is probably more accurate when large amounts of tissue are provided to the neuropathologist. We typically reserve biopsy for those cases in which resection of the lesion is not considered desirable, such as when a diffusely infiltrating lesion extends into the brainstem or when lesions are confined to eloquent brain regions.

Third, maximal resection may improve the control of symptoms, particularly seizure. Evidence from patients with large tumors and increased intracranial pressure suggests that patients who undergo gross total resection have better neurologic outcomes than do patients who undergo subtotal resection. It is our experience that partial resections often result in an exacerbation of edema and worsening of symptoms, whereas complete resections are associated with little or no postoperative edema and better palliation of symptoms.

Fourth, maximal resection for the purpose of reducing the tumor burden may prolong patient survival time. Two recent phase III studies have indicated that maximal resection of high-grade gliomas prolongs patient survival compared with biopsy or subtotal resection (Vuorinen et al, 2003; Stummer et al, 2006). Whether these results translate to diffuse LGGs is unknown, and there is no randomized trial of diffuse LGGs that specifically addresses this question.

Although the literature is replete with retrospective series analyzing the effect of surgical resection on patient outcome, critical to the discussion of cytoreductive surgery is a precise definition of "maximal or total resection." Whereas total resection of malignant gliomas such as glioblastoma multiforme implies removal of the contrast-enhanced portion of the tumor, total resection of diffuse LGGs that are not enhanced implies removal of all of the hypointense region on T1-weighted images or the hyperintense region on T2-weighted images. Thus, the decision to use total resection can be made only by comparing preoperative and postoperative MR images, ideally using volumetric computational analyses. Few studies have used postoperative imaging to evaluate the extent of resection. In one of the better studies in the literature, Berger et al (1994) used a computerized image analysis technique to assess the radiographic tumor volumes before and after surgery in a series of 53 patients with diffuse LGGs and found that the extent of resection significantly influenced the incidence of recurrence and the time to tumor progression. None of the 13 patients who had undergone a total resection had a recurrence during a mean follow-up of 54 months. In contrast, 14.8% of the 27 patients with a residual tumor volume less than 10 cm^3 and 46.2% of the 13 patients with a residual tumor volume greater than 10 cm^3 experienced recurrence.

In summary, current data suggest that both biopsy and attempts at maximal resection are appropriate options for treating patients with diffuse LGGs. However, in light of the potential advantages in terms of diagnosis, symptom control, and cytoreduction, we generally recommend removing as much of the tumor as possible, especially in patients who have large tumors that cause neurologic deficit, so long as neurologic function can be preserved. Effective surgery requires maximal use of surgical adjuncts for defining the spatial limits of the tumor (i.e., computer-assisted surgery and intraoperative ultrasonography) and for assessing functional brain (i.e., cortical and subcortical mapping techniques, usually with craniotomy while the patient is awake).

Radiotherapy

Similar to surgery, radiotherapy has been a mainstay of treatment for diffuse LGGs for decades, but much controversy has surrounded the actual implementation of this therapeutic modality. Several recently published phase III randomized studies have provided critical evidence regarding the timing and dosing of radiotherapy. These studies, organized by large cooperative groups with accrual continuing over 10 years, have greatly enhanced our understanding of the role of radiotherapy in diffuse LGGs and should serve as models for overcoming the difficulties associated with completing phase III trials of diffuse LGGs.

Radiation Dose. Two randomized trials, the EORTC 22844 study and a multigroup study led by the North Central Cancer Treatment Group, have addressed the role of a low versus high dose of radiation in diffuse LGGs (Table 5–2). Both studies concluded that there was no significant difference by dose for the 5-year overall and progression-free survival rates. These results were not affected by other factors that may influence survival (e.g., the percent surgical resection and the number of oligodendroglial tumors), as these variables were evenly distributed between the groups. Because high doses of radiation provide no significant advantage over lower doses but may increase toxicity, the standard radiation dose for diffuse LGGs is currently 50 to 54 Gy in fractions of 1.8 Gy.

Timing of Radiotherapy. Whether immediate radiotherapy offers any advantage over delayed radiotherapy is unknown. Some radiation oncologists follow a "wait and see" approach and initiate radiotherapy (and other therapies) at progression of the disease. Since radiotherapy is most effective against proliferating cells, these radiation oncologists reserve

Table 5–2. Randomized Phase III Radiotherapy Trials for Low-Grade Gliomas

Trial (Reference)	Radiation Dose (Gy)	Number of Patients	Rate of Gross Total Resection (%)	Non-astrocytomas* (%)	5-Year Survival Rate Overall (%)	5-Year Survival Rate Progression Free (%)
EORTC 22844 (Karim et al, 1996)	45.0	171	23	30	58	47
	59.4	172	26	31	59	50
North Central Cancer Treatment Group/RTOG/Eastern Cooperative Oncology Group (Shaw et al, 2002)	50.4	101	12	68	72	55
	64.8	102	17	69	64	52
EORTC 22845 Interim analysis (Karim et al, 2002)	0	140	42	33	66	37
	54	150	43	36	63	44[†]
Final analysis (van den Bent et al, 2005)	0	157	42	28	66	35
	54	154	47	25	68	55[†]

* Proportion of tumors that were not astrocytomas (i.e., that were oligodendrogliomas and oligoastrocytomas).
† Statistically significant difference vs 0-Gy radiation.

radiotherapy for tumors that progress to higher-grade lesions, which contain higher percentages of proliferative cells. Other radiation oncologists immediately initiate radiotherapy on the concept that early intervention eradicates the most proliferative and aggressive cells at their earliest stages, thereby reducing the population of cells most likely to progress to a higher grade.

To address this controversy, the EORTC and the Brain Tumor Working Group of the United Kingdom's Medical Research Council began a randomized trial in 1986 to assess the efficacy of early radiotherapy versus radiotherapy deferred until tumor progression (EORTC 22845). An interim analysis was reported in 2002 (Karim et al, 2002), and the long-term results were published in 2005 (van den Bent et al, 2005) (Table 5–2). In this study, patients with diffuse LGGs were randomly assigned to receive early radiotherapy (54 Gy in 6 weeks) within 8 weeks of the day of surgery (n = 154) or to receive no postoperative radiotherapy (n = 157). The 5-year progression-free survival rate was significantly higher in the radiotherapy group than in the control group (55% vs 35%). However, there was no difference in the 5-year overall survival rate (68% vs 66%) or in the median survival duration (7.2 vs 7.4 years). The absence of an overall survival benefit was probably due to the effectiveness of salvage radiotherapy in the control group, which was given to 65% of the patients at recurrence.

A major shortcoming of the EORTC 22845 trial was the absence of a quality-of-life assessment. Thus, it is unclear whether the capacity of radiotherapy to control tumor progression translates into a better quality of life and neurologic outcome for a longer period or whether the addition of radiotherapy impairs cognitive function and worsens quality of life. Without such data, we cannot be certain about the best approach. One interpretation of this phase III trial is that routine postoperative and early radiotherapy may be advisable for patients with diffuse LGGs because radiotherapy significantly extends the time to tumor progression. However, given our incomplete knowledge about the neurocognitive sequelae of radiotherapy, an equally valid interpretation of this study is that radiotherapy can be safely withheld until tumor progression without altering the overall patient survival duration. At M. D. Anderson, we tend to withhold radiotherapy in patients who are at low risk of rapid disease progression (i.e., who are younger than 40 years or who have undergone gross total resection). In addition, we often delay radiotherapy in patients with LOH 1p/19q and treat them with chemotherapy.

Chemotherapy

There have been limited studies examining the use of chemotherapy to treat diffuse LGGs. Although several retrospective studies have demonstrated that chemotherapy is not a prognostic factor for survival in patients with diffuse LGGs, recent studies have suggested a potential role for specific types of chemotherapy for the management of diffuse LGGs, either as an adjuvant or as first-line therapy.

To date, the only randomized phase III prospective trial that has evaluated the use of chemotherapy to treat diffuse LGGs showed no benefit from the addition of single-agent CCNU (the abbreviation of the chemical name of lomustine) to radiotherapy, but that study was closed early because of slow accrual. More recent evidence suggests that combination chemotherapy may be beneficial in treating diffuse LGGs, particularly oligodendrogliomas with LOH 1p/19q. Levin et al (1980) were among the first to demonstrate that the combination chemotherapy regimen of procarbazine, CCNU, and vincristine (PCV) is effective against malignant gliomas, including anaplastic (WHO grade III) oligodendrogliomas. Cairncross et al (1998) demonstrated that anaplastic oligodendrogliomas harboring LOH 1p/19q are particularly sensitive to PCV. However, the results from 2 phase III trials of patients with anaplastic oligodendrogliomas demonstrated that PCV has no effect on the overall survival rate (although it extends the progression-free survival rate) when given as adjuvant therapy after radiotherapy (EORTC 26951: Jaeckle et al, 2006; van den Bent et al, 2006) or when given before radiotherapy (Radiation Therapy Oncology Group [RTOG] 94-02: Jaeckle et al, 2006; Cairncross et al, 2006). Because most patients in the radiotherapy-only arms of these studies received PCV at recurrence, an interpretation of these trials is that PCV is as effective when given early as when given as salvage therapy in patients with anaplastic oligodendrogliomas. Although both the EORTC and RTOG trials showed that adding chemotherapy before or after radiotherapy was of little benefit in treating oligodendrogliomas, including those with LOH 1p/19q, they did not address whether tumors with LOH 1p/19q could be treated with chemotherapy alone. Thus, the role of chemotherapy in treating anaplastic oligodendrogliomas with LOH 1p/19q remains to be defined.

The role of chemotherapy in the treatment of low-grade oligodendrogliomas is even more unclear. Several retrospective and small phase II trials have suggested that low-grade oligodendrogliomas may respond favorably to PCV. However, these results should be interpreted with caution because most of the trials included contrast-enhanced tumors, which is an atypical feature of low-grade gliomas. On the basis of results from these early-phase trials, large phase III trials are needed to evaluate the role of PCV-based therapy in diffuse LGGs. The RTOG has initiated a phase III trial that is evaluating the use of adjuvant PCV in treating diffuse LGGs. In this trial (RTOG 98-02), patients at high risk of dying of their disease (i.e., those older than 40 years or who undergo surgical resection or biopsy) were randomly assigned to receive radiotherapy (54 Gy) alone or with 6 cycles of PCV (Table 5–3). This trial, which does not include stratification for LOH 1p/19q status, closed in 2002 and has enrolled more than 250 patients, but the results of this study are still maturing and have yet to be published.

Table 5–3. Current Phase III Chemotherapy Trials for Low-Grade Gliomas*

Trial	Trial Design	Stratification of LOH 1p/19q Status	Trial Status
RTOG 98-02	Arm 1: low-risk observation Arm 2: radiotherapy (54 Gy) Arm 3: radiotherapy (54 Gy) + PCV (6 cycles)	No	Accrual completed; data maturing
EORTC 22041	Arm 1: radiotherapy (50.4 Gy) Arm 2: temozolomide (75 mg/m^2/day for 4 weeks)	Yes	Accruing
RTOG	Arm 1: radiotherapy Arm 2: radiotherapy + temozolomide	Yes	Accruing

* All 3 trials include cases of astrocytomas, oligodendrogliomas, and mixed gliomas.

Temozolomide, an orally administered alkylating agent with a favorable toxicity profile, has recently been shown to be effective in treating anaplastic gliomas and glioblastomas, and interest has been generated in the potential role of this agent for treating diffuse LGGs. Responses to temozolomide have been seen in tumors before radiotherapy as well as in tumors that have progressed after radiotherapy. In the EORTC 26972 phase II trial, temozolomide has also been evaluated as second-line chemotherapy in recurrent oligodendrogliomas or oligoastrocytomas. Taken together, this information clearly supports the need for a randomized phase III trial comparing temozolomide with radiotherapy. The EORTC 22041 is such a study, and it includes stratification for LOH 1p/19q status (Table 5–3). The trial was recently opened to accrual.

At M. D. Anderson, there is no specific consensus regarding chemotherapy for newly diagnosed low-grade gliomas except that it is usually used only for patients with tumors showing LOH 1p/19q. In such patients, when only subtotal resection is achieved and there is a desire to avoid radiation toxicity (e.g., in patients younger than 40 years), chemotherapy with either PCV or temozolomide may be given.

CIRCUMSCRIBED LOW-GRADE GLIOMAS: "ASTROGLIAL VARIANTS"

Astroglial variants are less common, low-grade glial tumors that are classified as grade I or II by the WHO grading system. Astroglial variants are more circumscribed than diffuse LGGs and, most important, the tumor cells do not typically invade significantly within the brain. Therefore, these grade I and II lesions usually (but not invariably) do not progress to higher-grade lesions, and long-term survival after surgery alone is common. Although astroglial variants comprise several distinct tumor types (Table 5–1), the most common of which are pilocytic astrocytomas and gangliogliomas, all of the astroglial variants overlap in their clinical features, neuroimaging features, and relatively less invasive growth pattern compared with diffuse LGGs. Therefore, the clinical management of these various entities can be considered together. The practical keys to successful management of these lesions are that they not be misdiagnosed as diffusely infiltrating fibrillary astrocytomas, particularly high-grade gliomas (grade III or IV), and that patients are appropriately counseled about the better prognosis associated with these lesions and the potential for successful treatment.

Clinical Features

Unlike diffuse LGGs, astroglial variants generally occur in children and young adults. Pilocytic astrocytomas account for 20% of all brain tumors in children younger than 15 years; presentation in patients older than 30 years is uncommon. Gangliogliomas, which have a reported incidence of 0.4% to 11% of central nervous system neoplasms, are also more common in children. PXAs and SEGAs are rare tumors that arise most typically in the first and second decades of life. SEGAs occur exclusively in patients with tuberous sclerosis.

Pilocytic astrocytomas occur most commonly in the cerebellum (Figure 5–4) but also occur frequently in the cerebrum, suprasellar region (optic

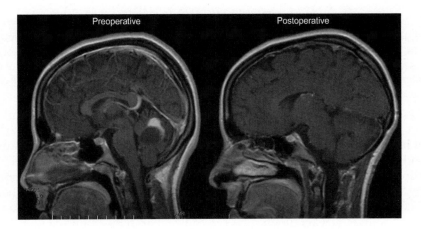

Figure 5–4. Preoperative and postoperative T1-weighted MR sagittal images of a classic cerebellar pilocytic astrocytoma in an 8-year-old girl. This lesion appeared as an enhanced mural nodule and cyst. Complete resection was performed.

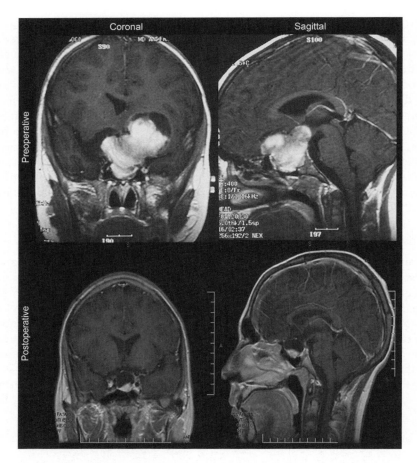

Figure 5–5. Preoperative and postoperative coronal and sagittal T1-weighted MR images of a giant suprasellar pilocytic astrocytoma in a 12-year-old boy. Total resection of the tumor was achieved. There is no evidence of recurrence 6 years later. Functionally, the patient is independent and has normal neurocognitive function on formal testing.

or hypothalamic pathway) (Figure 5–5), brainstem (Figure 5–6), thalamus, and spinal cord. However, in our experience at M. D. Anderson with 77 pilocytic astrocytomas, 26% were in the cerebellum, 38% in the brainstem, 26% in the suprasellar region, and 10% in the cerebrum (unpublished data). This difference is probably due to the pattern of patient referrals to M. D. Anderson. Gangliogliomas typically occur in the temporal lobe, but they also arise in the brainstem, spinal cord, and diencephalon. PXAs are typically subcortical supratentorial lesions. SEGAs invariably arise along the wall of the lateral ventricle near the foramen of Monro.

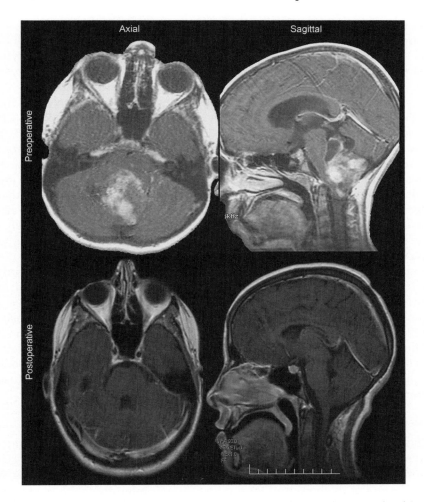

Figure 5–6. Preoperative and postoperative axial and sagittal T1-weighted MR images of a brainstem (cervicomedullary) pilocytic astrocytoma in an 8-year-old girl. The lesion was resected from the medulla without neurologic compromise. The patient is functioning normally 8 years later.

Neuroimaging Features

On computed tomography images, astroglial variants typically appear as well-circumscribed cystic lesions with solid mural nodules that are iso-dense compared with brain tissue and that are strongly enhanced after con-trast administration. On MR images, the solid tumor typically appears hypointense or isointense compared with brain tissue on T1-weighted images and hyperintense on T2-weighted images. The cyst is often isoin-tense with cerebrospinal fluid, but variation exists depending on the protein content of the cyst fluid. Although classic examples are cystic (Figure 5–4), astroglial variants also occur as predominantly solid masses with small or no cysts (Figures 5–5 and 5–6). In at least a third of patients with pilocytic astrocytomas, the masses are solid without a cyst or with only a small cyst, and examples of noncystic gangliogliomas are commonly found.

Unlike diffuse LGGs, which typically are not enhanced by contrast, the solid tumor in nearly all astroglial variants is brightly enhanced on T1-weighted MR images after gadolinium administration (Figures 5–4, 5–5, and 5–6). Although enhancement distinguishes astroglial variants from diffuse LGGs, it also often results in the misdiagnosis of astroglial variants as high-grade gliomas, particularly glioblastomas, which also are enhanced after contrast administration. A key radiographic feature that distinguishes astroglial variants (e.g., pilocytic astrocytomas) from diffusely infiltrating high-grade gliomas (e.g., glioblastoma multiforme) is the ratio of the volume of the enhanced mass on T1-weighted images to the volume of the hyperintense regions on T2-weighted images. This ratio is approximately 1 for pilocytic astrocytomas and other astroglial variants and less than 1 for glioblastomas. This ratio is particularly helpful in distinguishing brainstem and thalamic astroglial variants, which have a good prognosis and may be curable, from diffuse brainstem gliomas, which have a poor prognosis (median survival time, less than 2 years). Another distinguishing feature is that astroglial variants typically occur as dorsally exophytic or focal pontine lesions or occur outside the pons as cervicomedullary junction or tectal lesions, whereas most diffuse brainstem gliomas occur diffusely within the pons.

Histopathologic Characteristics

The most important and unifying histologic feature of the astroglial variants is that they are histologically low-grade tumors that are relatively circumscribed. Although there is no capsule, there is only a mild degree of infiltration at the border of the tumor where it interfaces with the brain. Unlike diffuse LGGs, which contain tumor cells juxtaposed to normal neurons, the solid portion of all astroglial variants is free of normal brain parenchyma. In their correlative studies, Kelly and colleagues (Daumas-Duport et al, 1987) showed that regions of contrast enhancement on MRI almost invariably correspond histologically to tumor tissue proper (i.e., tumor cells abutting each other without intervening brain). Because there is no brain tissue in enhanced astroglial variants, it follows that eradication of the enhanced lesion should not result in neurologic deficit, even if the lesion is located in eloquent brain regions such as the brainstem, speech cortex, motor cortex, and thalamus. This growth pattern is a critical difference between astroglial variants and diffuse LGGs, and it makes surgical resection a highly effective means of treating astroglial variants.

Although the details of the histologic classification of astroglial variants are beyond the scope of this chapter, several key elements define each of these lesions. Most important for the pathologist is distinguishing these lesions from high-grade gliomas, with which they are often confused, because the treatment and prognosis of patients with high-grade gliomas and of patients with astroglial variants are significantly different.

Key features of pilocytic astrocytomas are a characteristically biphasic pattern of alternating zones of loose spongy tissue and compact solid tissue with closely juxtaposed cells, bipolar spindly cells with elongated nuclei and thin hairlike (pilocytic) processes, numerous Rosenthal fibers or eosinophilic granular bodies, and well-delineated microcysts. Confusion with high-grade gliomas often occurs because of the cellular pleomorphism and significant vascular hyperplasia. However, unlike in high-grade gliomas, mitotic figures are inconspicuous and necrosis is not present. Progression of pilocytic astrocytomas to higher-grade gliomas is rare.

Gangliogliomas are composed of glial elements and neuronal elements. The glial elements, which stain positive for GFAP, are almost always astrocytic and often pilocytic, but fibrillary astrocytes are also common. The neurons in the tumor are neoplastic and are characteristically large and relatively mature (i.e., they have ganglion cells). Confirmation of neoplastic neurons is assisted by several immunostains, including those for neuron-specific enolase and synaptophysin. The glial elements dictate the grade of the lesion, and gangliogliomas can be grade I or II. The grade II lesions are often nonenhanced on MR images and behave as more localized diffuse LGGs. Progression of grade II lesions to a higher grade has been known to occur.

PXAs usually involve the cortex and the overlying leptomeninges but not the dura mater. Microscopically, they are composed of pleomorphic cells, including spindle cells intermingled with mononucleated or multinucleated giant cells, which invariably stain positive for GFAP, testifying to their astrocytic lineage. The most distinguishing feature is the presence of abundant lipid accumulations (the Greek term "xanthoma" means "yellow tumor") within the cytoplasm, which push the GFAP-stained elements to the periphery of the cell. PXAs are considered to be WHO grade II lesions. Although PXAs typically have a good prognosis, PXAs with anaplastic features have been reported. Confusion with glioblastomas is possible because lipid droplets are sometimes seen in glioblastomas near areas of necrosis. These "lipidized" glioblastomas can be distinguished from PXAs because the lipid-filled astrocytes of PXAs occur in areas without necrosis.

SEGAs are WHO grade I lesions composed of fibrillated spindle cells, gemistocytic cells, or giant ganglion-like cells. Both GFAP and neuron-specific enolase immunostaining has been observed in all 3 cell types. Mitoses and even necrosis may be present, but these histologic features do not portend an aggressive clinical behavior for SEGAs.

Therapeutic Options

Whereas the optimal treatment strategy for diffuse LGGs is quite controversial, the clinical management of astroglial variants is less so. Although there are no phase III trials confirming the advantage of one treatment approach over another, surgical resection is generally considered the optimal initial therapy, and radiotherapy is reserved for subtotally resected or recurrent cases. The role of chemotherapy is less well defined; it is used primarily in clinical trials.

Surgery

Surgical resection directed at removing the contrast-enhanced portion of the tumor is a rational approach to astroglial variants because the enhanced tumor mass contains tumors cells without intervening brain. So long as there is a safe corridor to the lesion, resection of most astroglial variants is achievable, including those in eloquent brain regions. Tumor recurrence and surgical morbidity relate to the juxtaposition of the tumor to the surrounding brain and to the degree of tumor invasion into functional neurons at the border of the tumor and the brain. Thus, although lesions located within eloquent brain regions are resectable, they represent significant surgical challenges because the border between tumor and functional brain may be difficult to define, even with the aid of modern surgical adjuncts such as microscopy, computer-assisted surgical guidance, and functional brainstem mapping.

Although no randomized phase III prospective studies have documented the superiority of surgery over other approaches (e.g., radiotherapy), for most astroglial variants, retrospective studies have indicated that gross total resection affords good long-term outcome. Most of the data available are for pilocytic astrocytomas. In a recent study of 80 pilocytic astrocytomas of the cerebellum, suprasellar region, brainstem, spinal cord, and thalamus, the 5-year survival rates were 100% and 92% after total and subtotal resection, respectively (Fernandez et al, 2003). The 5-year progression-free survival rates were 100% and 53% after gross total resection and subtotal resection, respectively. Resection of suprasellar tumors proved the most challenging in this series: they had the highest rate of recurrence and the lowest frequency of gross total resection.

At M. D. Anderson, surgical resection is generally the primary treatment for pilocytic astrocytomas, regardless of their location. In the series of 77 tumors operated on at our institution, most of which were located outside the cerebellum, gross total resection (i.e., removal of all the enhanced mass on postoperative images), which was achieved in nearly 60% of cases, afforded the best outcome and was associated with a 10-year disease-free survival rate of 100% (unpublished data). In contrast, the progression-free survival rate after subtotal resection was only 24% at 5 years. The value of total resection was most evident for tumors located in the brainstem and the suprasellar region: of the 29 brainstem tumors, 16 (55%) underwent gross total resection, and none of the tumors had recurred at last follow-up. Likewise, none of the 4 suprasellar tumors that had been treated with gross total resection recurred; however, complete removal was achieved in only 20% of the 20 tumors in this location (unpublished data).

These data suggest that total resection, if achievable, provides the best outcome for patients with pilocytic astrocytomas, regardless of the location of the tumors in the brain. Missing from the literature are good prospective studies analyzing the quality of life associated with aggressive resection of pilocytic astrocytomas, particularly when the lesions are located in the brainstem, thalamus, or suprasellar region. Prospective phase III randomized studies comparing total resection alone with subtotal resection followed by adjuvant therapy (e.g., radiotherapy) are warranted for tumors located in these surgically complex regions. Unfortunately, such studies are difficult to carry out because of the rarity of these lesions; to this author's knowledge, no such studies are planned.

For gangliogliomas, PXAs, and SEGAs, complete surgical resection is associated with long-term survival, although the studies in the literature are retrospective and few provide meaningful statistical analyses of patient outcome. Despite the good long-term outcome associated with surgery, grade II gangliogliomas and PXAs may recur and some patients do poorly. For gangliogliomas, the degree of astrocytic anaplasia appears to determine the prognosis of patients, and our experience at M. D. Anderson supports this notion. Likewise, despite their usually favorable biologic behavior, PXAs may recur after surgery, and metastases via cerebrospinal fluid seeding and transformation to more malignant forms, although rare, have been reported.

Radiotherapy

Because children's brains are more susceptible than adults' brains to the adverse effects of radiotherapy, there is a general desire to withhold radiotherapy for young people with astroglial variants. Nevertheless, radiotherapy remains a viable option, particularly for pilocytic astrocytomas. In light of the potential for surgical resection to cure most astroglial variants, radiotherapy is generally reserved for subtotally resected cases or for recurrences. There are no prospective randomized trials analyzing the role of radiotherapy in managing these tumors, although multiple retrospective series can be found on the need for radiotherapy after surgical treatment of astroglial variants. In our experience with 77 cases of pilocytic astrocytomas, radiotherapy after subtotal resection significantly improved the 5-year progression-free survival rate, from 27% for resection alone to 80% for radiotherapy after resection (unpublished data).

In view of the limited prospective data, radiotherapy at M. D. Anderson is generally reserved for lesions that recur despite repeat resection or for lesions in complex locations where further resection may result in significant morbidity. Careful studies are needed to analyze the benefits of tumor control versus the potential for causing unwanted cognitive adverse effects after radiotherapy for these astroglial variants.

Chemotherapy

The primary role of chemotherapy in the treatment of astroglial variants is to delay radiotherapy or other treatments, particularly for young children. Most studies in the literature have focused on suprasellar (optic or hypothalamic pathway) pilocytic astrocytomas because surgery for this disease often results in less than complete resection and because radiotherapy may contribute to progressive neurologic deterioration and even visual loss late in the course of the disease. In addition, moderate or severe cognitive dysfunction is common in children who survive long-term and who are treated early in life with radiotherapy to the suprasellar region. Chemotherapy is also used as salvage therapy when tumors recur after the failure of surgery and radiotherapy.

Although many studies report success with chemotherapy, complete responses are rare. Most researchers consider stabilization of the disease, rather than a complete tumor response, a successful outcome. Optimal chemotherapeutic regimens for astroglial variants have not been defined, although various chemotherapeutic regimens—including CCNU, PCV, and cisplatin—have been shown to be somewhat effective. Because most studies do not separate astroglial variants, such as pilocytic astrocytomas, from more diffuse low-grade gliomas (grade II astrocytomas), the interpretation of study results is difficult. At M. D. Anderson, chemotherapy is generally reserved for young children who have undergone subtotal resection and who demonstrate disease progression. In older patients with astroglial variants, chemotherapy is typically used as salvage therapy after the failure of surgery and radiotherapy.

CONCLUSION

Although there have been major advances recently in the management of diffuse LGGs and the more circumscribed astroglial variants, significant gaps remain in our basic knowledge of the biology of these tumors. The discovery of the prognostic implications of LOH 1p/19q in oligodendrogliomas gives hope for identifying similar molecular signatures in all low-grade gliomas so that rational and tailored therapies can be applied to individual patients. Continued advances in surgery, radiotherapy, and chemotherapy will be best achieved by studying newly acquired information in the context of well-designed, preferably phase III, clinical trials. These studies are difficult to conduct because of the rarity of these tumors, and progress will be made only if surgeons, oncologists, and radiation therapists diligently develop such trials and actively enroll patients with low-grade gliomas.

KEY PRACTICE POINTS

- Although considered low-grade tumors, diffusely infiltrating grade II astrocytomas, oligodendrogliomas, and mixed gliomas are not benign and typically progress to higher grades.

- Astroglial variants are less invasive and more circumscribed tumors. Grade I lesions, such as pilocytic astrocytomas, are benign tumors that can be cured with surgery.

- Diffuse LGGs appear as nonenhanced lesions in neuroimaging studies, whereas astroglial variants are typically enhanced. Because high-grade astrocytomas and anaplastic oligodendrogliomas are enhanced, they must be distinguished from low-grade astroglial variants on neuroimages. Clinicians and pathologists must avoid misdiagnosing an astroglial variant (e.g., a brainstem pilocytic astrocytoma) as a diffusely infiltrating high-grade glioma.

- For diffuse LGGs, we favor total resection to obtain adequate tissue for histologic diagnosis, assess for 1p/19q LOH, reduce symptoms, and potentially prolong patient survival.

- Surgical resection requires the use of a variety of adjuncts that improve tumor localization and define functionally important brain regions. Surgeons must be aware that nonenhanced tumors may contain functional neurons and that resecting these tumors can impair neurologic function.

- Complete resection of diffuse LGGs requires the removal of all areas of hyperintensity on T2-weighted images. Postoperative imaging is required to make this assessment because surgeons' assessments of complete resection are unreliable.

- Radiotherapy may be an effective treatment for diffuse LGGs, but when it is administered early after diagnosis or resection or at tumor progression, it does not alter the patient survival rate. The toxic effects of radiotherapy must be weighed against the benefits of tumor control. At M. D. Anderson, radiotherapy is often delayed for children and for patients who have undergone complete resection.

- Oligodendrogliomas with LOH 1p/19q have a better prognosis than do tumors without these chromosomal losses. Tumors with LOH 1p/19q may be more sensitive to chemotherapy than tumors with intact 1p/19q are.

- Whenever possible, patients with diffuse LGGs should be enrolled in clinical trials to help develop rational treatment algorithms for these difficult tumors.

- Most astroglial variants, even those in eloquent regions, can be safely resected because the enhanced tumor does not contain neuronal tissue. For this reason, total resection is the first-line treatment for most astroglial variants.

- Radiotherapy may be effective in treating astroglial variants, particularly pilocytic astrocytomas. Because these tumors often occur in young children, whose developing brains are susceptible to the adverse effects of radiotherapy, radiotherapy is generally delayed or avoided.

Suggested Readings

Berger, MS, Deliganis AV, Dobbins J, Keles GE. The effect of extent of resection on recurrence in patients with low grade cerebral hemisphere gliomas. *Cancer* 1994;74:1784–1791.

Bernstein M, Guha A. Biopsy of low-grade astrocytomas. *J Neurosurg* 1994;80: 776–777.

Cairncross G, Berkey B, Shaw E, et al. Phase III trial of chemotherapy plus radiotherapy compared with radiotherapy alone for pure and mixed anaplastic oligodendroglioma: Intergroup Radiation Therapy Oncology Group Trial 9402. *J Clin Oncol* 2006;24:2707–2714.

Cairncross JG, Ueki K, Zlatescu MC, et al. Specific genetic predictors of chemotherapeutic response and survival in patients with anaplastic oligodendrogliomas. *J Natl Cancer Inst* 1998;90:1473–1479.

Central Brain Tumor Registry of the United States. *Statistical Report: Primary Brain Tumors in the United States, 1998–2002.* Central Brain Tumor Registry of the United States; 2005.

Daumas-Duport C, Scheithauer BW, Kelly PJ. A histologic and cytologic method for the spatial definition of gliomas. *Mayo Clin Proc* 1987;62:435–449.

Fernandez C, Figarella-Branger D, Girard N, et al. Pilocytic astrocytomas in children: prognostic factors—a retrospective study of 80 cases. *Neurosurgery* 2003;53:544–553; discussion 554–555.

Jackson R, Fuller G, Abi-Said D, et al. Limitations of stereotactic biopsy in the initial management of gliomas. *Neuro-Oncology* 2001;3:193–200.

Jaeckle KA, Ballman KV, Rao RD, Jenkins RB, Buckner JC. Current strategies in treatment of oligodendroglioma: evolution of molecular signatures of response. *J Clin Oncol* 2006;24:1246–1252.

Karim AB, Afra D, Cornu P, et al. Randomized trial on the efficacy of radiotherapy for cerebral low-grade glioma in the adult: European Organization for Research and Treatment of Cancer Study 22845 with the Medical Research Council study BRO4: an interim analysis. *Int J Radiat Oncol Biol Phys* 2002;52:316–324.

Karim AB, Maat B, Hatlevoll R, et al. A randomized trial on dose-response in radiation therapy of low-grade cerebral glioma: European Organization for Research and Treatment of Cancer (EORTC) Study 22844. *Int J Radiat Oncol Biol Phys* 1996;36:549–556.

Kleihues P, Cavenee WK. *Pathology and Genetics of Tumors of the Nervous System.* Lyon, France: IARC Press: 2000.

Lang FF, Gilbert MR. Diffusely infiltrative low-grade gliomas in adults. *J Clin Oncol* 2006;24:1236–1245.

Levin VA, Edwards MS, Wright DC, et al. Modified procarbazine, CCNU, and vincristine (PCV 3) combination chemotherapy in the treatment of malignant brain tumors. *Cancer Treat Rep* 1980;64:237–244.

Pignatti F, van den Bent M, Curran D, et al. Prognostic factors for survival in adult patients with cerebral low-grade glioma. *J Clin Oncol* 2002;20:2076–2084.

Shaw E, Arusell R, Scheithauer B, et al. Prospective randomized trial of low- versus high-dose radiation therapy in adults with supratentorial low-grade glioma: initial report of a North Central Cancer Treatment Group/Radiation Therapy Oncology Group/Eastern Cooperative Oncology Group study. *J Clin Oncol* 2002;20:2267–2276.

Stummer W, Pichlmeier U, Meinel T, Wiestler OD, Zanella F, Reulen HJ. Fluorescence-guided surgery with 5-aminolevulinic acid for resection of malignant glioma: a randomised controlled multicentre phase III trial. *Lancet Oncol* 2006;7:392–401.

van den Bent MJ, Afra D, de Witte O, et al. Long-term efficacy of early versus delayed radiotherapy for low-grade astrocytoma and oligodendroglioma in adults: the EORTC 22845 randomised trial. *Lancet* 2005;366:985–990.

van den Bent MJ, Carpentier AF, Barndes AA, et al. Adjuvant procarbazine, lomustine, and vincristine improves progression-free survival but not overall survival in newly diagnosed anaplastic oligodendrogliomas and oligoastrocytomas: a randomized European Organisation for Research and Treatment of Cancer phase III trial. *J Clin Oncol* 2006;24:2715–2722.

Vuorinen V, Hinkka S, Färkkilä M, Jääskeläinen J. Debulking or biopsy of malignant glioma in elderly people—a randomised study. *Acta Neurochir (Wien)* 2003;145:5–10.

6   SURGICAL STRATEGIES FOR HIGH-GRADE GLIOMAS

Sujit S. Prabhu

Chapter Overview 121
Introduction 121
The Decision to Resect 122
Surgical Approaches to HGG 125
    Technical Adjuncts to Surgery 126
    Unresectable HGGs 129
    Recurrent HGGs 130
Conclusion 132
Key Practice Points 132
Suggested Readings 133

CHAPTER OVERVIEW

High-grade gliomas pose a formidable challenge for neurosurgeons. The propensity of these tumors to invade brain tissue makes surgical resection necessary yet complex. Only in the past 10 years has gross total resection been defined as a favorable first step in the management of these tumors. Minimizing neurologic morbidity should be the goal for every case of high-grade glioma. Defining safe anatomic corridors for resection is very important for safe surgery. Modern preoperative and intraoperative imaging techniques, including ultrasonography, can enhance the surgeon's ability to resect a tumor, as can electrophysiologic monitoring of speech and motor function in selected cases. The surgeon's expertise and experience play a very large role in the outcome. Rigorous outcome analyses should be developed in hospitals where glioma surgery is performed, both to promote objectivity about surgical results and to identify areas needing improvement. Specialized training in neuro-oncology will help younger neurosurgeons face the surgical challenges posed by these tumors.

INTRODUCTION

High-grade gliomas (HGGs) are malignant infiltrative tumors of the brain. The World Health Organization grading system classifies HGGs as grade III or IV tumors, the most malignant and most common of which is glioblastoma (grade IV). Grade III tumors are also called anaplastic tumors. Despite recent surgical and technologic advances and more intense chemotherapy regimens, the prognosis for patients with HGGs (particularly glioblastomas) has improved only minimally in the past 20 years. The best mean survival duration is 16 to 18 months for patients with glioblastoma multiforme. A long-standing controversy involves the efficacy of maximally resecting malignant gliomas. In other types of oncologic surgery, complete resection of a tumor with wide margins is critically important in controlling the disease; however, HGGs invade the surrounding brain, so wide resections are typically not possible because adjacent or nearby areas subserve important neurologic functions. Properly designed prospective studies have only recently been performed, and the results have demonstrated a beneficial relationship between the extent of resection of malignant gliomas and patient survival. With continued refinements in microsurgical techniques and with the use of adjunctive surgical technologies, major neurologic morbidity has been reduced to 8.5% and mortality to 1.7% for patients undergoing craniotomies for tumor resection (Sawaya et al, 1998). This chapter describes the factors used in deciding whether to resect an HGG, summarizes the surgical strategies for managing HGGs used at M. D. Anderson Cancer Center, and discusses some of the techniques and new technologies used to optimize resection of these tumors.

THE DECISION TO RESECT

At M. D. Anderson, we attach great relevance to patient selection in achieving good outcomes from surgery. The decision to resect or not to resect an HGG is always made after close collaboration between neurosurgeons, neuro-oncologists, and radiation oncologists. The surgeon must consider a number of critical factors before deciding to operate, including the patient's age and neurologic status, the location and size of the tumor, the number and extent of recurrences, and whether adjuvant treatment such as radiotherapy or chemotherapy would be suitable.

After deciding to operate, the surgeon must determine how much of the tumor to resect. Compared with patients who have undergone less extensive resection, those who have undergone gross total resection have a better long-term neurologic outcome and no added perioperative morbidity or mortality (Ammirati et al, 1987; Fadul et al, 1988; Sawaya et al, 1998). In a study of 416 consecutive patients with glioblastoma multiforme who were treated at M. D. Anderson, total resection of the main tumor mass (at least 98% by volumetric analysis) was an independent variable that significantly prolonged patient survival duration. The median survival time was 13.4 months for these patients and 8.8 months for patients who had undergone less extensive resection ($P < 0.0001$) (Lacroix et al, 2001). That study relied on prospective computerized measurement of the volume of the tumors, and the extent of resection was expressed as a percentage of the preoperative volume (Sawaya, 1999). The clinical variables of patient age and Karnofsky performance scale score, which have previously been found to influence survival, were included in the multivariate analysis to provide a sound statistical assessment of the link between the extent of tumor resection and patient survival. The multivariate analysis identified 5 independent predictors of survival, 3 of which were chosen for the outcome scale: tumor necrosis, patient age, and Karnofsky performance scale score (Table 6–1). With the use of that analysis, score groups were created to allow survival estimation based on the outcome scale according to the extent of tumor resection. For patients with the lowest (0) or highest (4 or 5) scores, a statistically significant advantage of more complete resection could not outweigh the importance of the 3 chosen predictors of survival in the determination of patient outcome (Table 6–2).

Overall, however, the results of the analysis by Lacroix et al (2001) showed that 90% resection or less did not significantly prolong the patient survival time and that the greatest survival benefit occurred when the extent of resection reached 98% or greater (Table 6–3). These data are particularly important because of their precision and because they avoid subjective terms such as "gross total" or "subtotal" to describe the degree of resection.

Table 6–1. **Clinical Outcome Scale for 416 Patients with Glioblastoma Multiforme***

Clinical Characteristic	Score*
Tumor necrosis on MR images†	
Yes	2
No	0
Patient age (years)	
<45	0
45–64	1
≥65	2
Karnofsky performance scale score	
<80	1
≥80	0

* The assignment of outcome scores relies on a multivariate analysis of predictors of survival.

† Presence of necrosis includes grades I–III, and absence of necrosis is equivalent to grade 0.

Adapted from Lacroix M, Abi-Said D, Fourney DR, et al. A multivariate analysis of 416 patients with glioblastoma multiforme: prognosis, extent of resection, and survival. *J Neurosurg* 2001;95:190–198 with permission from American Association of Neurological Surgeons.

S.S. Prabhu

Table 6–2.   Total Outcome Score and Median Survival Duration of 416 Patients with Glioblastoma Multiforme

			Median Survival Duration		
			Months (No. of Patients)		
Total Score	No. of Patients	Median Survival Duration, Months (95% CI)*	≥98% Resection	<98% Resection	P Value†
0	15	35.3 (not defined)	35.3 (8)	32.8 (7)	0.85
1 or 2	89	14.9 (11.7–18.0)	19.0 (49)	10.9 (40)	0.001
3	184	10.7 (9.2–12.2)	13.1 (79)	8.3 (105)	0.005
4 or 5	128	8.2 (6.6–9.8)	8.6 (61)	7.8 (67)	0.13

Abbreviation: CI, confidence interval.

* Log-rank test significant at $P < 0.0001$.

† Log-rank test for difference in median survival.

Adapted from Lacroix M, Abi-Said D, Fourney DR, et al. A multivariate analysis of 416 patients with glioblastoma multiforme: prognosis, extent of resection, and survival. *J Neurosurg* 2001;95:190–198 with permission from American Association of Neurological Surgeons.

Table 6–3.   Median Survival Time Relative to Degree of Tumor Resection in Patients with HGGs

Extent of Tumor Resection	Median Survival Duration, Months (95% CI)	Rate Ratio (95% CI)	P Value*
≥85%	10.90 (9.7–12.2)	1.11 (0.8–1.5)	0.5
≥90%	11.43 (10.1–12.7)	1.27 (1.0–1.7)	0.08
≥94%	11.90 (10.3–13.4)	1.31 (1.0–1.7)	0.03
≥96%	13.10 (11.3–14.9)	1.56 (1.2–2.0)	0.0004
≥98%	13.40 (12.0–14.9)	1.74 (1.4–2.2)	<0.0001
100%	13.60 (12.2–15.0)	1.78 (1.4–2.3)	<0.0001

Abbreviation: CI, confidence interval.

* Difference calculated for survival at each resection level versus combined data for all lesser levels of resection.

Adapted from Sawaya R. Fifty years of neurosurgery argue in favor of glioma resection. *Clin Neurosurg* 2001;48:10–19 with permission from Lippincott, Williams, and Wilkins.

The term "gross total resection" as used in the literature has at times referred to resections greater than 90% but less than 98%, thereby including values that we have shown to be insufficient to statistically affect the survival duration of patients with glioblastomas.

Beyond the extension of survival duration, several other benefits can result from more complete resection of a glioblastoma. In our experience, these additional benefits include (1) a diagnostic advantage in terms of better sampling of tumors and better quality of the tissue acquired for immunohistochemical and other analysis, (2) a symptomatic advantage through relief of mass effect, leading to improved performance status and enhanced tolerance to radiotherapy, (3) an oncologic advantage by reducing the number of neoplastic cells by almost 2 log orders of magnitude, and (4) a research advantage by harvesting of ample tissue material for molecular analysis and fingerprinting, with the eventual identification of novel and specific molecular targets that will form the basis of therapies of the future.

SURGICAL APPROACHES TO HGG

It is incumbent on the surgeon to understand that surgery is not necessarily the end point in treating patients with HGGs. Most of these patients undergo intensive external beam radiotherapy and chemotherapy, either of which can be debilitating. Hence, the preoperative management of chronic systemic conditions such as hypertension, diabetes mellitus, and various cardiovascular and pulmonary problems must be maximized. Medications that can affect bleeding and coagulation, such as aspirin, clopidogrel bisulfate, and warfarin, should be stopped well in advance of the planned surgery. The anesthetic and medical teams at M. D. Anderson are routinely involved in the preoperative assessment of patients.

It is a falsely held belief that maximal resection of malignant gliomas, even those in eloquent brain areas, results in a higher incidence of neurologic morbidity than lesser resections do. Therefore, rather than basing the decision to perform a craniotomy on the extent of resection, this decision is usually based on the characteristics of the tumor mass, as identified on good-quality MR images. At our institution, adjunctive imaging techniques such as functional MRI and MR spectroscopy also aid in clarifying the relationship of the tumor to eloquent areas and normal brain. The compactness of the mass and its accessibility dictate its resectability. Locating the mass, whether deep in the brain or close to eloquent areas, can be technically challenging; however, location by itself does not present a contraindication to surgery as long as the mass is accessible through nonfunctioning brain and its margin is reasonably defined. An example is shown in Figure 6–1. The basic surgical techniques used in performing a craniotomy are not detailed in this chapter, but we describe the techniques used at M. D. Anderson to accomplish maximal resection of an HGG.

For tumors that present on the cortical surface in non-eloquent areas of the brain, the superficial margins should be identified and dissection should begin at the margins. For tumors that do not present on the surface, an interhemispheric, trans-sulcal, or transcortical approach is used, depending on the size and location of the mass. When possible, a corticectomy facilitates

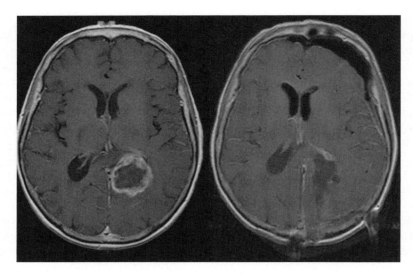

Figure 6–1. Preoperative axial image (T1-weighted, postcontrast) shows a glioblastoma situated in the deep left dominant temporal lobe adjacent to the choroidal fissure (*left*). A posterior approach to this lesion was chosen through non-eloquent cortex, and a gross total resection was accomplished (*right*). Patients with tumors in this location may have a visual field cut before resection and afterward will almost certainly have such a deficit.

removal of a large mass. Conversely, smaller masses, especially those located in functional areas, are better reached through an overlying sulcus. Regardless of the depth of the tumor and whenever possible, circumferential dissection of an HGG is recommended. This approach is obviously more easily accomplished when the tumor is superficial, but it is not limited to superficial tumors. Of course, in the attempt to remove more than 98% of the zone of enhancement by such a circumferential attack, the geographic relation of the tumor margin to white matter tracts of importance (e.g., the uncinate fasciculus and the corticospinal tract) must be studied and understood.

Technical Adjuncts to Surgery

Several technologic adjuncts to surgery are available to help localize the brain mass, identify zones of brain function, and help the surgeon maintain proper orientation in reference to the mass and surrounding anatomic structures. Of these techniques, intraoperative ultrasonography, is an inexpensive, readily accessible surgical tool that allows localization of the mass in real time and aids in the assessment of the completeness of tumor resection. Most malignant gliomas are hyperechoic with respect to normal brain and thus can be localized easily with an ultrasound probe. At M. D. Anderson, resection of HGGs is rarely performed without intraoperative ultrasonography.

Frameless stereotactic systems have provided significant assistance in many tasks, including the adequate placement and sizing of the bone flap, the identification of surface margins, the localization of the mass, and the navigational direction of dissection around or into the mass. The obvious drawback of such systems is their inability to provide a true assessment of residual tumor because of brain shifts that occur during surgery. Having experience with these systems and correlating imaging-derived data with ultrasound data and with what is visible in the operative field are necessary for using these techniques safely to obtain maximal tumor resection.

Neurophysiologic techniques are used primarily when the tumor is presumed to be in or adjacent to eloquent brain. The most commonly used techniques for cortical mapping are somatosensory evoked potential and direct cortical stimulation (Figure 6–2). For motor and sensory localization (Figure 6–3), the patient is usually under general anesthesia; for speech localization, however, an awake craniotomy is always necessary. Awake craniotomy involves waking up the patient during the most critical portion of the tumor resection. Initially, laryngeal mask intubation is carried out to facilitate extubation before the patient is woken up. The patient receives a scalp block using a long-acting anesthetic agent to minimize pain from the craniotomy. Before the tumor resection, brain stimulation is performed

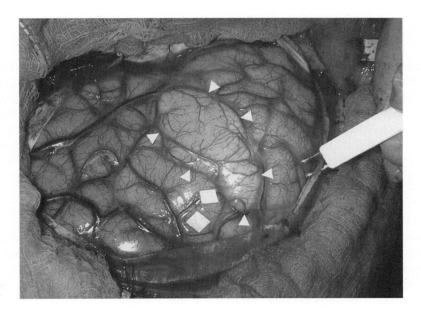

Figure 6–2. Intraoperative image of the left frontotemporal brain. The patient was awake for the procedure, and the Ojemann stimulator (at right) was used to stimulate the brain. Direct stimulation of the frontal speech areas at low intensities (1–5 mA) results in speech arrest with this technique. The tumor mass is outlined by triangles, and the 2 squares denote the site of speech arrest.

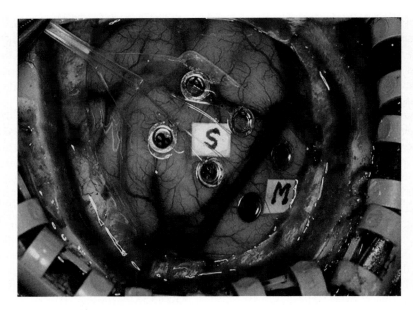

Figure 6–3. Intraoperative image shows grid mapping of the motor (M) and sensory (S) areas of the brain. A phase reversal obtained using this technique indicated the division between the motor and sensory cortices across the central sulcus (thick dark line).

using a bipolar stimulator to identify the speech centers. The patient is asked to perform reading tasks which activate both Broca's motor speech area and Wernicke's speech area. During the initial stimulation process and subsequent tumor resection, a "speech arrest" that occurs during the reading tasks alerts the surgeon to the proximity of the speech centers in the brain. In this manner, the speech centers can be mapped out and the tumor resection maximized while preserving neurologic function. The introduction of these techniques to surgery for malignant gliomas has made it possible to perform larger resections with increased safety.

Early MRI systems had low field strength, and as such they were less sensitive and provided less crisp images than the current generation of such equipment does. Intraoperative MRI has recently been introduced in several cancer treatment centers. This technique identifies residual tumor more accurately than any other method does (Figure 6–4). However, it has a major drawback: an expensive and sometimes cumbersome piece of equipment is needed, and before it can be installed, existing structures must be extensively modified.

Beyond the technical considerations, the most critical decision in glioma surgery is when to halt resection to avoid increasing preoperative deficits or inducing new ones. Surgical adjuncts such as intraoperative ultrasonography and systems for imaging guidance can aid in surgical decision making when the tumor border is not clearly distinguishable from

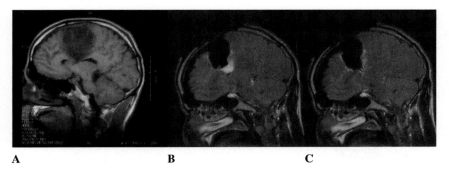

A   B   C

Figure 6–4. (A) Preoperative T1-weighted MR image reveals a large anaplastic glioma. (B) First intraoperative MR image (FLAIR sequence) reveals residual tumor inferiorly. (C) Postresection intraoperative MR image (also a FLAIR sequence) reveals complete tumor resection.

surrounding brain, but the ultimate decision resides with the surgeon, whose judgment and knowledge of neuroanatomy are needed to correlate the images with what is seen in the operative field (Hammoud et al, 1996; Toms et al, 1999). Extra care must be taken when the tumor is adjacent to eloquent cortex or near important subcortical white matter tracts.

Once the resection has been completed, the cavity must be inspected carefully for residual tumor. Hemostasis is necessary and can be checked by the Valsalva maneuver. The routine and excessive use of absorbable hemostatic agents is discouraged, but such agents may be placed selectively on areas that are raw, oozing, or difficult to control. The dura mater should be closed in a watertight fashion, if possible, to prevent cerebrospinal fluid leaks. Dural closure is especially important when the ventricular cavity has been entered or when the brain has been previously operated on and irradiated. After dural closure, intraoperative ultrasonography is used to ensure the absence of a hematoma in the resection cavity before the bone flap is replaced and secured.

Avoidance of surgical complications generally starts with proper patient selection. Modern neuroanesthetic techniques, prophylactic interventions, advanced imaging and localization devices such as ultrasound scanners, and a variety of surgical adjuncts—from microscopy to cortical mapping—contribute to low morbidity and mortality rates.

Unresectable HGGs

In general, malignant tumors are deemed unresectable if they widely infiltrate the brain (cerebral gliomas), brainstem, or basal ganglia (Figure 6–5); extend to both hemispheres through involvement of the corpus callosum; involve more than 1 lobe; or show multifocality or multicentricity. Both frame-based and frameless stereotactic procedures can be used with these tumors to obtain a biopsy sample with which to guide nonsurgical therapy. These procedures are usually done under local anesthesia with sedation

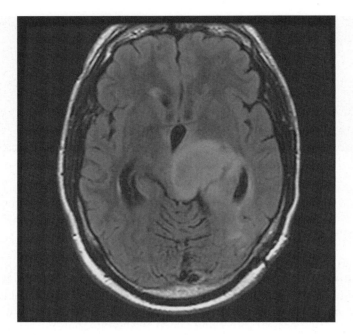

Figure 6–5. MR image (axial flair sequence) shows a diffuse glioblastoma of the left thalamus. Because of the high degree of potential morbidity, no surgical resection was advised for this patient, and a stereotactic biopsy was performed to establish the diagnosis.

and involve an overnight stay in the hospital. With the help of computer-assisted algorithms, the biopsy trajectory is chosen after an entry point and target are selected (Figure 6–6). Care should be taken to avoid penetration of a sulcus, pial interface, or vascular structure. Open biopsies are occasionally indicated if more tissue is required for establishing the diagnosis than a stereotactic biopsy can provide (typically 5–15 mm^3).

Recurrent HGGs

Because malignant gliomas tend to recur, reoperation is often contemplated and is often necessary. In the study by Sawaya et al (1998), 28% of the patients underwent 2 operations, and 10% had 3 or more craniotomies. There was no significant association between morbidity and the number of craniotomies, which is consistent with the observation by Fadul et al (1988) that the likelihood of neurologic deterioration or death was no greater for patients undergoing second or third operations for recurrent tumors than for those undergoing a first operation.

Recurrent tumors can sometimes be confused with changes consistent with radiation necrosis. Although small areas of necrosis after treatment may stabilize and repair over time, some require repeat resection to stop

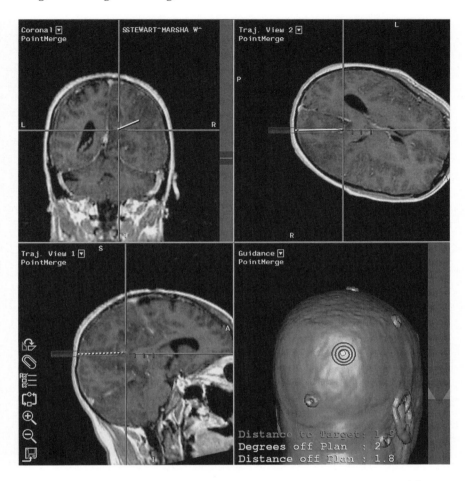

Figure 6–6. Imaging-guided stereotactic biopsy using a computer-assisted frameless technique of a diffuse right parieto-occipital mass. The entry point on the surface of the skin (bull's-eye in bottom right panel) and the target (tip of the crosshairs in the other 3 panels) are identified. A safe trajectory to the target is then selected, as indicated by the solid or dashed white lines. A biopsy needle is then passed in real time toward the target to obtain tissue samples.

these areas from propagating through adjacent brain. MR spectroscopy is a valuable tool for distinguishing between recurrent HGGs and radiation necrosis, but this examination is not entirely dependable, and the decision to operate must be made by the multidisciplinary team. Dynamic MR-guided or MR spectroscopy-guided stereotactic biopsy is sometimes useful in distinguishing between the 2 possibilities. With recurrent tumors, the overall goal at reoperation is to safely maximize the resection. Resection is more challenging with recurrent tumors than with the original HGGs because the recurrent tumors tend to be more invasive and have a less defined interface with normal brain. Special care should be taken with tumors close to eloquent brain, including the brainstem, and the cerebral arteries and veins should be preserved if possible. Although typically well preserved during initial resection, the pial boundaries tend to be compromised in recurrences due to postoperative gliotic reactions, radiotherapy, chemotherapy, and other factors. In recurrent tumors with a significant component of necrosis related to radiotherapy, the margins around the tumor are very ill defined, the mass is less easily seen on ultrasound images, and hence a gross total resection may not be achievable.

CONCLUSION

Existing data concerning the benefits of surgical resection suggest a survival advantage for patients with malignant gliomas who undergo a complete radiographic resection of the tumor mass (i.e., the contrast-enhanced portion of the tumor). Careful preoperative planning should allow for the gross total resection of most HGGs. Until convincing data to the contrary are presented, the goal of a neuro-oncologic operation should be resection of the tumor mass to the greatest degree possible that allows maintenance of neurologic function.

KEY PRACTICE POINTS

- Proper patient selection is important. If the operation carries a significant risk of neurologic injury (e.g., for patients with tumors within the basal ganglia or brainstem), surgical resection should not be offered.
- HGGs should be studied preoperatively with high-quality MR images. Particular attention should be given to T1-weighted images with contrast and fast fluid-attenuated inversion recovery (FLAIR) sequences (especially for nonenhanced tumors) because these images can accurately predict resectability. Postoperative scanning should be performed within 24 to 48 hours after surgery to determine the extent of resection.
- HGGs in eloquent brain areas should be considered for intraoperative monitoring, which is the gold standard for anatomically defining these areas and can prevent neurologic morbidity.
- Intraoperative ultrasonography and techniques using computerized navigational guidance should be part of a surgeon's arsenal during glioma surgery.
- A team of consultants, including neurosurgeons, neuro-oncologists, and radiation oncologists, should confer on the key issues of HGG management to achieve better outcomes.

SUGGESTED READINGS

Ammirati M, Vick N, Liao YL, Ciric I, Mikhael M. Effect of the extent of surgical resection on survival and quality of life in patients with supratentorial glioblastomas and anaplastic astrocytomas. *Neurosurgery* 1987;21:201–206.

Fadul C, Wood J, Thaler H, Galicich J, Patterson RH Jr, Posner JB. Morbidity and mortality of craniotomy for excision of supratentorial gliomas. *Neurology* 1988;38:1374–1379.

Hammoud MA, Ligon BL, ElSouki R, Shi WM, Schomer DF, Sawaya R. Use of intraoperative ultrasound for localizing tumors and determining the extent of resection: a comparative study with magnetic resonance imaging. *J Neurosurg* 1996;84:737–741.

Lacroix M, Abi-Said D, Fourney DR, et al. A multivariate analysis of 416 patients with glioblastoma multiforme: prognosis, extent of resection, and survival. *J Neurosurg* 2001;95:190–198.

Sawaya R. Extent of resection in malignant gliomas: a critical summary. *J Neurooncol* 1999;42:303–305.

Sawaya R, Hammoud M, Schoppa D, et al. Neurosurgical outcomes in a modern series of 400 craniotomies for treatment of parenchymal tumors. *Neurosurgery* 1998;42:1044–1056.

Toms SA, Ferson DZ, Sawaya R. Basic surgical techniques in the resection of malignant gliomas. *J Neurooncol* 1999;42:215–226.

7   RADIATION ONCOLOGY FOR TUMORS OF THE CENTRAL NERVOUS SYSTEM: IMPROVING THE THERAPEUTIC INDEX

Shiao Y. Woo

Chapter Overview 136
Introduction 136
Radiation Technologies 136
    Conventional Technology 136
    Modern Technologies 136
        Classic 3-Dimensional Conformal Radiotherapy 137
        Radiosurgery or Stereotactic Radiotherapy 138
        Intensity-Modulated Radiotherapy 139
        Brachytherapy 140
        Proton Therapy 140
Role of Radiotherapy in Malignant Tumors 141
    Malignant Gliomas 141
    WHO Grade II Astrocytomas 143
    Medulloblastomas and Primitive Neuroectodermal Tumors 143
    Intracranial Germ Cell Tumors 144
    Metastatic Tumors to the Brain 144
    Metastatic Tumors to the Spine 145
Role of Radiotherapy in Low-Grade or Benign Tumors 145
    WHO Grade I Astrocytomas 145
    Meningiomas 146
    Pituitary Adenomas 146
Adverse Effects of Radiotherapy 147
    Acute Adverse Effects 147
    Subacute Adverse Effects 147
    Late Adverse Effects 147
        Leukoencephalopathy 147
        Neurocognitive Deficit 148
        Neuroendocrine Dysfunction 148
        Brain Necrosis 148
Conclusion 149
Key Practice Points 149
Suggested Readings 149

CHAPTER OVERVIEW

Several advanced technologies in radiation oncology are being used to treat a variety of tumors of the central nervous system. These modern technologies include 3-dimensional conformal radiotherapy, radiosurgery or stereotactic radiotherapy, intensity-modulated radiotherapy, brachytherapy, and proton therapy. Radiotherapy is a potentially curative treatment for low-grade gliomas, medulloblastomas, primitive neuroectodermal tumors, intracranial germ cell tumors, meningiomas, and pituitary adenomas. Radiotherapy is used to prolong the survival time of patients with malignant gliomas, and it is an effective palliative treatment for metastatic tumors to the brain and spine. The acute and subacute adverse effects of radiotherapy are usually not severe and are transient. Although less common than acute adverse effects, certain late adverse effects can significantly affect the quality and even the quantity of life. When coupled with sophisticated imaging technologies, the advanced radiation planning and delivery technologies can surpass conventional technology in delivering high doses of radiation to tumors while sparing normal structures in the central nervous system, thereby improving the therapeutic index.

INTRODUCTION

Radiotherapy is an important modality for treating most tumors of the central nervous system, benign or malignant, primary or metastatic. It can be used as the sole treatment or to complement surgical resection, chemotherapy, or both. As a specialty, radiation oncology is technologically driven, and advancements in technology have allowed radiotherapy to be much more intricately planned and precisely delivered than previously, and they have probably helped to improve the therapeutic index.

RADIATION TECHNOLOGIES

Conventional Technology

In conventional radiotherapy, a limited number of portals (1 to 4) are usually used. Each portal can be shaped by a Cerrobend block or a multileaf collimator to shield important adjacent normal structures. The treatment planning is 2-dimensional in that the radiation dose distribution can be manipulated on only 1 plane across the isocenter of the portals.

Modern Technologies

The modern technology-driven concepts in radiotherapy are conformal radiotherapy and imaging-guided radiotherapy. Conformal radiotherapy is a general term that applies to a system of radiotherapy planning and delivery that aims to create high doses of radiation around the shape of the tumor and lower doses to the nearby normal structures. Imaging-guided radiotherapy uses various imaging techniques to help delineate the tumor and normal structures, to help determine the appropriate directions of the radiation beam or beams in the planning process, to display the radiation dose distribution, and to ensure the position of the patient and the tumor before the delivery of each dose of radiation. The different technologies available for conformal and imaging-guided radiotherapy are discussed below.

Classic 3-Dimensional Conformal Radiotherapy

In classic 3-dimensional technology, 3-dimensional images of the tumor and normal structures are reconstructed to aid in the selection of the directions of the radiation portals. The idea is to target the tumor while easily shielding the nearby normal tissue. The radiation portals are usually non-coplanar and are shaped by customized Cerrobend blocks or a multileaf collimator (Figure 7–1). The planning process is termed "forward planning," meaning that it is an experience-based trial-and-error process.

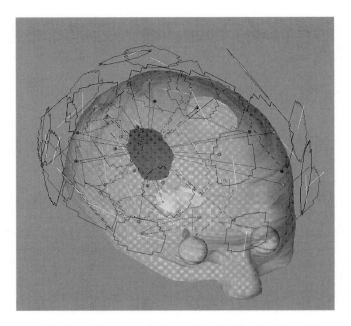

Figure 7–1.   Multiple radiation portals, each individually shaped by a multileaf collimator.

Radiosurgery or Stereotactic Radiotherapy

Radiosurgery refers to a single treatment with a relatively large dose of radiation by focusing many small beams of radiation from different directions onto a small tumor (up to 3 cm in diameter). The procedure generally requires invasive, rigid fixation of the head or an imaging-guided robotic delivery system. Using the same principle to deliver multiple fractions of radiation, stereotactic radiotherapy uses a noninvasive immobilization device coupled with a stereotactic system or an imaging-guided robotic delivery system.

Radiosurgery can be performed using the Gamma Knife, a linear accelerator (including the CyberKnife), or proton therapy equipment. The Gamma Knife is a rigid system in which 201 cobalt 60 sources are collimated at the head of the equipment so that the γ rays from all the sources are focused onto a small isocenter. Secondary collimation is done using 4 sets of removable helmets, each of which contains 201 precisely arranged collimators of increasing diameter (4, 8, 14, and 18 mm). The patient's head is attached to the treatment couch by an invasive Leksell stereotactic head frame and by using predetermined x, y, and z coordinates. The head is positioned so that the part of the tumor to be irradiated is at the isocenter of the γ beams. The new model has an automatic positioning device that can move the head from one position to another during the radiosurgical session.

A linear accelerator can also be adapted to perform radiosurgery. Circular collimators of various sizes or a micro-multileaf collimator can be attached to the head of the machine (Figure 7–2). The patient's head is rigidly fixed on the treatment couch using an invasive stereotactic head frame. The tumor is then positioned at the isocenter of the rotation of the gantry. By rotating the gantry with the couch at various positions, focused radiation can be delivered by several non-coplanar arcs. The end result is similar to that obtained with the Gamma Knife. With a micro-multileaf collimator, one can use multiple static non-coplanar individually shaped fields or an arc technique in which the leaves change the shape of the treatment field at every 10 degrees of rotation.

The CyberKnife is a specially designed imaging-guided system in which a small linear accelerator is moved around the patient by a programmable robotic arm. The position of each treatment field is verified by images, and the robotic arm makes the adjustments. An invasive head frame is therefore not required. In addition, the robotic arm has more positions and directions of radiotherapy delivery than a standard linear accelerator has. In addition to treating tumors of the brain, the Cyberknife can be used to treat tumors of the spine and other sites such as the head and neck, prostate, liver, lung, and kidney.

Proton therapy equipment can also be used to perform radiosurgery (see section Proton Therapy).

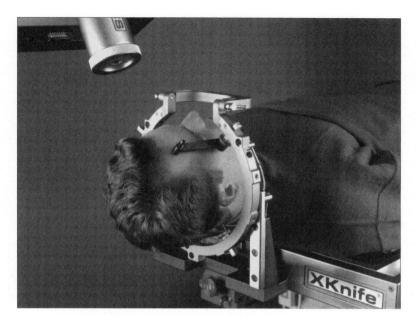

Figure 7–2.   Before linear accelerator–based stereotactic radiosurgery, a patient's head is rigidly fixed on the treatment couch using an invasive stereotactic head frame. The collimator attached to the linear accelerator can be seen at the top left of the photograph.

Intensity-Modulated Radiotherapy

Intensity-modulated radiotherapy (IMRT) is currently the most advanced technology for photon (x-ray) radiotherapy. Conceptually, it uses multiple small beamlets of radiation of different intensities (i.e., amounts) to build, like a 3-dimensional jigsaw puzzle, a composite high-radiation-dose "envelope" that conforms to the shape and size of the tumor. This envelope is compressible in that it can be "pinched" away from a nearby normal structure (Figure 7–3). The planning process is computationally complex, and an optimization algorithm is needed. As opposed to the forward planning process, IMRT planning is frequently referred to as "inverse planning" because the planner sets the parameters of the desired radiation dose to the tumor and the different dose limits to the various normal structures, and then the computer program, through multiple iterations, finds the solution that closely matches the goal. Because of its versatility, IMRT allows satisfactory delivery of radiotherapy in complex clinical situations that are beyond the capability of other photon-based technologies. A new dedicated IMRT machine, called the tomotherapy system, couples an accelerator with a helical computed tomography scanner so that a patient's body can be irradiated and imaged at the same time. Clinical testing with the tomotherapy system is currently under way.

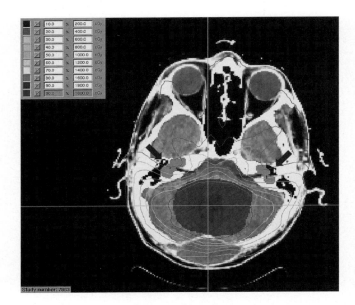

Figure 7–3. An IMRT plan showing radiation isodose lines curving around the auditory nerves and cochleas (arrows).

Brachytherapy

In brachytherapy, radioactive sources are placed in the tumor or in the tumor cavity after surgical resection. In the treatment of malignant brain tumors, radioactive sources such as iodine, iridium, or gold are inserted directly into the tumor or placed in removable catheters. The placement and the radiation strength of the sources are determined on the basis of the desired radiation dose, dose rate, and volume to be irradiated to the desired dose.

Brachytherapy is a form of conformal therapy because generally the radiation dose is the highest somewhere in the middle of the tumor and the dose falls rapidly away from the tumor. A removable balloon has recently been developed that can be inserted into the tumor cavity after resection (Figure 7–4). Liquid radioactive iodine can be instilled into the balloon. The surrounding brain that contains residual tumor molds around the balloon and is thus uniformly irradiated. When the desired dose is reached, the iodine solution is removed. Under the right circumstances, this balloon device is a convenient way to deliver brachytherapy to residual tumor after resection.

Proton Therapy

The proton is a positively charged particle that makes up the nucleus of a hydrogen atom. Protons entering the body deposit little energy along

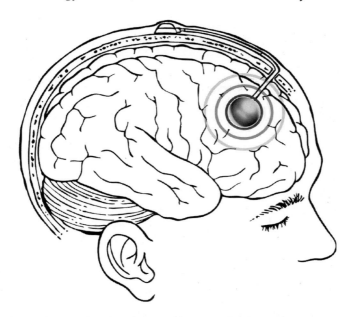

Figure 7–4. A drawing of the GliaSite balloon in a tumor cavity and the reservoir under the scalp. Image provided courtesy of Cytyc Corporation and affiliates.

their path; most of the energy is deposited at the end of the path—the Bragg peak—and virtually no radiation is delivered beyond this point. The distance between the point of entry into the body and the Bragg peak is determined by the initial energy of the protons. This physical characteristic of protons distinguishes them from photons (or x-rays) and allows highly conformal dose distributions to be generated around tumors. Because of the introduction of scanning proton beams, the ability of highly sophisticated and complex intensity-modulated proton therapy to spare normal tissue may surpass that of IMRT. Currently, there are about 25 treatment centers in the world that use proton therapy, and several more are under construction or being planned. Proton therapy will likely be an important radiotherapy technique for the treatment of central nervous system tumors in the near future.

ROLE OF RADIOTHERAPY IN MALIGNANT TUMORS

Malignant Gliomas

The benefit of radiotherapy in improving the survival duration of patients with malignant astrocytoma (World Health Organization [WHO] grade III or IV) after surgery was demonstrated in a prospective randomized trial conducted by the Brain Tumor Study Group. In that trial, patients who received postoperative radiotherapy either alone or with BCNU (the abbreviation for the chemical name of carmustine) had a significantly longer survival duration than those who underwent surgery either alone or with BCNU (without radiotherapy) (Walker et al, 1978). During the past 3 decades, many clinical trials have investigated the volume of radio-therapy (whole-brain vs local field irradiation), the timing of radiother-apy (preoperative vs postoperative), the total dose of radiation (greater than, less than, or equal to 60 Gy), and the fractionation schedule (con-ventional once-a-day vs hyperfractionation, accelerated fractionation, or hypofractionation) for malignant gliomas of the central nervous system. Results from some of the representative trials of radiation doses and frac-tionation schedules are shown in Table 7–1. These trials have led to the conclusion that there is not a radiotherapy regimen superior to one that delivers 60 Gy in 30 to 33 once-a-day fractions (1.8 to 2 Gy per fraction) 5 days a week to the tumor plus a defined margin. Therefore, this is cur-rently the standard radiotherapy regimen for newly diagnosed malignant gliomas.

For recurrent malignant gliomas and under certain circumstances, reir-radiation with radiosurgery, interstitial or intracavitary brachytherapy, or IMRT can prolong patient survival time, although usually not by much. Generally, the longer the interval is from the first course of radiotherapy,

Table 7–1. **Results from Representative Trials on Radiation Fractionation and Dose for Malignant Gliomas of the Central Nervous System**

Investigating Group (Reference)	Radiation Fractionation	Radiation Dose (Gy)	Median Patient Survival Duration
Radiation Therapy Oncology Group (Walker et al, 1979)	Conventional	50 55 60	28 weeks 36 weeks 42 weeks*
Radiation Therapy Oncology Group and Eastern Cooperative Oncology Group (Chang et al, 1983)	Conventional	60 60 + 10 boost	9.9 months 8.4 months
Radiation Therapy Oncology Group (Nelson et al, 1993)	Hyperfractionation (1.2 Gy twice a day)	64.8 72.0 76.8 81.6	11.4 months 12.8 months 12.0 months 11.7 months
Baylor College of Medicine (Floyd et al, 2004)	Hyperfractionation (5 Gy per fraction)	50	7 months

* $P = 0.004$ vs 28 weeks.

the smaller the recurrent tumor; and the farther the tumor is from eloquent areas of the brain, the lower the risk from reirradiation. Radiosurgery has been reported to produce a lower incidence of symptomatic necrosis (about 20% of patients) but a benefit equivalent to that obtained from brachytherapy (Shrieve et al, 1995). The updated analysis at M. D. Anderson Cancer Center showed a median survival time of 11 months after radiosurgery for selected patients with recurrent glioblastomas (Mahajan et al, 2005). However, the patients selected for radiosurgery had tumors that were 3 cm or less in diameter, whereas patients who underwent brachytherapy had tumors as large as 5 or 6 cm in diameter. Brachytherapy has been reported to produce symptomatic brain (and tumor) necrosis in about 50% to 60% of the patients, many of whom have required surgical removal of the necrotic mass. Leibel et al (1989) found that some patients who had undergone surgical resection of necrotic masses lived longer than those who had not developed symptomatic necrosis. IMRT has been used for reirradiation, but the data on its effect on patient survival are limited.

WHO Grade II Astrocytomas

A WHO grade II astrocytoma or ordinary low-grade astrocytoma, although not usually aggressive initially, has an increasing potential with time to degenerate into a malignant astrocytoma. A randomized study showed that patients who underwent radiotherapy immediately after surgery had a higher 5-year progression-free survival rate than did patients who underwent surgery alone (delaying radiotherapy until recurrence), but there was no difference in the overall survival rate (Karim et al, 2002). Two other randomized studies found no significant difference in tumor control when the radiation dose was 50.4 Gy versus 64.8 Gy (Shaw et al, 2002) or 45 Gy versus 59.4 Gy (Karim et al, 1996). Therefore, a dose of 45 to 50 Gy seems adequate for treating WHO grade II astrocytomas. Because these tumors are not very infiltrating, the treatment volume can be limited, and one of the modern conformal techniques is recommended to help minimize morbidity.

Medulloblastomas and Primitive Neuroectodermal Tumors

Medulloblastomas and primitive neuroectodermal tumors are more often encountered in children than in adults. Radiotherapy is the backbone of any potentially curative treatment program for these tumors. Since these tumors have a propensity to spread in the leptomeningeal space, irradiation of the entire craniospinal axis is usually required except in infants, for whom craniospinal irradiation is postponed until 3 or 4 years of age by using chemotherapy. Additional radiation is directed to the tumor bed after craniospinal irradiation. It has recently been shown that compared with the conventional technique, the use of IMRT to treat the tumor bed could significantly reduce the radiation dose to the cochlea. In children who also received *cis*-platinum chemotherapy, a known ototoxic agent, a decrease in the radiation dose to the cochlea led to a corresponding reduction in the incidence of severe hearing deficit (Huang et al, 2002). Investigation is ongoing to determine whether the dose of craniospinal irradiation can be lowered from 23.4 to 18 Gy in selected patients to reduce the long-term adverse effects of craniospinal irradiation, such as growth retardation, neuroendocrine deficit, thyroid dysfunction, and neurocognitive impairment. The use of proton therapy for spinal irradiation could essentially eliminate any significant radiation dose to organs and structures anterior to the spine and therefore could, in the long term, decrease organ dysfunction and the incidence of radiation-induced second malignancies (Miralbell et al, 2002).

Intracranial Germ Cell Tumors

Intracranial germ cell tumors are broadly categorized as germinomas, nongerminomatous germ cell tumors, or mixed germ cell tumors. Leptomeningeal dissemination is known to occur in varying frequencies, depending on the histologic type. Germinomas are very radiosensitive. For example, 18 to 20 Gy to the craniospinal axis followed by 20 to 25 Gy to the tumor bed has been reported to be curative for more than 90% of patients with minimal late sequelae (Maity et al, 2004). However, it is currently popular to give 2 to 4 cycles of platinum-based chemotherapy followed by local field irradiation to 30 to 40 Gy, with the radiation dose dependent on whether there is a complete response to the chemotherapy. The local field should include the suprasellar region extending from the pineal gland posteriorly to the frontal horns of the lateral ventricles anteriorly and encompassing the floor of the third ventricle. This combined modality approach has produced a cure rate similar to that obtained with craniospinal irradiation. Except for benign teratomas (which are treated by surgical resection), nongerminomatous germ cell tumors should generally be treated with 4 to 6 cycles of platinum-based chemotherapy and radiotherapy (generally craniospinal irradiation).

Metastatic Tumors to the Brain

Most cancers in the body can metastasize to the brain. The most common primary cancers that spread to the brain are lung cancer, breast cancer, melanoma, and renal cell carcinoma. Whole-brain irradiation is a commonly used palliative treatment, usually to 30 Gy delivered in 10 to 12 fractions. Although symptomatic improvement is frequently achieved, control of the tumor from whole-brain irradiation is usually not durable. Attempts have been made to improve the rate of tumor control by surgical resection or additional focal irradiation using radiosurgery. For patients with solitary brain metastases, surgical resection plus whole-brain irradiation has been shown to increase the duration of tumor control over whole-brain irradiation

(Patchell et al, 1998). For patients with recursive partitioning analysis class 1 or a favorable histologic status, the survival duration was prolonged when radiosurgery was added to whole-brain irradiation (Andrews et al, 2004). A recent trend has been the use of radiosurgery alone to treat brain metastases because of the perceived neurocognitive adverse effects of whole-brain irradiation in a minority of patients. In a randomized trial of radiosurgery alone versus radiosurgery plus whole-brain irradiation, the group of patients who had received both radiosurgery and whole-brain irradiation had a significantly lower rate of recurrence of radiosurgery-treated tumors and of tumors elsewhere in the brain, although the overall survival duration of the 2 patient groups was not statistically different (Aoyama et al, 2004). In practice, whether a patient receives whole-brain irradiation after radiosurgery is usually determined by the patient's preference and the physician's bias.

Metastatic Tumors to the Spine

Practically all cancers can metastasize to the bones, including the spine. The most common primary tumors are lung, breast, prostate, and kidney. Radiotherapy is commonly used to palliate pain or to treat spinal cord compression from the metastatic tumor in the vertebra. The common fraction scheme is 30 Gy delivered in 10 fractions, which does not exceed the tolerance of the spinal cord to radiation. Recent advances in imaging-guided radiotherapy and IMRT have allowed larger biologic doses to be delivered to the tumor in 1 to 5 fractions while keeping the dose to the spinal cord relatively low. Fractionations such as 6 Gy per fraction for 5 fractions, 9 Gy per fraction for 3 fractions, and 15 Gy delivered in a single fraction (similar to stereotactic radiosurgery) have been and are still being tested and thus far have been found to be safe. It is hoped that these larger fractions will result in better tumor control and longer symptom relief than the more conventional fractionation schema do.

ROLE OF RADIOTHERAPY IN LOW-GRADE OR BENIGN TUMORS

WHO Grade I Astrocytomas

For WHO grade I astrocytomas or juvenile pilocytic astrocytomas, surgical resection is the usual initial treatment. If a gross total resection is achieved, adjuvant radiotherapy is generally not necessary. If the resection is incomplete and the tumor is not in an eloquent area where recurrence could cause significant functional deficit, the patient can be observed; radiotherapy can then be considered if the tumor recurs and cannot be totally resected. This approach is more relevant for young children because the delay in radiotherapy allows for the further development of the young brain, potentially reducing the degree of neurocognitive deficits related to radiotherapy. If radiotherapy is used, a dose of about 50 Gy is sufficient with a tight margin around the tumor. It has been shown that for children, the margin can be reduced to 2 mm by using a fractionated stereotactic radiotherapy technique (Marcus et al, 2005). This limitation in the volume of normal brain irradiated is likely to reduce morbidity.

Meningiomas

The primary treatment for meningiomas is surgery. For incompletely resected meningiomas, the use of postoperative radiotherapy has been shown to improve the 10-year relapse-free patient survival rate from 45% (incomplete resection alone) (Mirimanoff et al, 1985) to 77% (Goldsmith et al, 1994). Meningiomas located at the skull base are more difficult to resect completely. For meningiomas located in the cavernous sinus, primary radiotherapy is frequently the treatment of choice. With modern conformal radiotherapy techniques, an overall actuarial 10-year survival rate of 96% and a low morbidity rate have been reported for patients with meningiomas at the base of the skull (Debus et al, 2001). The usual dose of radiation is 50 to 54 Gy delivered in 25 to 30 fractions. However, unlike after surgery, the tumor does not disappear, as seen on follow-up magnetic resonance images after radiotherapy. A lack of growth over time is the measure of tumor control.

Meningiomas affecting the optic nerve sheath deserve special mention. Patients with these tumors usually present with a visual defect. Attempts at resection or even biopsy have historically been associated with a high risk of further visual loss, probably because of injury to the vascular supply of the optic nerve. On the other hand, primary radiotherapy without biopsy has resulted in rapid gain of visual function in many cases, sometimes even during the middle of the radiotherapy. An analysis of the visual outcome of 4 groups of patients with optic nerve sheath meningiomas treated by observation, surgery alone, surgery plus radiotherapy, or radiotherapy alone showed that patients treated with radiotherapy alone had the best visual outcome (Turbin et al, 2002). Again, one of the modern conformal radiotherapy techniques is recommended. A dose of 50.4 Gy delivered in 1.8-Gy fractions appears to strike the balance between efficacy and possible risk of radiation injury to the optic nerve.

Pituitary Adenomas

Surgery is the primary treatment for pituitary adenomas. Residual tumor (macroscopic or microscopic) can be present if the tumor invades 1 or both of the cavernous sinuses, has a large suprasellar extension, or significantly erodes the bony floor of the sella. Postoperative radiotherapy in doses of 45 to 50.4 Gy has produced a 10-year relapse-free survival rate higher than 90% (Brada et al, 1993). The modern conformal techniques have generally produced little morbidity except for a degree a hypopituitarism.

For secretory pituitary tumors, although fractionated radiotherapy is effective in stopping the growth of the tumor, it is less effective in correcting the overproduction of the specific hormone. Generally, after conventional fractionation radiotherapy, the hypersecretion of the specific hormone normalizes in only 50% to 65% of secretory tumors. Whether radiosurgery or proton therapy could produce a higher hormonal response rate remains to be seen.

ADVERSE EFFECTS OF RADIOTHERAPY

Acute Adverse Effects

Acute adverse effects occur during radiotherapy. Besides skin reaction, hair loss, and fatigue, neurologic adverse effects are related to increased edema around the tumor, usually as a result of tumor cell death from the treatment. These neurologic effects include headache and exacerbation of existing or presenting neurologic symptoms and are controlled with steroids.

Subacute Adverse Effects

Subacute adverse effects usually appear 4 to 8 weeks after radiotherapy and resolve within weeks. A well-known subacute effect after whole-brain irradiation is the somnolence syndrome, which is more common in children than in adults. Patients with this syndrome can present with drowsiness, excessive sleepiness, irritability, apathy, nausea, and dizziness. The use of steroids may hasten recovery. The underlying mechanism is transient demyelination. Another manifestation of transient demyelination after spinal irradiation is Lhermitte's sign, which is an electric shock–like sensation radiating down the spine. This sensation may be precipitated by flexion of the neck and is self-limiting.

Late Adverse Effects

Late morbidity due to radiotherapy occurs in a small percentage of patients, usually 6 months or longer from the completion of treatment. The known late adverse effects include leukoencephalopathy, neurocognitive deficit, neuroendocrine dysfunction, and brain necrosis.

Leukoencephalopathy

Leukoencephalopathy is a condition in which there is destruction of the white matter of the brain, leading to cerebral atrophy and ventricular enlargement. Intracerebral calcification may be detected on computed tomography scans. Both cranial radiotherapy and treatment with methotrexate are known contributing factors. Cranial irradiation and intrathecal methotrexate have each been reported to cause less than 1% of cases of leukoencephalopathy; however, various combinations of these treatments have resulted in an incidence of 5% to 45%. The highest incidence results from a combination of cranial radiotherapy, intrathecal methotrexate, and intravenous methotrexate (Griffin, 1980).

Neurocognitive Deficit

Neurocognitive deficit in a patient with a brain tumor is a complex, multifactorial phenomenon. The contributing factors include genetic make-up, age at diagnosis and at treatment, tumor type and location, presence of hydrocephalus, complications associated with surgery, radiation volume and dose, systemic agents, depression, and social factors. When appropriate, cranial irradiation should be avoided for children younger than 3 years old, and the volume of brain outside the tumor receiving high doses of radiation should be limited by using modern conformal technologies.

Neuroendocrine Dysfunction

Pituitary growth hormone production is very sensitive to radiation. The sensitive target is the hypothalamus. A radiation dose of about 18 to 25 Gy is sufficient to decrease growth hormone secretion. The higher the radiation dose received is, the earlier the onset of growth hormone deficiency. The deficiency of other hypothalamic-pituitary hormones after radiotherapy is less common, probably because the threshold is higher at about 40 to 70 Gy. A study at St. Jude Children's Research Hospital evaluated neuroendocrine function by stimulation tests of children with brain tumors before cranial irradiation. Overall, 66% of the children had evidence of endocrinopathy: 38% had growth hormone deficiency, 45% had thyroid-stimulating hormone deficiency, 25% had abnormal corticotropin reserve, and 13% had abnormal age-dependent gonadotropin secretion (Merchant et al, 2002). A surprising finding was that 47% of the children with posterior fossa tumors had endocrinopathy. The investigators concluded that the incidence of radiation-induced endocrinopathy may be overestimated.

Brain Necrosis

Neurons are generally resistant to radiation because they do not divide. However, the oligodendrocytes and the endothelial cells of the vasa vasorum of the arteries in the brain do divide, albeit slowly, and can therefore be killed by radiation. Hence, the pathogenesis of radiation-induced brain necrosis is either a depletion of the supporting oligodendrocytes at the irradiated area or sclerosis of an artery that leads to hypoxic cell death. The incidence of parenchymal brain necrosis after brain irradiation has been reported to be 5% to 20% and is related to the total radiation dose to the brain, radiation fraction size, volume of brain irradiated, presence of radiation-sensitizing drugs, and genetic susceptibility. On magnetic resonance images, radiation necrosis can resemble tumor recurrence, although a "soap bubble" appearance has been ascribed to radiation-induced brain necrosis. Other imaging studies such as magnetic resonance spectroscopy, positron emission tomography, thallium single-photon emission computerized tomography, and dynamic magnetic resonance may be helpful in distinguishing tumor recurrence from necrosis, but none of these techniques is completely reliable (see chapter 3). Surgical resection may be necessary both for confirmation of diagnosis and for treatment.

CONCLUSION

The treatment of most brain tumors is complex and frequently multi-modal. The outcomes, in terms of tumor control and morbidity, are determined by many factors, not the least of which are the characteristics and extent of the tumor. For tumors that infiltrate into normal brain parenchyma, the therapeutic window for most treatment modalities is small. The current technologic advances in radiotherapy can improve the therapeutic index to only a limited extent. Continued research into the fundamental biology of brain tumors is essential so that more effective and less morbid therapies can be discovered.

KEY PRACTICE POINTS

- Radiotherapy is an effective treatment for primary brain tumors and metastatic tumors to the brain.
- When a brain tumor is being treated, one of the technologies for conformal radiotherapy should be used to reduce radiotherapy-related morbidity.
- Advanced imaging techniques are helpful in the planning and delivery of conformal radiotherapy for brain tumors.
- The optimal treatment of most brain tumors is generally decided by a multidisciplinary team of experts in brain tumor therapy.

SUGGESTED READINGS

Andrews DW, Scott CB, Sperduto PW, et al. Whole brain radiation therapy with or without stereotactic radiosurgery boost for patients with one to three brain metastases: phase III results of the RTOG 9508 randomised trial. *Lancet* 2004;363:1665–1672.

Aoyama H, Shirato H, Nakagawa K, Taga M. Interim report of the JROSG99-1 multi-institutional randomized trial, comparing radiosurgery alone vs. radiosurgery plus whole brain irradiation for 1-4 brain metastases. [Abstract] *ASCO Annual Meeting Proceedings* 2004;23:108.

Brada M, Rajan B, Traish D, et al. The long-term efficacy of conservative surgery and radiotherapy in the control of pituitary adenomas. *Clin Endocrinol (Oxf)* 1993;38:571–578.

Chang CH, Horton J, Schoenfeld D, et al. Comparison of postoperative radiotherapy and combined postoperative radiotherapy and chemotherapy in the multidisciplinary management of malignant gliomas. *Cancer* 1983;52:997–1007.

Debus J, Wuendrich M, Pirzkall A, et al. High efficacy of fractionated stereotactic radiotherapy of large base-of-skull meningiomas: long-term results. *J Clin Oncol* 2001;19:3547–3553.

Floyd NS, Woo SY, The BS, et al. Hypofractionated intensity-modulated radiotherapy for primary glioblastoma multiforme. *Int J Radiat Oncol Biol Phys* 2004;58:721–726.

Goldsmith BJ, Wara WM, Wilson CB, Larson DA. Postoperative irradiation for subtotally resected meningiomas. A retrospective analysis of 140 patients treated from 1967 to 1990. *J Neurosurg* 1994;80:195–201.

Griffin TW. White matter necrosis, microangiopathy and intellectual abilities in survivors of childhood leukemia. Association with central nervous system irradiation and methorexate therapy. In: Gilbert HA, Kagan AR, eds. *Radiation Damage to the Nervous System*. New York, NY: Raven Press; 1980:155–174.

Huang E, The BS, Strother DR, et al. Intensity-modulated radiation therapy for pediatric medulloblastoma: early report on the reduction of ototoxicity. *Int J Radiat Oncol Biol Phys* 2002;52:599–605.

Karim AB, Afra D, Cornu P, et al. Randomized trial on the efficacy of radiotherapy for cerebral low-grade glioma in the adult: European Organization for Research and Treatment of Cancer Study 22845 with the Medical Research Council study BRO4: an interim analysis. *Int J Radiat Oncol Biol Phys* 2002;52:316–324.

Karim AB, Maat B, Hatievoll R, et al. A randomized trial on dose-response in radiation therapy of low-grade cerebral glioma: European Organization for Research and Treatment of Cancer (EORTC) Study 22844. *Int J Radiat Oncol Biol Phys* 1996;36:549–556.

Leibel SA, Gutin PH, Wara WM, et al. Survival and quality of life after interstitial implantation of removable high-activity iodine-125 sources for the treatment of patients with recurrent malignant gliomas. *Int J Radiat Oncol Biol Phys* 1989;17:1129–1139.

Mahajan A, McCutcheon IE, Suki D, et al. Case control study of stereotactic radiosurgery for recurrent glioblastoma multiforme. *J Neurosurg* 2005;103:210–217.

Maity A, Shu HG, Janss A, et al. Craniospinal radiation in the treatment of biopsy-proven intracranial germinomas: twenty-five years' experience in a single center. *Int J Radiat Oncol Biol Phys* 2004;58:1165–1170.

Marcus KJ, Goumnerova L, Billett AL, et al. Stereotactic radiotherapy for localized low-grade gliomas in children: final results of a prospective trial. *Int J Radiat Oncol Biol Phys* 2005;61:374–379.

Merchant TE, Williams T, Smith JM, et al. Preirradiation endocrinopathies in pediatric brain tumor patients determined by dynamic tests of endocrine function. *Int J Radiat Oncol Biol Phys* 2002;54:45–50.

Miralbell R, Lomax A, Cella L, Schneider U. Potential reduction of the incidence of radiation-induced second cancers by using proton beams in the treatment of pediatric tumors. *Int J Radiat Oncol Biol Phys* 2002;54:824–829.

Mirimanoff RO, Dosoretz DE, Linggood RM, Ojemann RG, Martuza RL. Meningioma: analysis of recurrence and progression following neurosurgical resection. *J Neurosurg* 1985;62:18–24.

Nelson DF, Curran WJ Jr, Scott C, et al. Hyperfractionated radiation therapy and bis-chlorethyl nitrosourea in the treatment of malignant glioma—possible advantage observed at 72.0 Gy in 1.2 Gy B.I.D. fractions: report of the Radiation Therapy Oncology Group Protocol 8302. *Int J Radiat Oncol Biol Phys* 1993;25:193–207.

Patchell RA, Tibbs PA, Regine WF, et al. Postoperative radiotherapy in the treatment of single metastases to the brain: a randomized trial. *JAMA* 1998;280: 1485–1489.

Shaw E, Arusell R, Scheithauer B, et al. Prospective randomized trial of low- versus high-dose radiation therapy in adults with supratentorial low-grade glioma: initial report of a North Central Cancer Treatment Group/Radiation Therapy Oncology Group/Eastern Cooperative Oncology Group Study. *J Clin Oncol* 2002;20:2267–2276.

Shrieve DC, Alexander E 3rd, Wen PY, et al. Comparison of stereotactic radiosurgery and brachytherapy in the treatment of recurrent glioblastoma multiforme. *Neurosurgery* 1995;36:275–282.

Turbin RE, Thompson CR, Kennerdell JS, Cockerham KP, Kupersmith MJ. A long-term visual outcome comparison in patients with optic nerve sheath meningiomas managed with observation, surgery, radiotherapy, or surgery and radiotherapy. *Ophthalmology* 2002;109:890–899.

Walker MD, Alexander E Jr, Hunt WE, et al. Evaluation of BCNU and/or radiotherapy in the treatment of anaplastic gliomas. A cooperative clinical trial. *J Neurosurg* 1978;49:333–343.

Walker MD, Strike TA, Sheline GL. An analysis of dose-effect relationship in the radiotherapy of malignant gliomas. *Int J Radiat Oncol Biol Phys* 1979;5: 1725–1730.

8 CYTOTOXIC CHEMOTHERAPY FOR DIFFUSE GLIOMAS

Ivo W. Tremont-Lukats and Mark R. Gilbert

Chapter Overview 153
Introduction 154
Challenges in Developing Effective Treatments for
Malignant Brain Tumors 154
    Neuroimaging 155
    Blood-Brain Barrier and Tumor Heterogeneity 155
    Drug–Drug Interactions 156
    Tumor Resistance 156
    Determination of Tumor Response and Treatment Efficacy 157
    Effect of Prognostic Factors on the Outcome and
    Interpretation of Studies 158
Chemotherapy for Glioblastomas 159
    Treatment of Newly Diagnosed Glioblastomas 159
    Concurrent Chemotherapy and Radiotherapy for Glioblastomas 160
    Local Delivery of Chemotherapy for Glioblastomas 161
    Treatment of Recurrent Glioblastomas 162
Chemotherapy for Anaplastic Astrocytomas 163
Chemotherapy for Anaplastic Oligodendrogliomas 165
Chemotherapy for Low-Grade Gliomas 166
Key Practice Points 167
Suggested Readings 167

CHAPTER OVERVIEW

The prognosis for patients with malignant gliomas is poor. However, increasing efforts in the areas of basic, translational, and clinical research will likely lead to significant therapeutic advances over the next several years. Recent clinical trial results confirming the benefit of chemotherapy for malignant gliomas have prompted the increased enthusiasm to explore new therapeutic approaches as well as laboratory investigations. Studies of gliomagenesis and molecular profiling of glial tumors are resulting in novel therapeutic targets and new combination therapies involving specific signaling pathways or their use with conventional cytotoxic therapies. Innovative clinical trial designs are enhancing the efficiency of determining efficacy, and international collaborations are augmenting research efforts.

This chapter reviews the pathways of gliomagenesis, discusses the unique therapeutic challenges in developing new brain tumor treatments, summarizes the results of important cytotoxic chemotherapeutic clinical trials, and provides an overview of new signal transduction-modulating agents and clinical trial designs, underscoring the increasing research efforts in this area.

INTRODUCTION

In this chapter we review the chemotherapy of diffuse gliomas. Under this term we include glioblastoma (GBM; World Health Organization [WHO] grade IV astrocytoma), anaplastic astrocytoma (AA; WHO grade III astrocytoma), anaplastic oligodendroglioma (AO; WHO grade III oligodendroglioma), and the low-grade gliomas (WHO grade II oligodendrogliomas, astrocytomas, and oligoastrocytomas). Over the past several decades, there have been major advances in neurosurgery and radiation oncology. As a consequence, more extensive resections of brain tumors are now possible with less morbidity and often improved neurologic function. In addition, radiotherapy can now be delivered with greater precision to the area of interest, thereby permitting higher doses of radiation with less risk of injury to the surrounding normal brain tissue.

In contrast, there is a perception that chemotherapy for malignant gliomas has lagged far behind neurosurgical and radiotherapeutic advances and even chemotherapy treatments for other solid tumors. In fact, until recently there was no level 1 evidence that chemotherapy provides a survival advantage for patients with malignant gliomas.

The difficulty in finding effective therapies may be due to the inherent invasiveness of tumor cells and their genotypic and phenotypic heterogeneity within the tumor mass. Laboratory studies have confirmed that high-grade tumors undergo rapid change because of a high rate of mutation, leading to heterogeneity and the rapid development of treatment resistance. Furthermore, the interpretation of clinical trials has been complicated by the inclusion of different histologic types in a single trial, the limitations of the outcome measurements currently in use, the lack of screening tests for prevention and early diagnosis, the existence of a blood-brain barrier, the interference of anticonvulsants with cytotoxic drugs, and the relatively poor accrual of patients into clinical trials. All of these factors have slowed the determination of treatment efficacy.

CHALLENGES IN DEVELOPING EFFECTIVE TREATMENTS
FOR MALIGNANT BRAIN TUMORS

As outlined above, several issues persist that interfere with the development of effective treatment strategies. These issues range from problems in determining tumor response to failure to develop treatments that can be adequately delivered and demonstrate cytotoxic (cell-killing) or cyto-static (growth-arresting) effects on the tumor.

Neuroimaging

The development of computed tomography and magnetic resonance imaging of the brain markedly improved our ability to diagnose brain tumors much earlier in the course of the disease. These neurodiagnostic tests, particularly magnetic resonance imaging, provide the navigational information that is critical for both tumor resection and radiation delivery. Such tests are also essential for evaluating the tumor response to therapy and the course of the disease. However, many studies have clearly demonstrated that computed tomography scans and magnetic resonance images provide incomplete information about the size and location of gliomas because the contrast enhancement occurs only in regions of blood-brain barrier disruption. Surrounding brain parenchyma often con-tains infiltrating tumors cells, but the scans and images may show only changes that are most consistent with peritumoral edema. Studies have also clearly demonstrated that glioma cells are present far from the areas of enhancement, even beyond the regions with hyperintense signaling. Moreover, the intensity of enhancement can increase with irradiation or decrease with glucocorticoid use even if the tumor status does not change, thereby making the interpretation of tumor response more difficult. Further, radiotherapy can cause alterations in the blood-brain and blood-tumor barriers that may increase the uptake of contrast agents, and it can even cause tissue necrosis, mimicking tumor growth. Finally, a lack of specificity of enhancement after the initial treatment complicates the determination of true tumor relapse or progression.

Blood-Brain Barrier and Tumor Heterogeneity

In the normal brain, the blood-brain barrier is a continuous membrane that protects the central nervous system from potentially harmful molecules. This continuity of a healthy, normal barrier is provided by tight junctions of capillary endothelial cells, lack of fenestrations within normal endothelial cells, limited pinocytosis, normal astrocytes, and the presence of P-glycoprotein. The latter is a 170-kDa membrane glycoprotein encoded by a multidrug resistance gene (*MDR*) that serves as a pump to prevent unwanted molecules from crossing the blood-brain barrier.

The intimate relationship between capillary permeability, the molecu-lar weight of a drug, and lipophilicity modulates the penetration of drugs into the brain. The molecular weight of a drug is critical because highly lipophilic drugs cannot penetrate the blood-brain barrier if their molecu-lar weight is greater than 450 kDa. After a drug has penetrated this bar-rier, the transcapillary flow of the drug into the tumor is a process difficult to predict because of the heterogeneity within the tumor mass. The tumor cells may be in different phases of the cell cycle or in varied degrees of malignant transformation, thereby altering sensitivity to the treatment. Factors related to the heterogeneity of the vascular supply to the tumor may also have a large effect on treatment efficacy because of the unpredictability of drug delivery. These factors include the efficiency of the capillary networks formed during angiogenesis, local blood flow, extent of the blood-brain barrier disruption, and capillary permeability in the area adjacent to the tumor. Animal models have limited applicability because of differences in blood-brain barrier characteristics across species. Direct measurements from surgically derived tissues are complicated by contamination of the drug from intratumoral blood and by the inability to sample all components of a tumor, such as the core and the nonenhanced infiltrating component.

Drug–Drug Interactions

The widely used anticonvulsants phenytoin, carbamazepine, and phenobarbital are potent inducers of hepatic cytochrome p450 enzymes, which are frequently involved in the metabolism of systemic chemotherapy. Recent studies have revealed that concurrent use of these anticonvulsants with chemotherapy markedly alters and increases the metabolism and clearance of anticancer drugs. With conventional doses of chemotherapy, this drug–drug interaction results in suboptimal treatment and potentially loss of therapeutic efficacy. This discovery suggests that many patients may receive an insufficient chemotherapeutic regimen.

Tumor Resistance

Inherent tumor resistance to chemotherapy has been recognized for many years. As a consequence, most studies report an objective response rate of less than 10% for GBM. AAs tend to have a moderately higher response rate, and some AOs, particularly those with chromosomal alterations characterized by loss of heterozygosity of chromosome arms 1p and 19q (LOH 1p/19q), have an unusually high response rate. However, even in the responsive tumors the benefit is often short-lived, and in many studies the 6-month progression-free survival rate is the primary end point. Such a short progression-free interval implies that there is often a population of resistant tumor cells or that this resistance develops rapidly. Ongoing research is uncovering the mechanisms of resistance that exist or develop in a glioma cell exposed to a cytotoxic or cytostatic drug, although our knowledge is still far from complete. The sensitivity of gliomas to chemotherapy depends on a complex interaction between (1) the presence or absence of genetic changes (i.e., loss of *PTEN* or mutation or loss of *p53*), which may influence resistance to apoptosis even in the setting of DNA damage, (2) the existence of multiple intracellular and intercellular signaling pathways that prevent cell death due to inhibition of a single pathway, (3) the proportion of cells in the G_0 phase of the cell cycle, which is when cells are the least susceptible to most chemotherapeutic agents, and (4) the existence of enzymes that inactivate drugs (e.g., methylated O^6-methylguanine-DNA methyltransferase [MGMT]).

Determination of Tumor Response and Treatment Efficacy

Traditionally, the determination of tumor response in cancer clinical trials relied on direct measurement of the tumor size, typically a cross-sectional area, which was established as a reliable measurement for brain tumor studies by MacDonald and colleagues (1990). In 1999, the National Cancer Institute introduced new response criteria based on unidimensional measurements, the Response Evaluation Criteria in Solid Tumors (RECIST). This system has been adopted for all solid tumors except those of the central nervous system because of the irregular shape of gliomas and the possible inaccuracies that may result from unidimensional measurements. In addition, radiotherapy can cause changes on computed tomography scans or magnetic resonance images that mimic tumor progression. Therefore, accurate delineation of the tumor and the treatment response may be difficult when a large component of the visible mass consists of treatment-associated necrosis or gliosis. For this reason, measures of progression-free end points have been adopted, particularly for evaluating chemotherapeutic regimens after radiotherapy. Many recent studies have successfully used such measures and have based trial-sized power calculations and the measure of success on the results compiled and reported by Wong and colleagues (1999), who analyzed the overall and progression-free survival at 6 months of 225 patients with recurrent GBMs who were enrolled in phase II trials. The rates calculated by Wong and colleagues provided a useful and more appropriate benchmark than had previously been available against which progression-free survival rates from new phase II trials could be measured and have provided the framework for deriving a sample size that adequately powers phase II trials. All phase II trials conducted by M. D. Anderson Cancer Center and the North American Brain Tumor Consortium (NABTC) use this progression-free survival rate from this database to judge whether a new therapy is promising enough to warrant a phase III trial. The Radiation Therapy Oncology Group (RTOG), the North Central Cancer Therapy Group (NCCTG), and other cooperative consortia use their own databases, but this methodology has been adopted as a meaningful measure of efficacy across cooperative groups. In contrast to evaluating progression-free end points, survival end points are often used for large phase III trials. Treatment efficacy as measured by improved survival is considered the "gold standard," but differences among subsequent therapies for disease relapse may reduce the ability to compare the study regimens.

The advent of targeted therapy with cytostatic drugs has brought new challenges to clinical trial design. Researchers at M. D. Anderson have proposed some modifications to the design of phase II trials to allow (1) adequate numbers of patients participating in such trials, (2) determination of a biologically active dose in contrast to a maximal tolerated dose, (3) molecular analysis of tissue samples from treated and untreated patients to measure the activity of cytostatic drugs, (4) examination of response (defined as progression-free survival, changes in quality-of-life measures, toxicity, etc.), and (5) implementation of factorial designs and Bayesian approaches to increase the efficiency of identifying promising drugs or drug combinations in the shortest time. These innovations would also be applicable to trials that combine traditional cytotoxic drugs with cytostatic agents.

Effect of Prognostic Factors on the Outcome and Interpretation of Studies

Careful examination of many phase III trials of brain tumor treatments conducted in the past reveals serious design flaws related to the absence of appropriate stratification of prognostic variables that affect patient survival, thereby introducing potential imbalance and inaccurate results. Patient age at diagnosis, WHO histologic grade, Karnofsky performance scale score, and duration of symptoms can profoundly affect patient survival (Table 8–1). Other factors, such as extent of tumor resection and tumor location, can also influence outcome.

There is also evidence that the survival of patients with GBMs, AAs, or AOs is intertwined with genetic abnormalities, which can be unfavorable or favorable to survival. For GBM, poorer patient survival has been

Table 8–1. **Effect of Prognostic Variables on Death Rate of Patients with Brain Tumors**

Variable*	Death Rate (Hazard Ratio)
Age at diagnosis	
<45 years	0.36
>65 years	1.27
WHO histologic grade	
GBM	0.76
AA	0.43
Karnofsky performance scale score	
>80	0.44
≤40	1.31
Duration of symptoms	
<6 months	0.81
>6 months	0.41

* Categories are not mutually exclusive because the results were obtained from different studies.
Source: Shapiro WR. Toward a changing paradigm in glioma biology. Presented at: Advances in Neuro-Oncology meeting; October 21–22, 2005; New York, NY.

associated with losses in chromosome arms 6q and 10q (the latter is the locus for the *PTEN* gene) and gains in chromosome arm 19q. In high-grade astrocytomas, aberrant methylation of the *MGMT* gene promoter increases the patient survival duration; this benefit has been hypothesized to be due to increased chemosensitivity to alkylating agents compared with gliomas with the unmethylated *MGMT* gene promoter. Patients aged 45 years or older with AAs tend to have mutations in chromosome 7, whereas younger patients without detectable chromosome 7 abnormalities survive longer. Patients with AOs who have LOH 1p/19q are more responsive to therapy and survive longer than patients without these mutations. About 30% of gliomas overall have mutations in the *TP53* gene, but the prognostic importance of a mutated *TP53* gene in gliomas is not clear yet. Genetic abnormalities in cancer is an area of active research, and recent results suggest that more complex interactions of molecular pathways may also have a tremendous influence on patient prognosis and on tumor response to specific treatment regimens.

CHEMOTHERAPY FOR GLIOBLASTOMAS

The treatment of GBM with chemotherapy has been very challenging. Despite an extensive series of clinical trials over the past 30 years, until recently there was no level 1 evidence that demonstrated a benefit for adding chemotherapy to radiotherapy. A large meta-analysis of aggregate data from 16 trials with random allocation of patients into treatment arms found an increase in the overall survival rate of only 10% at 1 year and 9% at 2 years (Fine et al, 1993). This study was the first serious effort to collect, pool, and analyze data from trials that individually did not have enough statistical power to rule out Type I errors with confidence, but it also had the limitations that can flaw any meta-analysis: dependence on published data that cannot be verified, inclusion of other glioma types, and lack of sensitivity analyses with which to investigate bias and heterogeneity. Nine years later, a more rigorous meta-analysis based on individual data from 3,004 patients in 12 randomized studies found a small but clear and statistically significant treatment effect (Stewart, 2002). The results agreed with the main conclusion of the first meta-analysis, but the treatment effect was smaller: the absolute increase in the survival rate at 1 year was 6% (95% confidence interval, 3% to 9%). Both meta-analyses demonstrated that the benefit from nitrosourea-based chemotherapy was very small and that better agents and clinical trials were needed.

Treatment of Newly Diagnosed Glioblastomas

Efforts to improve the prognosis for patients with glioblastomas have included several chemotherapeutic strategies, including administration of chemotherapy before radiotherapy (i.e., neoadjuvant chemotherapy),

**Table 8–2. Fully Published Phase I and II Trials of Neoadjuvant
Chemotherapy for Glioblastoma**

Regimen	Reference	Number of Patients	Median Survival Duration (Months)
BCNU	Brandes et al, 1996	24	13.5
BCNU + cisplatin	Rajkumar et al, 1998	18	14
BCNU + cisplatin	Grossman et al, 1997	52	13
Cisplatin + etoposide, with or without tamoxifen	Diaz et al, 2005	44	11.3
Gemcitabine + treosulfan	Wick et al, 2002	17	12
Fotemustine + cisplatin + etoposide	Frenay et al, 2000	33	10
Temozolomide	Brada et al, 2005	162	10
Temozolomide	Gilbert et al, 2002	36	13.2
Temozolomide + BCNU*	Barrie et al, 2005	40	12.7

* Inoperable tumors.

concurrent chemoradiotherapy, and local administration of chemotherapy. The neoadjuvant use of chemotherapy has the appeal of identifying active drugs as well as useless agents or regimens. However, the evidence available from completed trials does not support the use of neoadjuvant chemotherapy. Table 8–2 lists some of the regimens used in the neoadjuvant setting that have been tested in phase I and II studies.

Because some of these studies reported objective response rates that ranged between 21% and 54% and a survival rate of 19% at 2 years, the Eastern Cooperative Oncology Group (ECOG) and the Southwest Oncology Group (SWOG) conducted a joint phase III trial comparing neoadjuvant BCNU (the abbreviation of the chemical name of carmustine) and cisplatin followed by radiotherapy with standard radiotherapy followed by adjuvant BCNU (Grossman et al, 2003). Although the earlier phase II trial showed promising data (Grossman et al, 1997), the phase III trial did not find a statistical difference between the 2 treatment arms for patient survival.

Concurrent Chemotherapy and Radiotherapy for Glioblastomas

Several investigators have used chemotherapy concurrently with external beam radiotherapy to treat GBM. A series of phase II studies did not demonstrate an increase in patient survival time until a phase II study conducted by Stupp and colleagues (2002), who used a treatment protocol that included temozolomide at 75 mg/m^2 orally for 42 days concurrently with external beam radiotherapy (Table 8–3). The participants had a median survival time of 16 months, a clear outlier compared with the other study results. These preliminary findings prompted a large multiinstitutional phase III trial comparing this chemoradiotherapeutic

Table 8–3. Representative Phase I and II Trials of Concurrent Chemotherapy and Radiotherapy for Newly Diagnosed Supratentorial GBMs

Chemotherapeutic Regimen	Reference	Number of Patients	Median Survival Duration (Months)
Cisplatin + BCNU	Kleinberg et al, 1999	49	13.8
Carboplatin + teniposide, followed by BCNU	Brandes et al, 1998	56	12.5
Carboplatin, followed by PCV	Levin et al, 1995	83	12.7
Etoposide	Beauchesne et al, 2003	26	12
Paclitaxel	Glantz et al, 1996	48	9.2
Intra-arterial cisplatin	Fountzilas et al, 1997	22	13.5
Intra-arterial carboplatin + 5-fluorouracil	Larner et al, 1995	19	9.2
BCNU + intra-arterial cisplatin + peripheral blood stem cells	Fernandez-Hildago et al, 1996	34	16
Tirapazamine (150 mg/m^2), followed by 6 months of adjuvant temozolamide	Del Rowe et al, 2000	55	10.8
Tirapazamine (260 mg/m^2)	Del Rowe et al, 2000	69	9.5
Topotecan	Fisher et al, 2002	87	9.3
Paclitaxel	Schuck et al, 2002	81	12
Temozolomide (75 mg/m^2)	Stupp et al, 2002	64	16

regimen with radiotherapy alone. This study, which was conducted by the European Organization for Research and Treatment of Cancer (EORTC) and the National Cancer Institute of Canada, demonstrated a statistically significant advantage to the combination regimen (median survival time, 14.6 vs 12.1 months; 2-year survival rate, 26% vs 10%). This phase III study was the first to provide level 1 evidence of the effect of systemic chemotherapy for GBM. As a consequence, concurrent temozolomide and radiotherapy followed by 6 cycles of temozolomide given for 5 days every 28 days is the standard of care for this disease.

Local Delivery of Chemotherapy for Glioblastomas

Biodegradable polymer wafers containing BCNU (Gliadel wafers) are designed to release the drug over 2 to 3 weeks after placement in the surgical cavity. Gliadel wafers were more effective than placebo wafers in a phase III trial for patients with recurrent gliomas, including GBMs (Brem et al, 1995). Another phase III trial of Gliadel wafers with a double-blind design enrolled 207 patients with GBMs who were randomly allocated to the treatment arm or the placebo arm (Westphal et al, 2003). The group treated with Gliadel wafers had a longer median survival duration (13.5 vs 11.4 months; risk reduction, 24%; $P = 0.10$). Because the trial included other histologic types of gliomas, a multivariate analysis was necessary to determine whether the treatment effect for GBMs was statistically significant. Therefore, the results for the GBM subgroup were less solid than the overall result of the trial.

Although Gliadel wafers are approved by the U.S. Food and Drug Administration for use in patients with newly diagnosed GBMs, they are not indicated for multifocal, deep, or bilateral disease; juxtaventricular lesions; or tumors in eloquent areas. Even so, the phase III trial of Gliadel wafers is relevant because for the first time, local delivery of chemotherapy was shown to have some efficacy against newly diagnosed GBMs. In addition, it set the stage for trials using Gliadel wafers in combination with other cytotoxic or cytostatic drugs in an attempt to improve outcomes. However, very few studies with Gliadel wafers have been conducted since. Only 2 are registered in the Clinical Trial Register of the National Institutes of Health: the PRECISE trial, which is a phase III trial comparing IL13-PE38QQR with Gliadel wafers (accrual is completed and results are pending), and a phase II study of temozolomide during and after radiotherapy for patients with GBMs who will undergo surgery and placement of Gliadel wafers (accrual is completed and results are pending).

Treatment of Recurrent Glioblastomas

There are no established treatments for patients with recurrent glioblastomas. Often, patients who previously received temozolomide as frontline treatment will undergo therapy with a nitrosourea such as BCNU or CCNU (the abbreviation of the chemical name of lomustine). Other treatments include irinotecan (also called CPT-11), carboplatin, and cisplatin. Patients with good performance status should be encouraged to participate in clinical trials that are designed to test novel agents or treatment combinations that might be more efficacious than currently available therapies.

Combination regimens for treating patients with recurrent glioblastomas have been under extensive investigation. Many studies have combined temozolomide with another agent because of the excellent toxicity profile of temozolomide and its oral bioavailability. An example of efficient testing of treatment regimens is illustrated by a series of phase II trials performed by the North American Brain Tumor Consortium or as an institutional study by M. D. Anderson. These studies had identical eligibility criteria and used the 6-month progression-free survival rate as the end point. Although many other phase II trials have had negative results, this methodology identified promising regimens, such as isotretinoin with temozolomide and marimastat with temozolomide. Similar trial

Table 8–4. Ongoing Phase II Trials for Recurrent GBMs at M. D. Anderson Cancer Center

Study Identifier	Drug Combination
2003-0600	6-Thioguanine + capecitabine + celecoxib + temozolomide
DM01-528	Pegylated interferon α-2b + temozolomide
2005-0285	Carboplatin + erlotinib
DM02-595	Thalidomide + irinotecan

design strategies using the 6-month progression-free survival rate are currently being used to study other drug combinations and new agents. M. D. Anderson has several phase II trials of temozolomide-containing regimens for treating recurrent GBMs that are open to accrual (Table 8–4).

Nitrosoureas in combination therapy are also used to treat recurrent glioblastomas after radiotherapy or after failure with temozolomide. Well-known combinations that include a nitrosourea are procarbazine, CCNU, and vincristine (PCV) and its variant, procarbazine and CCNU. Despite the popularity of PCV, there is no evidence that it is better than BCNU alone, although no randomized controlled trial has yet been conducted to compare these treatment regimens.

Besides PCV and temozolomide, other second-line drugs used for recurrent glioblastomas are carboplatin, etoposide, and irinotecan. Several studies have used carboplatin alone, although a phase II trial conducted at M. D. Anderson of carboplatin plus the tyrosine kinase inhibitor erlotinib is currently recruiting patients (Table 8–4). Irinotecan alone or with cytostatic or cytotoxic drugs is another drug under intense investigation, including in combination with bevacizumab. Hydroxyurea is used as a radiosensitizer and as a cell cycle-specific cytotoxic agent in recurrent glioblastomas. A recent phase II trial that combined hydroxyurea and imatinib to treat recurrent GBMs resulted in a median survival duration of 19 weeks and a progression-free survival duration of 14 weeks (Reardon et al, 2005). However, the role of hydroxyurea in the treatment of gliomas remains as unclear as it was in 1992 when Levin first reviewed the use of this agent for the treatment of gliomas.

CHEMOTHERAPY FOR ANAPLASTIC ASTROCYTOMAS

Early studies that evaluated the role of adjuvant chemotherapy for patients with AAs only demonstrated a trend toward longer survival duration. However, these studies, which were conducted by the Brain Tumor Study Group, assessed both AAs and the more prominent GBMs and did not analyze them separately. Because of the higher response rate of AAs than GBMs to chemotherapy, the benefit of adding chemotherapy to radiotherapy for patients with AAs may have been masked in those studies.

Neoadjuvant chemotherapy for AA has just begun to be adequately tested. An NCCTG phase II trial using BCNU, cisplatin, and etoposide before radiotherapy for AA did not find evidence of efficacy (Rajkumar et al, 1998). Adjuvant PCV after radiotherapy and surgery was widely used in the treatment of AA after a randomized trial of 73 patients demonstrated the superiority of PCV after radiotherapy over single-agent BCNU for patients with anaplastic gliomas (Levin et al, 1990). In contrast, a retrospective comparison of 257 patients with AAs from 3 RTOG studies who were treated with BCNU as an adjuvant to radiotherapy and 175 patients with AAs from the RTOG 9404 study who were treated with adjuvant PCV found similar survival outcomes between the 2 treatment arms.

Several trials that assessed variations or additions to adjuvant PCV did not show any substantial difference in patient survival, with the exception of 2 studies. In 2001, the Medical Research Council of the United Kingdom published the results of a randomized trial in which 113 patients with AAs were allocated to receive adjuvant PCV after radiotherapy or no PCV. Although the survival benefit in patients treated with PCV was small and nonsignificant, the poor 12-month and 24-month survival rates (53% and 36%, respectively) were striking compared with other published data on adjuvant PCV. In 2003, Levin and associates reported the results of a randomized controlled trial of 249 patients with anaplastic gliomas treated with adjuvant PCV and DFMO (an ornithine decarboxylase inhibitor) or with adjuvant PCV alone. The median survival duration was 63.9 months for the PCV plus DFMO group and 41.1 months for the PCV-alone group ($P = 0.11$), and the corresponding progression-free survival times were 42.9 months and 17.0 months, respectively ($P = 0.15$).

BCNU is frequently used in the adjuvant setting as well. Prados and associates (1999) reported the results of a single-arm trial in which 110 patients with anaplastic gliomas (103 patients had AAs) received hydroxyurea with radiotherapy followed by 6-thioguanine and BCNU after completion of radiotherapy. The median time to progression was 64.9 months, the median survival duration had not yet been reached after a median follow-up interval of 68.6 months, and the 2- and 4-year survival rates were 80% and 66%, respectively. Despite the extensive testing of adjuvant chemotherapy (PCV or BCNU) for AA, there is no consensus on the benefit.

The outcome of patients with recurrent AAs is poor. The median survival time of such patients is 47 weeks despite aggressive treatment. The most frequently used chemotherapeutic agents for AA are the nitrosoureas; however, their use for recurrent disease is limited by the development of resistance and cumulative toxicities such as myelosuppression and pulmonary fibrosis. A study of 97 patients with recurrent AAs treated with temozolomide showed some efficacy: the median progression-free survival time was 5.5 months, the 6-month progression-free survival rate was 49%, and the median survival time was 14.2 months (Yung et al, 1999). In that study, the complete or partial response rate was 35%, even though 60% of the patients had prior exposure to nitrosoureas.

Single agents such as procarbazine and combinations of carboplatin with etoposide and of 6-thioguanine with hydroxyurea, CCNU, and procarbazine have demonstrated limited efficacy for recurrent AAs. Irinotecan was recently shown to have some activity against recurrent malignant gliomas in a phase II trial: among the 10 patients with recurrent AAs, 1 had a partial response, and the overall median time to progression was 12 weeks (Friedman et al, 1999). Several trials with irinotecan used alone or with other agents (e.g., temozolomide) are in progress.

CHEMOTHERAPY FOR ANAPLASTIC OLIGODENDROGLIOMAS

The treatment of patients with AOs is undergoing intensive evaluation. A small series of studies in the early 1990s reported that patients with AOs could have a high response rate to chemotherapy, most commonly the PCV regimen. Further research determined that most of the tumors that were responsive to chemotherapy had a distinct molecular signature: LOH 1p/19q. In addition, prognosis as assessed by median survival duration was positively associated with these chromosomal changes. Although the mechanism responsible for these molecular changes resulting in increased responsiveness to treatment is unknown, several series of studies found this association.

Two major clinical trials have been completed in an effort to define the role of chemotherapy in patients with AOs. These randomized phase III studies compared the combination of chemotherapy and radiotherapy with radiotherapy alone. Both studies included patients with "pure" AOs as well as anaplastic oligoastrocytomas. The study conducted jointly by the RTOG, ECOG, SWOG, and NCCTG compared the outcome of patients treated with conventional external beam radiotherapy alone or with up to 4 cycles of PCV before radiotherapy (Cairncross et al, 2006). The study conducted by the EORTC compared the outcome of patients treated with radiotherapy alone or followed by up to 6 cycles of PCV (van den Bent et al, 2003b). Remarkably, both studies showed almost identical results: neither demonstrated a significant difference in overall survival duration, whereas time to tumor progression was significantly longer in the groups treated with PCV. However, a high percentage of patients who initially received only radiotherapy subsequently underwent chemotherapy treatment at relapse. These studies suggest that chemotherapy at relapse is as effective as neoadjuvant or adjuvant chemotherapy. The effect of delaying tumor progression on neurologic function and quality of life remains undetermined.

Subsequent laboratory correlative studies of tumor tissues from patients enrolled in both of these trials have provided important information. Tumor tissue was available from approximately 70% of the patients enrolled in the intergroup trial, permitting analysis of LOH 1p/19q, which was noted in 46% of samples. The prognosis was significantly better for this group of patients than for patients with no LOH or only a single deletion, thereby validating the prognostic significance of this marker. Interestingly, both trials demonstrated that overall survival was not substantially different among patients with LOH 1p/19q who received chemoradiotherapy and patients with LOH 1p/19q who received only radiotherapy.

Early reports described the treatment of patients who had AOs with radiotherapy alone; only recurrent disease was treated with chemotherapy, usually PCV. However, the use of PCV in the neoadjuvant or adjuvant setting subsequently became the standard of care. The use of temozolomide for managing AO had a similar evolution. Temozolomide was used for patients with tumor recurrence and then as a first-line drug in newly diagnosed disease. Although no clinical trial has compared temozolomide with PCV, both regimens are thought to have similar response rates but temozolomide has a better toxicity profile. For patients with tumor recurrence after temozolomide treatment, PCV may be an effective salvage therapy.

CHEMOTHERAPY FOR LOW-GRADE GLIOMAS

The role of chemotherapy for the treatment of patients with low-grade gliomas (WHO grade II oligodendrogliomas, astrocytomas, and oligoastrocytomas) is currently being scrutinized. Most studies that have evaluated chemotherapeutic regimens included all WHO grade II histologic types. Some studies have found that most oligodendrogliomas have LOH 1p/19q, which suggests that this loss is an early event in oligodendroglial transformation. LOH 1p/19q is as frequent in oligodendrogliomas and oligoastrocytomas as it is in their grade III (anaplastic) counterparts, and tumors with LOH 1p/19q are associated with better overall and progression-free survival than tumors without LOH 1p/19q are. Several trials using PCV or temozolomide for recurrent or previously untreated oligodendrogliomas and oligoastrocytomas have reported high tumor response rates. Several of the issues regarding the treatment of patients with low-grade gliomas have been addressed by the large intergroup study RTOG 98-04. In that study, patients younger than 40 years who underwent gross total tumor resection were observed. All others were randomly allocated to receive radiotherapy or radiotherapy plus 6 cycles of PCV. The study completed accrual in 2002, and the results are expected to be published soon. Future studies defining the role of chemotherapy for patients with low-grade gliomas who have a good prognosis, such as patients who have tumors with LOH 1p/19q, are being considered.

Although level 1 evidence is not available, practice patterns show that chemotherapy for low-grade gliomas is limited to oligodendrogliomas with LOH 1p/19q in patients older than 40 years and to patients who have incompletely resected tumors, recurrent tumor after resection and radio-therapy, or oligodendrogliomas with or without LOH 1p/19q where there is extensive tumor infiltration (i.e, infiltration in more than 3 brain regions) in an effort to delay extensive exposure to radiation. For patients with newly diagnosed low-grade gliomas who are younger than 40 years and undergo gross total resection, observation is recommended (see chapter 5).

KEY PRACTICE POINTS

- Concurrent temozolomide and external beam radiotherapy followed by at least 6 cycles of temozolomide has become the standard of care after surgery for GBM. However, the contribution of adjuvant temozolomide and the optimal treatment duration need to be defined.
- For recurrent GBMs, any drug or combination of drugs with a track record against GBM can be used. Cytotoxic drugs (e.g., temozolomide, carboplatin, and irinotecan) combined with small-molecule drugs (e.g., imatinib and erlotinib) are effective, although more clinical research is needed to quantify the real treatment effect.
- We encourage participation in clinical trials for newly diagnosed and recurrent gliomas that implement the concepts of biologically active doses, tissue sampling to measure response, and Bayesian or other adaptive methods to enroll patients quickly and effectively into the most promising regimens.
- Multicenter trials of new drugs that are potentially effective specifically against AA are needed. The trend in almost all phase II studies was to include AA with GBM. Although AO occurs less frequently, many cooperative groups have launched clinical trials only for patients with AOs.
- The molecular biology of oligodendrogliomas will guide the management of these tumors. Consistent and reliable molecular or genetic markers for astrocytic tumors will likely be accessible to daily clinical practice in the future.
- Temozolomide has replaced PCV as the chemotherapy of choice in anaplastic, low-grade oligodendrogliomas and in mixed tumors. The optimal timing and the best regimen have not been determined yet.
- For oligodendrogliomas with LOH 1p/19q, whether chemotherapy alone is as effective as radiotherapy alone needs to be determined. Large, international cooperative group studies are being planned to address this question.

SUGGESTED READINGS

Barrie M, Couprie C, Dufour H, et al. Temozolomide in combination with BCNU before and after radiotherapy in patients with inoperable newly diagnosed glioblastoma multiforme. *Ann Oncol* 2005;16:1177–1184.

Beauchesne P, Soler C, Boniol M, Schmitt T. Response to a phase II study of concomitant-to-sequential use of etoposide and radiation therapy in newly diagnosed malignant gliomas. *Am J Clin Oncol* 2003;26:e22–e27.

Brada M, Ashley S, Dowe A, et al. Neoadjuvant phase II multicentre study of new agents in patients with malignant glioma after minimal surgery. Report of a cohort of 187 patients treated with temozolomide. *Ann Oncol* 2005;16:942–949.

Brandes AA, Rigon A, Zampieri P, et al. Carboplatin and teniposide concurrent with radiotherapy in patients with glioblastoma multiforme: a phase II study. *Cancer* 1998;82:355–361.

Brandes AA, Rigon A, Zampieri P, et al. Early chemotherapy and concurrent radio-chemotherapy in high grade glioma. *J Neurooncol* 1996;30:247–255.

Brem H, Piantadosi S, Burger PC, et al. Placebo-controlled trial of safety and efficacy of intraoperative controlled delivery by biodegradable polymers of chemotherapy for recurrent gliomas. The Polymer-brain Tumor Treatment Group. *Lancet* 1995;345:1008–1012.

Cairncross G, Berkey B, Shaw E, et al. Phase III trial of chemotherapy plus radiotherapy alone for pure and mixed anaplastic oligodendrogliomas: Intergroup Radiation Therapy Oncology Group Trial 9402. *J Clin Oncol* 2006;24:2707–2014.

Del Rowe J, Scott C, Werner-Wasik M, et al. Single-arm, open-label phase II study of intravenously administered tirapazamine and radiation therapy for glioblastoma multiforme. *J Clin Oncol* 2000;18:1254–1259.

Diaz R, Jorda MV, Reynes G, et al. Neoadjuvant cisplatin and etoposide, with or without tamoxifen, prior to radiotherapy in high-grade gliomas: a single-center experience. *Anticancer Drugs* 2005;16:323–329.

Fernandez-Hidalgo OA, Vanaclocha V, Vieitez JM, et al. High-dose BCNU and autologous progenitor cell transplantation given with intra-arterial cisplatinum and simultaneous radiotherapy in the treatment of high-grade gliomas: benefit for selected patients. *Bone Marrow Transplant* 1996;18:143–149.

Fine HA, Dear KB, Loeffler JS, Black PM, Canellos GP. Meta-analysis of radiation therapy with and without adjuvant chemotherapy for malignant gliomas in adults. *Cancer* 1993;71:2585–2597.

Fisher B, Won M, Macdonald D, Johnson DW, Roa W. Phase II study of topotecan plus cranial radiation for glioblastoma multiforme: results of Radiation Therapy Oncology Group 9513. *Int J Radiat Oncol Biol Phys* 2002;53:980–986.

Fountzilas G, Karavelis A, Makrantonakis P, et al. Concurrent radiation and intracarotid cisplatin infusion in malignant gliomas: a feasibility study. *Am J Clin Oncol* 1997;20:138–142.

Frenay M, Lebrun C, Lonjon M, Bondiau PY, Chatel M. Up-front chemotherapy with fotemustine (F)/cisplatin (CDDP)/etoposide (VP16) regimen in the treatment of 33 non-removable glioblastomas. *Eur J Cancer* 2000;36:1026–1031.

Friedman HS, Petros WP, Friedman AH, et al. Irinotecan therapy in adults with recurrent or progressive malignant glioma. *J Clin Oncol* 1999;17:1516–1525.

Gilbert MR, Friedman HS, Kuttesch JF, et al. A phase II study of temozolomide in patients with newly diagnosed supratentorial malignant glioma before radiation therapy. *Neuro-oncology* 2002;4:261–267.

Glantz MJ, Choy H, Kearns CM, et al. Phase I study of weekly outpatient paclitaxel and concurrent cranial irradiation in adults with astrocytomas. *J Clin Oncol* 1996;14:600–609.

Grossman S. Management of glioblastoma multiforme. In: Perry MC, ed. *ASCO 2005 Educational Book*. Alexandria, VA: American Society of Clinical Oncology; 2006;180–186.

Grossman SA, Wharam M, Sheidler V, et al. Phase II study of continuous infusion carmustine and cisplatin followed by cranial irradiation in adults with newly diagnosed high-grade astrocytoma. *J Clin Oncol* 1997;15:2596–2603.

Grossman SA, O'Neill A, Grunnet M, et al. Phase III study comparing three cycles of infusional carmustine and cisplatin followed by radiation therapy with radiation therapy and concurrent carmustine in patients with newly diagnosed supratentorial glioblastoma multiforme: Eastern Cooperative Oncology Group Trial 2394. *J Clin Oncol* 2003;21:1485–1491.

Groves MD, Puduvalli VK, Hess KR, et al. Phase II trial of temozolomide plus the matrix metalloproteinase inhibitor, marimastat, in recurrent and progressive glioblastoma multiforme. *J Clin Oncol* 2002;20:1383–1388.

Hegi ME, Diserens AC, Gorlia T, et al. MGMT gene silencing and benefit from temozolomide in glioblastoma. *N Engl J Med* 2005;352:997–1003.

Ino Y, Betensky RA, Zlatescu MC, et al. Molecular subtypes of anaplastic oligodendroglioma: implications for patient management at diagnosis. *Clin Cancer Res* 2001;7:839–845.

Jaeckle KA, Hess KR, Yung WK, et al. Phase II evaluation of temozolomide and 13-*cis*-retinoic acid for the treatment of recurrent and progressive malignant glioma: a North American Brain Tumor Consortium study. *J Clin Oncol* 2003;21: 2305–2311.

Kleinberg L, Grossman SA, Piantadosi S, Zeltzman M, Wharam M. The effects of sequential versus concurrent chemotherapy and radiotherapy on survival and toxicity in patients with newly diagnosed high-grade astrocytoma. *Int J Radiat Oncol Biol Phys* 1999;44:535–543.

Lang FF, Gilbert MR, Puduvalli VK, et al. Toward better early-phase brain tumor clinical trials: a reappraisal of current methods and proposals for future strategies. *Neuro-Oncology* 2002;4:268–277.

Larner JM, Phillips CD, Dion JE, Jensen ME, Newman SA, Jane JA. A phase 1-2 trial of superselective carboplatin, low-dose infusional 5-fluorouracil and concurrent radiation for high-grade gliomas. *Am J Clin Oncol* 1995;18:1–7.

Levin VA. The place of hydroxyurea in the treatment of primary brain tumors. *Semin Oncol* 1992;19:34–39.

Levin VA, Hess KR, Choucair A, et al. Phase III randomized study of postradiotherapy chemotherapy with combination α-difluoromethylornithine-PCV versus PCV for anaplastic gliomas. *Clin Cancer Res* 2003;9:981–990.

Levin VA, Maor MH, Thall PF, et al. Phase II study of accelerated fractionation radiation therapy with carboplatin followed by vincristine chemotherapy for the treatment of glioblastoma multiforme. *Int J Radiat Oncol Biol Phys* 1995;33: 357–364.

Levin VA, Silver P, Hannigan J, et al. Superiority of post-radiotherapy with CCNU, procarbazine, and vincristine (PCV) over BCNU for anaplastic gliomas: NCOG 6G61 final report. *Int J Radiat Oncol Biol Phys* 1990;18:321–324.

Macdonald DR, Cascino TL, Schold SC Jr, Cairncross JG. Response criteria for phase II studies of supratentorial malignant glioma. *J Clin Oncol* 1990;8: 1277–1280.

Medical Research Council Brain Tumor Working Party. Randomized trial of procarbazine, lomustine, and vincristine in the adjuvant treatment of high-grade astrocytoma: a Medical Research Council trial. *J Clin Oncol* 2001;19:509–518.

Mellinghoff IK, Wang MY, Vivanco I, et al. Molecular determinants of the response of glioblastomas to EGFR kinase inhibitors. *N Engl J Med* 2005;353:2012–2024.

Perry JR, DeAngelis LM, Schold SC Jr, et al. Challenges in the design and conduct of phase III brain tumor therapy trials. *Neurology* 1997;49:912–917.

Prados MD, Scott C, Curran WJ Jr, et al. Procarbazine, lomustine, and vincristine (PCV) chemotherapy for anaplastic astrocytoma: a retrospective review of radiation therapy oncology group protocols comparing survival with carmustine or PCV adjuvant chemotherapy. *J Clin Oncol* 1999;17:3389–3395.

Rajkumar SV, Buckner JC, Schomberg PJ, et al. Phase I and pharmacokinetic study of preirradiation chemotherapy with BCNU, cisplatin, etoposide, and accelerated radiation therapy in patients with high-grade glioma. *Int J Radiat Oncol Biol Phys* 1998;42:969–975.

Reardon DA, Egorin MJ, Quinn JA, et al. Phase II study of imatinib mesylate plus hydroxyurea in adults with recurrent glioblastoma multiforme. *J Clin Oncol* 2005;23:9359–9368.

Schuck A, Muller SB, Kohler A, et al. Combined radiochemotherapy with paclitaxel in the treatment of malignant glioma. *Strahlenther Onkol* 2002;178:486–490.

Stewart LA. Chemotherapy in adult high-grade glioma: a systematic review and meta-analysis of individual patient data from 12 randomised trials. *Lancet* 2002;359:1011–1018.

Stupp R, Dietrich PY, Ostermann Kraljevic S, et al. Promising survival for patients with newly diagnosed glioblastoma multiforme treated with concomitant radiation plus temozolomide followed by adjuvant temozolomide. *J Clin Oncol* 2002;20:1375–1382.

Stupp R, Mason WP, van den Bent MJ, et al. Radiotherapy plus concomitant and adjuvant temozolomide for glioblastoma. *N Engl J Med* 2005;352:987–996.

van den Bent MJ, Chinot O, Boogerd W, et al. Second-line chemotherapy with temozolomide in recurrent oligodendroglioma after PCV (procarbazine, lomustine and vincristine) chemotherapy: EORTC Brain Tumor Group phase II study 26972. *Ann Oncol* 2003a:14:599–602.

van den Bent MJ, Taphoorn MJ, Brandes AA, et al. Phase II study of first-line chemotherapy with temozolomide in recurrent oligodendroglial tumors: the European Organization for Research and Treatment of Cancer Brain Tumor Group Study 26971. *J Clin Oncol* 2003b:21:2525–2528.

Walker MD, Green SB, Byar DP, et al. Randomized comparisons of radiotherapy and nitrosoureas for the treatment of malignant glioma after surgery. *N Engl J Med* 1980;303:1323–1329.

Westphal M, Hilt DC, Bortey E, et al. A phase 3 trial of local chemotherapy with biodegradable carmustine (BCNU) wafers (Gliadel wafers) in patients with primary malignant glioma. *Neuro-oncology* 2003;5:79–88.

Wick W, Hermisson M, Kortmann RD, et al. Neoadjuvant gemcitabine/treosulfan chemotherapy for newly diagnosed glioblastoma: a phase II study. *J Neurooncol* 2002;59:151–155.

Wong ET, Hess KR, Gleason MJ, et al. Outcomes and prognostic factors in recurrent glioma patients enrolled onto phase II clinical trials. *J Clin Oncol* 1999;17:2572–2578.

Yung WK, Prados MD, Yaya-Tur R, et al. Multicenter phase II trial of temozolomide in patients with anaplastic astrocytoma or anaplastic oligoastrocytoma at first relapse. Temodal Brain Tumor Group. *J Clin Oncol* 1999;17:2762–2771.

9 INNOVATIVE TREATMENT STRATEGIES FOR HIGH-GRADE GLIOMAS

Charles A. Conrad and Amy B. Heimberger

Chapter Overview 171
Introduction 172
Chemotherapy Options 173
Potential Targets in Gliomas 174
Signal Transduction Inhibitors in Current Clinical Trials 174
New Delivery Techniques 179
Immunotherapy for Gliomas 179
    Cellular Immunotherapy 182
    Antibody-Guided Therapy 184
    Vaccination 185
    Next Generation of Immunotherapy 186
Conclusion 187
Key Practice Points 187
Suggested Readings 187

CHAPTER OVERVIEW

The extrapolation of treatments for high-grade gliomas from treatments for other solid tumors may not necessarily be successful because of inherent biologic differences. In high-grade gliomas, compartmentalization of gliomas within the central nervous system with exceedingly rare systemic metastasis, residual infiltrative components that are not surgically accessible, heterogeneity, elaboration of immunosuppressive cytokines, parallel signaling pathways, and antigenic diversity present additional treatment challenges. With evolving findings from molecular biology and immunology, more specific targeted therapies have been devised. However, these targeted therapies will likely need to be combined in novel ways so that multiple synergistic targets can affect the growth, invasiveness, angiogenesis, and immunologic reactivity of high-grade gliomas. This chapter delineates this exciting field and focuses on the treatment modalities and the future outlook.

INTRODUCTION

Viable treatment options for refractory tumors such as malignant gliomas are extremely limited, and the clinical outcome of these tumors has traditionally been dismal. In the United States, malignant gliomas have an annual incidence of 6.4 cases per 100,000 population (McCarthy et al, 2002). These neurologically devastating tumors are the most common subtype of primary brain tumors and are one of the deadliest types of human cancer. In its most aggressive manifestation, glioblastoma multiforme (GBM), the median patient survival duration ranges from 9 to 14 months despite aggressive treatment. Current surgical, chemotherapeutic, and radiotherapeutic techniques have done little to extend patient survival time. The lack of agents that specifically target the molecular biology of gliomas significantly reduces the likelihood of finding an effective therapy. Understanding the molecular biology of these tumors and the tumor–host interactions is necessary to develop alternative methods of treatment.

As with other solid tumors, the heterogeneity of malignant gliomas has been confirmed at the morphologic, biologic, genetic, and antigenic levels. This diversity renders these tumor cells differentially susceptible to various therapeutic modalities and offers a biologic explanation for therapeutic resistance. Genetic alterations occurring within gliomas include *TP53* mutations, epidermal growth factor receptor (EGFR) amplification, inactivation of the *CDKN2A* gene (on chromosome 9p21), overexpression of platelet-derived growth factor (PDGF), *p16* deletion, and loss of heterozygosity on chromosomes 13q, 19q, 17p, and 10 (Kleiheus et al, 1997). These alterations provide specific targets, some of which can be identified immunologically. Antigenic targets that have been exploited in gliomas include the extracellular matrix-associated antigens GP240 and tenascin, the membrane-associated ganglioside molecules, and the overexpressed deletion variant of EGFR (EGFRvIII) (Kurpad et al, 1995). The implication of tumor heterogeneity is profound and must be recognized to promote the design of rational therapeutic approaches, which may require an individualized approach or targeting with multiple agents. Furthermore, because malignant gliomas can arise from lower grade gliomas and because chemotherapy and radiotherapy are generally more efficacious against malignant dividing cells than against less proliferative cells, vaccinations for patients with low-grade gliomas to prevent progression to more malignant phenotypes may be developed in the future. Currently, treatment for high-grade gliomas is centered on surgical resection and radiotherapy. This chapter focuses on the evolving innovative treatments that use small-molecule signal transduction inhibitors and immunotherapy.

CHEMOTHERAPY OPTIONS

Chemotherapy for high-grade gliomas has traditionally included agents such as BCNU (the abbreviation of the chemical name of carmustine), CCNU (the abbreviation of the chemical name of lomustine), and combinations of procarbazine, CCNU, and vincristine (PCV). All of these agents have limited efficacy in a small proportion of patients (Prados and Levin, 2000). PCV was preferred for a number of years on the basis of a study comparing PCV and BCNU in patients with anaplastic astrocytomas, which demonstrated that the former provided a significantly longer median survival duration (37.8 vs 20.5 months) (Levin et al, 1990). However, temozolomide essentially replaced PCV after its approval following a pivotal phase II study comparing temozolomide and procarbazine (Yung et al, 1999). At M. D. Anderson Cancer Center, the use of PCV is typically restricted to patients with oligodendrogliomas that have demonstrated loss of chromosomes 1p and 19q. Patients with oligodendrogliomas can also be treated with temozolomide initially and then switched to PCV if a good response is not seen within 2 to 4 cycles of temozolomide. This practice, however, is somewhat controversial because no published studies have directly compared temozolomide and PCV in patients with oligodendrogliomas. Temozolomide is used instead of PCV to treat anaplastic astrocytomas largely because significant myelosuppression is commonly seen with BCNU- and CCNU-containing regimens.

Recently, Stupp et al (2005) reported the results of a large, multiinstitutional study performed by the European Organization for Research on the Treatment of Cancer and by the National Cancer Institute of Canada in which patients with GBMs were treated with a 6-week course of radiotherapy alone or with 75 mg/m^2 temozolomide on a continuous daily basis during radiotherapy plus 6 courses of adjuvant 200 mg/m^2 temozolomide. In that study, the addition of temozolomide significantly increased the percentage of patients with GBMs who survived 2 years or longer (26% vs 10%) and the median survival duration (14.6 vs 12.1 months). This combined regimen is now the standard of care at M. D. Anderson.

The routine use of other cytotoxic chemotherapeutic agents is difficult to justify because few large clinical trials have definitively proven their utility. In addition, the number of relatively small clinical trials has frequently confused rather than clarified the role of chemotherapeutic drugs both as adjuvants and for treating recurrent cancer. One of the difficulties in determining their usefulness is that many clinical trials lack the statistical power to confirm a small gain of benefit or a gain for a small subpopulation. To illustrate this point, for a study to have an 80% chance of detecting a modest 25% gain in median survival duration, 250 patients would be needed in each arm of a comparative study. Consequently, agents such as nitrosourea, irinotecan, carboplatin, and capecitabine have only limited anecdotal support as salvage therapy.

POTENTIAL TARGETS IN GLIOMAS

Like other malignant solid tumors, malignant gliomas have a number of dysregulated or mutated gene products that have transforming and pro-liferative properties. As described by Hanahan and Weinberg (2000), tumor cells need to be able to replicate without limit, avoid apoptotic sig-nals, be independent of external growth factors, invade surrounding nor-mal tissue, stimulate angiogenesis, and avoid immune surveillance. These features are enabled by dysregulated genetic pathways, which can be used to target these tumors. In the case of malignant gliomas, a number of com-mon pathways can be exploited. For instance, gliomas tend to have dys-regulated Rb/p16/E2F pathway members (Ueki et al, 1996) that drive an unchecked cell cycle; p53/mdm2 dysfunction, thereby creating failure to undergo apoptosis; and growth factor amplification or mutations in genes coding for EGFR, PDGF receptor, and insulin-like growth factor receptor. Survival, invasion, and stimulated angiogenesis seem to be commonly driven by the phosphoinositide 3-kinase (PI3K)/PTEN/AKT/mammalian target of rapamycin (mTOR) pathways as well as the activated signal transducers and activators of transcription 3 (STAT3) pathways (Talapatra and Thompson, 2001). Because these dysfunctional pathways appear in a large proportion of high-grade gliomas, the opportunity exists to target them with novel approaches. We believe that cytotoxic chemotherapy is often ineffective predominantly because of the intrinsic resistance of glioma cells and parallel pathways, which are mediated through induction of cell survival and anti-apoptotic signals. The major pathways that medi-ate these survival signals include the PI3K/AKT axis, the Janus kinase (Jak)/STAT pathway, and the Ras/MEK/ERK pathway (Figure 9–1).

SIGNAL TRANSDUCTION INHIBITORS IN CURRENT CLINICAL TRIALS

Several newer signal transduction inhibitors are being evaluated at M. D. Anderson and by the National Association of Brain Tumor Consortium (NABTC). These clinical trials are either currently enrolling patients or have recently completed enrollment. Many of the first clinical trials used drugs that, although not specifically designed for treating gliomas, targeted some components of the pathways important for glioma growth and maintenance.

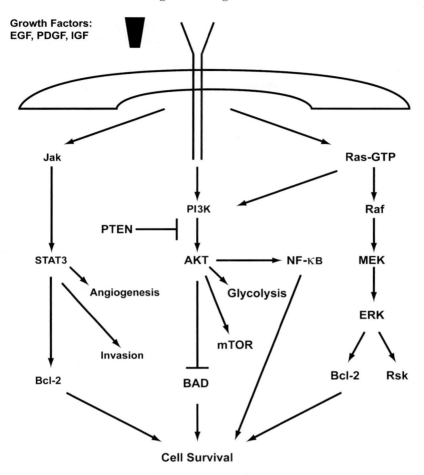

Figure 9–1.   The major pathways that mediate the survival signals in high-grade gliomas. EGF, epidermal growth factor; IGF, insulin-like growth factor.

An example is the matrix metalloproteinase inhibitor known as marimastat, which was evaluated in a phase II clinical trial of GBM in combination with temozolomide (Groves et al, 2002). The trial demonstrated 6-month progression-free and overall survival rates of 39% and 73%, respectively. A recent subgroup analysis demonstrated efficacy for this combination if the patients were stratified into those who had developed arthralgia and those who had been taking enzyme-inducing antiepileptic drugs: the progression-free survival time was 2.3 months for patients without arthropathy who had not been taking these drugs, 6 months for patients with arthropathy who had not been taking these drugs, and a striking 17.3 months for patients with arthropathy who had been taking these drugs (Groves et al, 2005). These results suggest that the pharma-cokinetic and pharmacodynamic properties of marimastat with temo-zolomide need to be better defined and should be correlated with characteristics of responsive patients. Because of these findings, there is a renewed interest in matrix metalloproteinase in combination with temo-zolomide. However, subsequent clinical trials may need to push the lev-els of the drug to the point of producing arthropathy in enrolled patients.

Many cell surface or membrane-linked growth factor receptors appear to be unregulated or constitutively activated in gliomas (Rasheed et al, 1999), thereby resulting in cell proliferation, survival of the tumor cells, and stimulation of downstream events. The PDGF/PDGF receptor path-way seems to be turned on in the early stages of glioma, and it is often associated with *p53* alterations (von Deimling et al, 1992). These observa-tions have led some investigators to suggest that this pathway might be a common early pathway for the genesis of low-grade gliomas. At M. D. Anderson, a single-agent evaluation of imatinib mesylate, which inhibits the receptor tyrosine kinases for PDGF and Bcr/Abl, was performed in cooperation with the NABTC. Although the study did not show a signif-icant improvement in patients' overall or 6-month progression-free sur-vival time, interest in this compound has continued based on a recent European trial with imatinib mesylate and hydroxyurea. That study demonstrated a very high response rate of more than 40% (Dresemann, 2005). On the basis of the results from that trial, a comparative trial of these 2 agents is being planned in the United States.

The fact that patients with GBMs overexpress EGFR has been known for some time and has generated a great amount of interest in this receptor as a potential therapeutic target (Wikstrand et al, 1992). Overexpression of EGFR occurs in approximately 50% to 60% of patients with GBMs and is more commonly seen in those with high-grade gliomas and in elderly patients. One form of EGFR, called EGFRvIII, is a tumor-specific antigen with a truncated extracellular domain and a constitutively active internal kinase domain. The small-molecule inhibitors targeting EGFR that are being evaluated by the NABTC are gefitinib and erlotinib. Another com-pound, AEE788 (Traxler et al, 2004), inhibits both EGFR and the vascular endothelial growth factor (VEGF) receptor. The single-agent phase I trial with AEE788 is almost complete, and so far the results have demon-strated toxicity similar to other EGFR inhibitors. The combination of any of these agents with cytotoxic chemotherapy or other signal transduction inhibitors may be synergistic because of the number of potential parallel pathways involved in cellular signal transduction of tumor development and maintenance.

Signals downstream of growth factor receptors are also potential targets. One of the important signaling molecules is Ras, which is a G-protein that binds both GDP and GTP. When Ras binds GTP, it is enzymatically active. For Ras to transmit its activating signal to downstream elements, it must localize to the plasma membrane. The process that allows membrane localization is the addition of a prenylation group to Ras, which is catalyzed by the enzyme farnesyl transferase. At M. D. Anderson, there are 2 ongoing phase II trials evaluating the efficacy of farnesyl transferase inhibitors in combination with temozolomide. Although the studies are not yet complete, early indications suggest that this drug combination is effective in patients with GBMs and may represent an exciting therapeutic strategy.

Another central pathway activated by membrane growth factor receptors is the PI3K/Akt axis. This critical pathway promotes cell survival, angiogenesis, and invasion. The tumor suppressor serine phosphatase (PTEN/MMAC) was codiscovered at M. D. Anderson (Steck et al, 1997). Loss of PTEN function in glioma cells tends to constitutively activate the PI3K/Akt pathway. Direct inhibitors of PI3K or Akt appear attractive (Lu et al, 2003), although these agents seem to be toxic in animal models. A downstream molecule from this pathway, mTOR, is phosphorylated by activated Akt. Activation of mTOR in turn significantly alters protein translation from mRNA. An orally bioavailable ester analog of rapamycin, named RAD001, is currently in phase I clinical trials in combination with AEE788. This combination is based partly on promising preclinical animal model data suggesting an additive antitumor effect against orthotopic and subcutaneous gliomas (Goudar et al, 2005).

The process of angiogenesis, which most high-grade solid tumors briskly stimulate, has been an attractive target since the pioneering work of Judah Folkman (Folkman, 1974, 2002, 2003). Angiogenesis appears to be necessary for solid tumors to grow more than a few millimeters in size. However, the relationship between angiogenesis and brain tumor invasion into surrounding tissue in the absence of neovascularization is not completely understood. There are many stages to the development of vascular structures to feed a growing tumor, which include the secretion of angiogenic growth factors such as VEGF by the malignant tumor and degradation of the intercellular matrix by matrix metalloproteinases. The endothelial cells must migrate into the tumor to begin forming a leading vessel. These processes rely on multiple growth factor receptors, including VEGF receptor and neuropilin-1. In addition, other cells such as pericytes need to be recruited into this process. New inhibitors of the VEGF receptors FLT-1 and FLK-1/KDR, such as PTK787 and AEE788, are being evaluated in clinical trials. Although AEE788 is in early phase I clinical trial testing, PTK787, which potently inhibits both VEGF receptor and PDGF receptor, has been in phase I and phase II clinical trials as a single agent and in combination with temozolomide or CCNU. These clinical trials commonly use imaging surrogates of tumor vascular perfusion, such as dynamic contrast-enhanced magnetic resonance imaging, to capture the drug's or drugs' effect on the treated tumor. Dramatic reductions in contrast enhancement on magnetic resonance imaging have been seen with PTK787 (Figure 9–2). These early and dramatic effects on gadolinium

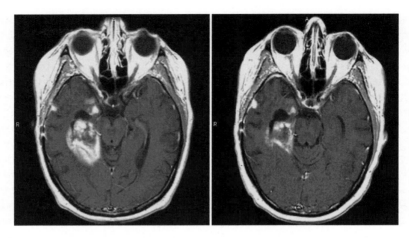

Figure 9–2. Axial magnetic resonance images showing gadolinium enhancement of a high-grade glioma before (*left*) and after (*right*) treatment with PTK787.

enhancement in patients tend to predict which patients will have more prolonged responses to this agent.

Increased expression of a number of integrins must occur during endothelial cell migration. The compound cilengitide contains the amino acid sequence arginine-glycine-aspartic acid, which binds the integrins α-vβ3 and β5 (Tucker, 2003). This binding disrupts the normal adhesion molecule cell signaling and ultimately disrupts angiogenesis. A phase II clinical trial with cilengitide conducted by M. D. Anderson and the NABTC is currently under way.

Membrane-associated growth factor receptors can also stimulate a parallel pathway involving Jak, which ultimately phosphorylates a number of STATs. On phosphorylation, STAT members will dimerize, translocate to the nucleus of the cell, bind to a number of promoters, and ultimately stimulate the production of various target proteins. These proteins play a major role in stimulating angiogenesis, invasion, and importantly, cell survival (Vinkemeier, 2004). M. D. Anderson has recently developed a number of unique small-molecule inhibitors of STAT3. One of these inhibitors, WP1066, has initially shown promising results within glioma xenograft models and appears to have good central nervous system (CNS) penetration. The preclinical data are of sufficient merit to justify a phase I clinical trial.

Although much emphasis has been placed on tissue invasion, angiogenesis, and avoidance of apoptotic signals within tumor cells, an old observation that tumor cells significantly alter their metabolism to preferentially use glucose through the process of glycolysis is under renewed scrutiny. The tumor cell's preference of metabolizing glucose through glycolysis even in the presence of sufficient oxygen (i.e., aerobic glycolysis; also known as the "Warburg effect" [Warburg, 1956]) appears to be a general phenomenon within many solid tumors, including malignant gliomas. In fact, malignant gliomas appear to have very high rates of aerobic glycolysis. For this reason, ongoing investigative efforts at M. D. Anderson include the use of glycolytic inhibitors for the treatment of high-grade gliomas. Two such inhibitors, 2-deoxyglucose and 3-bromopyruvate, have recently been shown to be active in mouse glioma xenograft models.

NEW DELIVERY TECHNIQUES

Because there is a residual infiltrating component even after a "gross total resection" of a malignant glioma, the suppression or eradication of these isolated cells is a therapeutic goal. Convection-enhanced delivery was developed as a way to deliver an agent under constant volumetric flow to a greater distribution area than could normally be achieved by simple diffusion. Because the administration is localized to the CNS compartment, higher concentrations of a therapeutic agent can be administered with this technique than with systemic administration. At M. D. Anderson, a multi-institutional phase III clinical trial sponsored by NeoPharm is open that uses convection-enhanced delivery of interleukin-13, which binds to the surface of gliomas, conjugated to a *Pseudomonas* exotoxin, a bacterial protein that causes tumor cells to die once it is internalized by the cells. This randomized trial compares convection-enhanced delivery of the interleukin-13–*Pseudomonas* exotoxin with that of Gliadel wafers (a BCNU formulation). This trial is being conducted on the basis of a study that showed an improved median survival duration from time of treatment for patients with recurrent GBMs compared with historical controls (Kunwar, 2003).

IMMUNOTHERAPY FOR GLIOMAS

The goal of immunotherapy in treating gliomas is to eradicate or suppress the residual infiltrative component of these tumors without incurring the significant toxicities associated with other treatment modalities. Although there is clinical evidence for cell-mediated and humoral antiglioma activity, immunotherapy has to overcome a striking state of immunosuppression mediated, in part, by the glioma secreting tumor growth factor β, interleukin-10, and prostaglandin E_2. The immunosuppression-related defects in patients with gliomas include low peripheral lymphocyte counts, reduced delayed-type hypersensitivity reactions to recall antigens, impaired mitogen-induced blastogenic responses by peripheral mononuclear cells, increased $CD4^+$ suppressor T cell counts within the

CD4$^+$ compartment, decreased CD4 T-cell activity in vitro, diminished immunoglobulin synthesis by B cells, and impaired transmembrane signaling through the T-cell receptor/CD3 complex. Other impairments that have recently been identified include the induction of anergy, failure of costimulation, lack of sufficient numbers of functional effector T cells, and T suppressor cells within the tumor microenvironment (Fecci et al, 2006; Hussain et al, 2006) (Table 9–1). Although attempts have been made to block the immunosuppressive factors in patients with gliomas, the results have been disappointing. The failure of immunosuppressive blockade is compounded by the fact that gliomas usually express a variety of immunosuppressive cytokines: the blockade of a solitary cytokine would not be expected to significantly affect the overall immunosuppressive milieu. Even so, immunosuppressive blockade represents a potential therapy to use in combination with systemic activation.

Immune responses are initiated by uptake of a protein by antigen-presenting cells, processing of that protein, and its presentation on class I or II major histocompatibility complexes (MHC) (i.e., adaptive immunity). T cells recognize the antigen within the context of these MHC-antigen complexes via cell surface receptors, specifically T-cell receptors. More specifically, CD4$^+$ helper T cells recognize peptide-MHC class II complexes, whereas CD8$^+$ cytotoxic T cells recognize peptide-MHC class I complexes. Full activation of a T cell requires costimulation, which results in the clonal expansion of the naive T cell. The absence of costimulation or the presence of costimulatory inhibition markers can lead to a state of unresponsiveness or anergy in the effector T cell. The stimulated cytotoxic immune effector cells (CD8$^+$) can destroy tumor cells via perforin-induced cell lysis or Fas/APO-1 receptor-mediated apoptosis. Another immune mechanism involved in glioma eradication is antibody-dependent cellular cytotoxicity (Sampson et al, 2000; Heimberger et al, 2003).

Table 9–1.   Potential and Known Mechanisms of Resistance to Immunotherapy in High-Grade Gliomas

Loss of antigen
Decrease in β_2-microglobulin or human leukocyte antigen level
Inadequate antigen processing and presentation
Inadequate T cell responses:
  Insufficient number
  Resistance of the tumor to killer T cells
  T cell anergy or inactivation
  Induction of inappropriate T helper function
Elaboration of immunosuppressive cytokines (e.g., tumor growth factor β and interleukin-10)
Depletion of essential nutrients (e.g., tryptophan and arginase)
Recruitment of regulatory or suppressive T cells
Elaboration of immunosuppressive microvesicles

Lymphocytes in the CNS of healthy humans are rare except during inflammatory responses, when they are abundant. Lymphocytes generally require activation before entry into the CNS (Hickey et al, 1991), but antigen specificity is not necessary for entry. T-cell infiltrates are common within the parenchyma of human gliomas (von Hanwehr et al, 1984). Several studies have attempted to correlate the intensity of infiltration with patient survival duration. Most (Brooks et al, 1978; Palma et al, 1978; von Hanwehr et al, 1984) but not all (Safdari et al, 1985) have reported that survival duration is positively associated with lymphocytic infiltration. These activated lymphocytes can be therapeutically efficacious against intracerebral tumors. However, the activity of these T cells is impaired on entry into the tumor microenvironment (Hussain et al, 2006).

The brain has been characterized as "immunologically privileged" because of the protection provided by the brain's environment to allografts and xenografts. A number of vaccination strategies in experimental animals have been quite effective against tumors outside the CNS but completely useless against tumors within the CNS. Furthermore, patients successfully treated with biomodulators have tumor relapses within the brain despite extracranial remissions. One explanation for the immunologic privilege of the brain is the absence of conventional lymphatics; however, proteins, lymphocytes, and macrophages can drain from the cranial subarachonoid space into the deep cervical lymph nodes (Cserr et al, 1992). The blood-brain barrier might explain the immunologic privilege, except that it is broken down during inflammatory processes. A final possible explanation relates to the presumed paucity of antigen-presenting cells within the CNS; however, antigens draining to the cervical lymph nodes could be presented there. What remain unresolved are whether antigen processing occurs within the CNS and how the tumor microenvironment affects the immunologic responses. However, there is ample evidence that immune recognition of gliomas does occur.

One concern about using immunotherapy for patients with gliomas is the possibility of inducing fatal autoimmunity. However, in previous immunotherapy trials of humans with brain tumors, there were only 2 possible cases of autoimmunity (Bloom et al, 1973; Trouillas, 1973). Autoimmunity remains a consideration, but it is likely related to the use of strong adjuvants (Wikstrand and Bigner, 1981). The rationale for selecting the tumor-specific antigen approach in immunotherapy is based on the fact that the targeting antigen preparation does not contain CNS antigens that could possibly induce an autoimmune response; furthermore, the tumor-specific immune response can be monitored. However, the disadvantage of using a tumor-specific antigen is secondary to the heterogeneity of gliomas: a single antigen is unlikely to produce a durable response because a clonal negative population is likely to arise (Heimberger et al, 2003).

The advent of immunotherapy for malignant gliomas began in the late 1950s, when patients with gliomas received tumor homogenate mixed with a variety of adjuvants. Since then, immunotherapy has used cytokine-based approaches (which result in adverse effects such as induction of acute inflammatory responses, thereby resulting in cerebral edema), a variety of adoptive cellular immunotherapies, active immunization, immunotoxins, monoclonal antibodies, and viral transfection techniques. Many immunotherapy trials lack appropriate control groups, include a variety of tumor grades and types, use various additional treatment types, or use too few patients to draw conclusions from. Ongoing immunotherapy for gliomas can be categorized as cellular immunotherapy, antibody-guided therapy, or vaccination.

Cellular Immunotherapy

Cellular immunotherapy involves the isolation of immune effector cells from a patient, their expansion and activation in vitro, and then their infusion back into the patient. Examples of this type of therapy include lymphokine-activated natural killer cells, lymphokine-activated lymphocytes or tumor-infiltrating lymphocytes, and dendritic cells. The most recent cellular immunotherapies to have demonstrated therapeutic efficacy involve dendritic cells, which are potent antigen-presenting cells. Multiple clinical trials have recently been completed with promising results at the University of California–Los Angeles and the Duke University Medical Center (Table 9–2). The dendritic cells are loaded with acid-eluted peptides, tumor homogenates, or the tumor-specific antigen EGFRvIII after being stimulated and matured with granulocyte-macrophage colony-stimulating factor and interleukin-4. The patients are then systemically vaccinated with the dendritic cell preparations. In 1 phase I clinical trial, 9 patients with newly diagnosed high-grade gliomas received 3 separate vaccinations spaced 2 weeks apart (Yu et al, 2001). A robust infiltration of T cells was detected in tumor specimens, and the median survival time was 15.1 months (vs 8.6 months for the control population). A subsequent trial using the same vaccination protocol with 8 patients with GBMs resulted in a median survival time of 33.3 months (vs 7.5 months of a comparable set of patients receiving other treatment protocols) (Yu et al, 2004).

In a phase I clinical trial using an antigen-specific approach to EGFRvIII with dendritic cells, the median survival time was a remarkable 20.0 months in patients with GBMs (vs 7 months for the control population), and tumor-specific cytotoxic responses were generated (Archer et al, 2003) (Table 9–2). These results are notable because the patients were not screened for expression of EGFRvIII, and the clinical efficacy could have been even more pronounced in this subset of patients because EGFRvIII is expressed on only approximately 30% of GBMs (Heimberger et al, 2005).

Researchers at Cedars-Sinai Medical Center reported the results of a clinical trial using chemotherapy after patients received the dendritic cell

Table 9–2.   Recent and Ongoing Immunotherapy Clinical Trials for High-Grade Gliomas*

Immunotherapy Type and Agent Delivered	Trial Phase	Sponsor or Center Involved	Trial Status	Median Survival Duration (Months)
Cellular immunotherapy				
Dendritic cells + CMV + PEP-3-KLH	I/II	Duke University Medical Center	Open	
Dendritic cells + tumor lysate/ acid-eluted peptides	I, II	University of California–Los Angeles	Open	14.9–30.6
Dendritic cells + PEP-3-KLH	I	Duke University Medical Center	Closed	20.0
Dendritic cells + glioma lysate + IL-4	I	University of Pittsburgh	Closed	Data not released
Antibody-guided therapy				
Pegylated interferon α-2b	II	National Cancer Institute	Open	
Anti-tenascin antibody 81C6	I/II, III	Duke University Medical Center	Open	22.2
Vaccination				
Poly-ICLC	II	NABTC	Open	19.2
GM-CSF + PEP-3-KLH	II	M. D. Anderson and Duke University Medical Center	Open	

* Site was intracavitary in the anti-tenascin antibody 81C6 trial and systemic for all other trials.

vaccination protocol. The mean survival duration and 2-year survival rate were 18 months and 8% for patients who received only the vaccine and 26 months and 42% for patients who received both the vaccine and chemotherapy (Wheeler et al, 2004). The authors hypothesized that the improved outcome was attributable to the vaccine having primed the apoptotic machinery of the cancer cells and the ability of the chemotherapy to then trigger the apoptotic pathway. However, an alternative explanation exists: the immunotherapy may have selected the more aggressive, infiltrative tumor cells and left behind the more chemosensitive cells. Regardless, this study indicates that a synergy may exist between immunotherapy and chemotherapy and needs to be explored.

An alternative immunologic approach amplifies the T cells generated by the patient in response to tumor cells. Glioblastoma tumor cells gathered during surgery were cultured with growth factors and then injected subcutaneously back into the patients (Plautz et al, 2000). After development of an immune reaction, the lymph nodes draining the location of the injection were resected to obtain lymphocytes directed against the tumor cells and were stimulated with staphylococcal toxin and interleukin-2. This procedure generated a large number of activated T cells, which were then infused back into the patient. Of 10 patients, 2 had tumor regression but 8 had progressive disease (Plautz et al, 2000). It is unknown whether these T cells were functional once they were in the tumor microenvironment. Techniques to maintain T-cell activation despite immunosuppressive factors are under development.

An inherent problem with cellular immunotherapy is the ex vivo manipulation of cells. These ex vivo techniques can be labor intensive, require special facilities for generating a product that can be infused into human patients, and will probably only be available at specialty treatment centers.

Antibody-Guided Therapy

Monoclonal antibodies can be used to induce apoptosis or mediate immune responses, or they can be used as delivery vehicles for chemotherapeutic agents, toxins, or radionucleotides. Unconjugated antibodies may have potential for future clinical trials if delivered via convection-enhanced delivery (Sampson et al, 2000). One of the most exploited targets has been tenascin, which is an extracellular matrix glycoprotein ubiquitously expressed in malignant gliomas but not by normal brain. The monoclonal antibody 81C6 binds an epitope within the alternatively spliced fibronectin type III region of tenascin. In a phase II clinical trial, iodine 131-labeled murine 81C6 was injected into patients' surgically created resection cavities (Reardon et al, 2002). The median survival duration was 19.9 months for patients with newly diagnosed GBMs and 12 months for patients with recurrent GBMs. These durations significantly surpassed the historical control values even when established prognostic factors such as age and Karnofsky performance scale score were accounted for. Patient-specific dosing in patients with newly diagnosed GBMs further extended the median survival time to 23 months (Reardon et al, 2002) (Table 10–2). A multi-institutional phase III clinical trial of 81C6 antibody treatment for newly diagnosed GBM is being planned to open in 2007 at M. D. Anderson.

Vaccination

Vaccination would ultimately induce the patient's own immune system to react against high-grade gliomas and is the theoretical ideal of immunologic approaches to cancer. A phase II clinical trial is investigating poly-ICLC, which is a double-stranded RNA that is a nonspecific activator of the immune system. In this trial, poly-ICLC is administered intramuscularly 2 or 3 times weekly for up to 56 months and is well tolerated. In the initial clinical trial with poly-ICLC, the overall median survival duration was 96 months for patients with anaplastic astrocytomas, in contrast to the expected survival duration of 22 months with conventional chemotherapy (Salazar et al, 1996). However, vaccination with poly-ICLC was notably less effective for patients with GBMs: for them, the median survival time was 19 months. A second clinical trial with recurrent glioma patients is currently under way (Table 10–2).

The vaccination trial that is demonstrating the most clinical promise was designed at M. D. Anderson (Table 10–2). This trial, called ACTIVATE, uses the tumor-specific antigen EGFRvIII as an immune target. Preclinical data demonstrated that when mice with established intracerebral tumors were vaccinated with a single dose of PEP-3-KLH, they had significantly increased long-term and median survival durations (Heimberger et al, 2003). Newly diagnosed GBM patients with tumors that express EGFRvIII who have undergone gross total resection and radiotherapy are eligible to receive the intradermal vaccination, which consists of a 14-mer peptide (PEP-3) encompassing the EGFRvIII mutation with granulocyte-macrophage colony-stimulating factor. During an induction period, patients receive the vaccine every 2 weeks for 6 weeks and thereafter shift to a monthly maintenance dose until evidence of tumor progression appears. Immunologic evaluation includes the determination of EGFRvIII-specific humoral and cytotoxic responses and the appraisal of mechanisms of treatment failure. Preliminary data have demonstrated a time to tumor progression and a median survival duration that significantly exceed that expected with standard care (Stupp et al, 2005). The preliminary results are even more striking when one considers the fact that the expression of EGFRvIII on GBMs is a negative prognosticator for patients who survive longer than 1 year. Typically, the median survival duration is 12.8 months for patients with EGFRvIII-expressing tumors, and no patient survives longer than 18 months (Heimberger et al, 2005). The ACTIVATE trial is ongoing at M. D. Anderson and the Duke University Medical Center.

Next Generation of Immunotherapy

The next generation of immunotherapy is directed at synergy with systemic activation. Two specific areas can be addressed, the effector T cell and the tumor microenvironment. Regarding the former, future therapeutic techniques include the increase of adhesion molecule and integrin expression on T cells to increase trafficking to the tumor, maintenance of T-cell activation by constitutive activation of costimulator molecules or CD3 receptor, bone marrow ablation and reconstitution with clonotypic glioma-specific T cells to amplify the T-cell response (the durability of this technique is currently being investigated), and inhibition of systemic T suppressor cells. Proposed techniques with which to modulate the local tumor microenvironment include the use of small-molecule inhibitors of immunosuppressive molecules, inhibition of tumor T suppressor cells, up-regulation of costimulatory molecules, and induced maturation of immature dendritic cells.

In the future, we expect that immunotherapy will be tailored to the antigen expression and genetic makeup of the individual patient's glioma. Multimodality treatments will include systemic activation with intrinsic immunosuppressive blockade or modulation of the local tumor microenvironment, and the synergistic effects of chemotherapy and radiotherapy with immunotherapy will be explored. In addition, insight will be gained into the immune cells within gliomas and the CNS, and modalities that increase the local traffic of cytotoxic T cells and their function will be investigated. Finally, greater emphasis will be placed on the design of clinical trials for mechanisms of treatment failure, such as antigen mismatch, generation of antigen-negative revertants, lack of sufficient activation, and the interference of T suppressor cells.

Various immunotherapies for gliomas appear promising, but the unique characteristics of CNS tumors will need to be considered for rational design of these therapies. Novel approaches to antitumor immunotherapy will need to be independently and thoroughly evaluated against tumors within the CNS regardless of their success against tumors outside the CNS. Recent identification of tumor-associated antigens such as EGFRvIII may provide selective targeting to the gliomas and decrease the risk of inducing autoimmunity. Many of the previous attempts to treat glioma patients with immunotherapies such as lymphocyte transfer, vaccination with glioma cells, and the use of some cytokines have not met with significant success. Emerging concepts in immunology, advances in molecular techniques, and a greater understanding of the interaction between the CNS and the immune system provide the background for more rational and, we hope, more efficacious treatments.

CONCLUSION

A number of mechanisms are being explored to improve the treatment possibilities of patients at M. D. Anderson who have high-grade gliomas in the CNS. Because of the heterogeneity, antigenic diversity, parallel signaling pathways, and duplicated autocrine stimulation of these tumors, combination therapies will need to be designed. For example, multiple signal transduction inhibitors with chemotherapy or multiple immunologic modulation techniques may offer advantages that were not available previously. We are trying to not only prolong the survival duration of patients with gliomas but also improve their quality of life. For example, a pilot study currently open at M. D. Anderson is evaluating the efficacy of indomethacin to reduce CNS inflammation during radiotherapy. The inflammatory response mediated by cytokines inhibits neurogenesis, which contributes to memory impairment and cognitive decline. This trial was designed to evaluate whether indomethacin can prevent this decline in patients with GBMs who are undergoing radiotherapy. We are hopeful that this and other types of intervention as well as the evolving findings in molecular biology, genetics, and immunology will improve treatment outcomes for our patients. Our philosophy is to actively enroll patients who have not responded to other standard forms of therapy.

KEY PRACTICE POINTS

- Successful strategies against gliomas will likely involve multiple targets, such as cell proliferation, angiogenesis, and invasion. A single agent is unlikely to be successful.

- Signal transduction inhibitors will likely need to be combined because there are parallel pathways in gliomas.

- Convection-enhanced delivery is a way to significantly increase the amount and concentration of an agent administered directly to a glioma while minimizing systemic toxicity.

- Although theoretically very appealing, immunotherapy has to overcome significant hurdles (including antigenic diversity, immunosuppression mediated by cytokines and T suppressor cells, and tumor microenvironment downregulation of those immune responses while not inducing cerebral edema and autoimmunity) before it can become a viable treatment strategy.

SUGGESTED READINGS

Archer GE, Bigner DD, Friedman AH, Heimberger AB, Sampson J. Induction of CD4 and CD8 T cells to the tumor-specific antigen EGFRvIII. 15th International Conference on Brain Tumor Research and Therapy. Sorrento, Italy. May 24–27, 2003. [Abstract] *Neuro-Oncology* 2003;5:5.

Bloom HJ, Peckham MJ, Richardson AE, Alexander PA, Payne PM. Glioblastoma multiforme: a controlled trial to assess the value of specific active immunotherapy in patients treated by radical surgery and radiotherapy. *Br J Cancer* 1973;27: 253–267.

Brooks WH, Markesbery WR, Gupta GD, Roszman TL. Relationship of lymphocyte invasion and survival of brain tumor patients. *Ann Neurol* 1978;4:219–224.

Cserr HF, DePasquale M, Harling-Berg CJ, Park JT, Knopf PM. Afferent and efferent arms of the humoral immune response to CSF-administered albumins in a rat model with normal blood-brain barrier permeability. *J Neuroimmunol* 1992; 41:195–202.

Dresemann G. Temozolomide/pegylated liposomal doxorubicin (PLD) in progressive glioblastoma multiforme (GBM). In: *Abstracts from the World Federation of Neuro-Oncology Second Quadrennial Meeting and the Sixth Meeting of the European Association for Neuro-Oncology. May 5–8, 2005. Edinburgh, United Kingdom.* [Abstract 112] Society of Neuro-Oncology, 2005:310.

Fecci PE, Mitchell DA, Whitesides JF, et al. Increased regulatory T-cell fraction amidst a diminished CD4 compartment explains cellular immune defects in patients with malignant glioma. *Cancer Res* 2006;66:3294–3302.

Folkman J. Tumor angiogenesis. [Review] *Adv Cancer Res* 1974;19:331–358.

Folkman J. From the lab to the clinic: one investigator's journey. *J Law Med Ethics* 2002;30:361–366.

Folkman J. Fundamental concepts of the angiogenic process. [Review] *Curr Mol Med* 2003;3:643–651.

Goudar R, Shi Q, Hjelmeland M, et al. Combination therapy of inhibitors of epidermal growth factor receptor/vascular endothelial growth factor receptor 2 (AEE788) and the mammalian target of rapamycin (RAD001) offers improved glioblastoma tumor growth inhibition. *Mol Cancer Ther* 2005;4:101–112.

Groves M, Puduvalli V, Conrad CA, et al. Matrix metalloproteinase inhibitor-induced joint-related toxicity predicts prolonged progression-free survival in recurrent high-grade glioma trials. In: *Abstracts from the World Federation of Neuro-Oncology Second Quadrennial Meeting and the Sixth Meeting of the European Association for Neuro-Oncology. May 5–8, 2005. Edinburgh, United Kingdom.* [Abstract 143] Society of Neuro-Oncology, 2005:318.

Groves M, Puduvalli V, Hess K, et al. Phase II trial of temozolomide plus the matrix metalloproteinase inhibitor, marimastat, in recurrent and progressive glioblastoma multiforme. *J Clin Oncol* 2002;20:1383–1388.

Hanahan D, Weinberg R. The hallmarks of cancer. *Cell* 2000;100:57–70.

Heimberger A, Hlatky R, Suki D, et al. Prognostic effect of epidermal growth factor receptor and EGFRvIII in glioblastoma multiforme patients. *Clin Cancer Res* 2005;11:1462–1466.

Heimberger AB, Crotty LE, Archer GE, et al. Epidermal growth factor receptor VIII peptide vaccination is efficacious against established intracerebral tumors. *Clin Cancer Res* 2003;9:4247–4254.

Hickey WF, Hsu BL, Kimura H. T-lymphocyte entry into the central nervous system. *J Neurosci Res* 1991;28:254–260.

Hussain SF, Yang D, Suki D, Aldape K, Grimm E, Heimberger AB. The role of human glioma-infiltrating microglia/macrophages in mediating antitumor immune responses. *Neuro-Oncology* 2006;8:261–279.

Kleiheus P, Burger P, Plate K, Ohgaki H, Cavenee W. Astrocytic tumors. In: Kleihues P, Cavenee W, eds. *Pathology and Genetics: Tumors of the Nervous System*. Vol. 1. Lyon, France: International Agency for Research on Cancer; 1997.

Kunwar S. Convection enhanced delivery of IL13-PE38QQR for treatment of recurrent malignant glioma: presentation of interim findings from ongoing phase 1 studies. *Acta Neurochir Suppl* 2003;88:105–111.

Kurpad SN, Zhao XG, Wikstrand CJ, Batra SK, McLendon RE, Bigner DD. Tumor antigens in astrocytic gliomas. [Review] *Glia* 1995;15:244–256.

Levin V, Silver P, Hannigan J, et al. Superiority of post-radiotherapy adjuvant chemotherapy with CCNU, procarbazine, and vincristine (PCV) over BCNU for anaplastic gliomas: NCOG 6G61 final report. *Int J Radiat Oncol Biol Phys* 1990;18:321–324.

Lu Y, Wang H, Mills G. Targeting PI3K-AKT pathway for cancer therapy. *Rev Clin Exp Hematol* 2003;7:205–228.

McCarthy B, Surawicz T, Bruner J, Kruchko C, Davis F. Consensus Conference on Brain Tumor Definition for registration. *Neuro-oncology* 2002;4:134–145.

Palma L, Di Lorenzo N, Guidetti B. Lymphocytic infiltrates in primary glioblastomas and recidivous gliomas. Incidence, fate, and relevance to prognosis in 228 operated cases. *J Neurosurg* 1978;49:854–861.

Plautz G, Miller D, Barnett G, et al. T cell adoptive immunotherapy of newly diagnosed gliomas. *Clin Cancer Res* 2000;6:2209–2218.

Prados M, Levin V. Biology and treatment of malignant glioma. *Semin Oncol* 2000;27:1–10.

Rasheed BK, Wiltshire RN, Bigner SH, Bigner DD. Molecular pathogenesis of malignant gliomas. [Review] *Curr Opin Oncol* 1999;11:162–167.

Reardon DA, Akabani G, Coleman RE, et al. Phase II trial of murine ^{131}I-labeled antitenascin monoclonal antibody 81C6 administered into surgically created resection cavities of patients with newly diagnosed malignant gliomas. *J Clin Oncol* 2002;20:1389–1397.

Safdari H, Hochberg F, Richardson E. Prognostic value of round cell (lymphocyte) infiltration in malignant gliomas. *Surg Neurol* 1985;23:221–226.

Salazar A, Levy H, Ondra S, et al. Long-term treatment of malignant gliomas with intramuscularly administered polyinosinic-polycytidylic acid stabilized with polylysine and carboxymethylcellulose: an open pilot study. *Neurosurgery* 1996;38:1096–1103; Discussion 1103–1104.

Sampson JH, Crotty LE, Lee S, et al. Unarmed, tumor-specific monoclonal antibody effectively treats brain tumors. *Proc Natl Acad Sci U S A* 2000;97: 7503–7508.

Steck PA, Pershouse MA, Jasser SA, et al. Identification of a candidate tumour suppressor gene, *MMAC1*, at chromosome 10q23.3 that is mutated in multiple advanced cancers. *Nat Genet* 1997;15:356–362.

Stupp R, Mason W, van den Bent M, et al. Radiotherapy plus concomitant and adjuvant temozolomide for glioblastoma. *N Engl J Med* 2005;352:987–996.

Talapatra S, Thompson C. Growth factor signaling in cell survival: implications for cancer treatment. *J Pharmacol Exp Ther* 2001;298:873–878.

Traxler P, Allegrini P, Brandt RM, et al. AEE788: a dual family epidermal growth factor receptor/ErbB2 and vascular endothelial growth factor receptor tyrosine kinase inhibitor with antitumor and antiangiogenic activity. *Cancer Res* 2004;64:4931–4941.

Trouillas P. Immunology and immunotherapy of cerebral tumors. Current status. *Rev Neurol (Paris)* 1973;128:23–38.

Tucker GC. Alpha v integrin inhibitors and cancer therapy. *Curr Opin Investig Drugs* 2003;4:723–731.

Ueki K, Ono Y, Henson JW, Efird JT, von Deimling A, Louis DN. CDKN2/p16 or RB alterations occur in the majority of glioblastomas and are inversely correlated. *Cancer Res* 1996;56:150–153.

Vinkemeier U. Getting the message across, STAT! Design principles of a molecular signaling circuit. *J Cell Biol* 2004;167:197–201.

von Deimling A, Eibl R, Ohgaki H, et al. p53 mutations are associated with 17p allelic loss in grade II and grade III astrocytoma. *Cancer Res* 1992; 52:2987–2990.

von Hanwehr RI, Hofman FM, Taylor CR, Apuzzo ML. Mononuclear lymphoid populations infiltrating the microenvironment of primary CNS tumors. Characterization of cell subsets with monoclonal antibodies. *J Neurosurg* 1984;60:1138–1147.

Warburg O. On the origin of cancer cells. *Science* 1956;123:309–314.

Wheeler CJ, Das A, Liu G, Yu J, Black K. Clinical responsiveness of glioblastoma multiforme to chemotherapy after vaccination. *Clin Cancer Res* 2004;10: 5316–5326.

Wikstrand CJ, Bigner DD. Hyperimmunization of non-human primates with BCG-CW and cultured human glioma-derived cells. Production of reactive antisera and absence of EAE induction. *J Neuroimmunol* 1981;1:249–260.

Wikstrand CJ, Fredman P, Svennerholm L, Humphrey PA, Bigner SH, Bigner DD. Monoclonal antibodies to malignant human gliomas. [Review] *Mol Chem Neuropathol* 1992;17:137–146.

Yu J, Liu G, Ying H, Yong WH, Black KL, Wheeler CJ. Vaccination with tumor lysate-pulsed dendritic cells elicits antigen-specific, cytotoxic T-cells in patients with malignant glioma. *Cancer Res* 2004;64:4973–4979.

Yu J, Wheeler C, Zeltzer P, et al. Vaccination of malignant glioma patients with peptide-pulsed dendritic cells elicits systemic cytotoxicity and intracranial T-cell infiltration. *Cancer Res* 2001;61:842–847.

Yung WK, Prados MD, Yaya-Tur R, et al. Multicenter phase II trial of temozolomide in patients with anaplastic astrocytoma or anaplastic oligoastrocytoma at first relapse. Temodal Brain Tumor Group [published erratum appears in *J Clin Oncol* 1999;17:3693], *J Clin Oncol* 1999;17:2762–2771.

10 PITUITARY TUMORS IN ONCOLOGY

Ian E. McCutcheon

Chapter Overview 191
Introduction 192
Pathology 193
Clinical Presentation 194
    Signs and Symptoms of Compression of the Pituitary Gland 194
    Signs and Symptoms of Excess Secretion of Hormone 195
    Changes in Vision 196
    Headache 197
Laboratory Investigation 197
Radiologic Evaluation 198
Treatment 199
    Why Treat Pituitary Tumors? 199
    Overview of Surgical Treatment of Pituitary Tumors 200
    Specific Tumor Types 202
        Prolactin-Secreting Adenomas 202
        GH-Secreting Adenomas 204
        ACTH-Secreting Adenomas 207
        TSH-Secreting Adenomas 209
        Clinically Nonfunctional Adenomas 210
    Pituitary Tumors Needing No Treatment 212
Malignant Pituitary Tumors 212
Metastases to the Pituitary Gland from Systemic Cancer 215
Special Situations 217
    Cystic Lesions of the Sella Turcica 217
        Cystic Pituitary Adenomas 218
        Rathke's Cleft Cysts 218
        Pars Intermedia Cysts 218
        Craniopharyngiomas 218
    Pituitary Tumors Associated with Tumor Syndromes 219
Key Practice Points 220
Suggested Readings 221

CHAPTER OVERVIEW

Patients with pituitary tumors present to oncologists because their tumors may be causing hormonal disturbance, may be compressing or threatening adjacent critical neural structures, or may pose the possibility of metastasis to the pituitary fossa in those with known cancer elsewhere. This chapter addresses tumors intrinsic to or metastatic to the pituitary gland as well as cystic lesions occurring within the sella turcica. A tumor of the pituitary gland must be distinguished from a tumor intrinsic to the brain because this distinction carries important implications for treatment. Pituitary tumors are common in the general population and are no less common in patients being assessed and treated for malignant neoplasms in other organ systems. In clinical medicine, the pituitary gland and the diseases that afflict it sit at the nexus between the fields of endocrinology and neurosurgery and frequently involve the fields of ophthalmology and radiotherapy. Thus, treating these diseases is somewhat complex and requires a broad understanding of these various fields. In most instances, pituitary tumors are relatively benign and can be controlled; however, invasive or malignant tumors of the pituitary gland pose great challenges to the physician and patient alike.

INTRODUCTION

Tumors of the sella turcica are typically pituitary adenomas and are among the most common intracranial neoplasms. Pituitary tumors are anatomically distinct from tumors of the brain by virtue of their location in the sella turcica beneath the brain. In addition, their clinical behaviors are very different. Although pituitary tumors are much less likely than brain tumors to be malignant, they are located in a sensitive area adjacent to a number of important structures. The currently accepted prevalence of pituitary tumors is 14% in the population at large, although many of these tumors are clinically insignificant and never need medical attention (Ezzat et al, 2004). Pituitary adenomas may cause syndromes of endocrine hypersecretion through tumoral secretion of hormone, cause hypopituitarism by compressing the anterior lobe of the pituitary gland (from which these tumors typically arise), or remain small and cause neither hormonal disturbance nor compression of adjacent critical neural structures.

Modern treatment of pituitary tumors depends on 3 signal advances in medicine that have occurred in the past 40 years. First, increasingly sensitive tests can now measure picomolar levels of the entire panoply of pituitary hormones and can therefore be used to create a profile of pituitary function that indicates whether the gland is functioning properly or secreting excessively. Second, surgical techniques long in abeyance were revived in North America by the energy and drive of Jules Hardy, who in the late 1960s was the first surgeon to report the successful removal of a microadenoma (a pituitary tumor smaller than 10 mm in diameter) (Hardy, 1969). Hardy also developed many of the instruments used in modern transsphenoidal surgery and repopularized this approach to a point that it is now used for 95% of pituitary tumor resections. Third, the introduction of and ongoing improvements in magnetic resonance imaging (MRI) have made increasingly earlier diagnosis of such tumors possible. Microadenomas as small as 2 to 3 mm in diameter can now be detected with this technique.

As recently as 30 years ago, most patients who underwent pituitary surgery had visual loss due to delays in diagnosis that allowed the tumor to extend significantly into the suprasellar space and compress the optic chiasm or optic nerves. Such circumstances still arise occasionally, but the average tumor size at the time of surgery is smaller today, which contributes to the more complete resections now achieved by experienced surgeons. Early detection has also allowed more prompt interruption of the debilitating physiologic changes induced by small endocrinologically active tumors, especially those seen in Cushing's disease.

PATHOLOGY

Most tumors of the pituitary gland are pituitary adenomas. These typically benign lesions arise from the anterior portion of the gland (the adenohypophysis). They grow within a pseudocapsule that sharply separates them from adjacent normal gland, which may be compressed by the tumor to a point that it is invisible on scans, although it is almost always visible during surgery. Most pituitary adenomas arise within the pars distalis of the gland, but some have been reported to arise within the pars tuberalis, a superior extension of the anterior lobe on the anterior surface of the pituitary stalk. In pituitary adenomas, there is loss of the normal acinar pattern of cells and the intervening reticulin network. Pituitary tumor cells are relatively uniform and show small nuclei and scanty cytoplasm.

The current pathologic classification of pituitary adenomas is based on immunohistochemical staining patterns (Asa, 1998). The 6 major hormones of clinical relevance produced by the anterior lobe (prolactin, growth hormone [GH], adrenocorticotropic hormone [ACTH; also called corticotropin], thyrotropin [TSH], follicle-stimulating hormone [FSH], and luteinizing hormone [LH]; the relative incidence of the hormonal types is shown in Table 10–1) can be detected by the application of polyclonal or monoclonal antibodies to tumor sections. Positive immunostaining implies hormone production, but it does not always correlate with actual hormone secretion.

"Nonsecreting" or clinically nonfunctional adenomas make up 40% of pituitary tumors. A significant minority of nonsecreting tumors do synthesize FSH or LH, but these hormones are not secreted or are secreted inefficiently. Indeed, serum levels of FSH and LH are rarely elevated by pituitary tumors. In addition, pituitary tumors occasionally produce hormone that is detectable in serum but biologically inactive in the patient. Despite these caveats, in most patients, the clinical endocrine status correlates quite well

Table 10–1. **Relative Incidence of Sporadic Pituitary Adenomas, by Predominant Hormone Secreted**

Predominant Hormone Secreted	Relative Incidence (%)
Clinically nonfunctional	43
Null cell	70
FSH	15
LH	15
Prolactin	30
GH	14
ACTH	12
TSH	<1

with serum hormone levels and with the levels shown qualitatively within the tumor through immunohistochemical analysis. Tumors that are truly hormonally inactive are called null cell adenomas. Such tumors show negative immunostaining and lack hormone granules when examined by electron microscopy. Additional staining targets that are occasionally used to identify pituitary adenomas are α subunit (which is common to all glycoprotein hormones), chromogranin (which is produced by a variety of neuroendocrine tumors), and synaptophysin.

CLINICAL PRESENTATION

The signs and symptoms seen across the spectrum of pituitary tumors can be classified as those due to compression of an adjacent normal gland, those due to hypersecretion of hormone, changes in optic function, and headache due to dural compression or infiltration. Completely asymptomatic tumors (i.e., incidentalomas) are increasingly found in this era of easy access to MRI. In patients with incidentalomas and indeed in any patient with a pituitary tumor, the standard workup includes high-quality MRI focused on the sella turcica, a complete panel of pituitary hormones, and a comprehensive ophthalmologic evaluation.

Signs and Symptoms of Compression of the Pituitary Gland

The hormone system most vulnerable to extrinsic pressure is the pituitary-gonadal axis. In this axis, minor disturbances of the pulsatile rhythms of FSH or LH production can affect fertility and libido in either sex and can disrupt the menstrual cycle in women. Depression of the pituitary-thyroid and pituitary-adrenal axes may also occur, which in severe cases may induce myxedema or addisonian crisis, respectively.

Other hormone systems can also become inefficient when the anterior lobe of the pituitary gland is compressed. Low levels of prolactin and GH have not traditionally been considered clinically significant. However, over the past 10 years, endocrinologists have reexamined their attitude toward GH replacement (Toogood, 2005). The current consensus is that replacement is reasonable, although quite expensive, if persistently low GH level is detected in association with an overall syndrome of malaise and low energy levels. In patients older than 50 years, close monitoring is necessary to ensure that the exogenous GH does not encourage the growth of other tumors dependent on insulin-like growth factor I (IGF-I) as a primary growth factor (colon cancer being the prime example thereof) (Jenkins et al, 2006).

Tumors arising within the anterior lobe automatically compress the posterior lobe to some extent by virtue of its proximity. The main product of the posterior lobe is vasopressin, the lack of which induces a syndrome of diabetes insipidus with polyuria, polydipsia, hypernatremia, and hyperosmolality. However, patients with pituitary adenomas very rarely present with diabetes insipidus, even when the tumors are large and the compression is great against the posterior lobe. Patients with a newly diagnosed sellar mass and diabetes insipidus generally have either granulomatous involvement of the pituitary stalk or metastasis to the pituitary gland from a systemic cancer.

Signs and Symptoms of Excess Secretion of Hormone

The clinical syndrome seen with pituitary tumors producing excess hormone depends on the hormone produced. The most common syndrome is due to excessive prolactin secreted by a prolactinoma, which causes galactorrhea in both men and women, menstrual irregularity in women, and in many cases infertility and loss of libido in both sexes. Osteoporosis is also an issue if the excess production of prolactin is prolonged.

Tumors secreting GH cause acromegaly, which is characterized by enlargement of the hands and feet, coarsening of facial features, insulin intolerance (leading to diabetes mellitus), and cardiac dysfunction. Acromegaly shortens life expectancy, and the observed-to-expected mortality ratio is 1.6 to 3.3 (Holdaway and Rajasoorya, 1999).

Cushing's disease arises in patients who have tumors that secrete ACTH. In such patients, cortisol excess secondary to overstimulation of the pituitary-adrenal axis has diverse manifestations, reflecting the importance of cortisol in regulating many organ systems. Patients with Cushing's disease show changes in body habitus caused by excess fat deposits; the buffalo hump and moon face are hallmarks. Other signs are abdominal striae, osteoporosis, diabetes mellitus, proximal muscle weakness, and emotional or psychiatric disturbances. The spectrum of the ACTH effect is quite variable from person to person, and some patients present without the characteristic weight gain, show only mild arterial hypertension, or show changes only in skin texture and color.

The least common secretory tumors are those releasing TSH or gonadotropins. TSH-secreting tumors cause hyperthyroidism in many patients. This state is characterized by heat intolerance, tremor, and disturbances of cardiac rhythm. Tumors secreting FSH or LH rarely do so to a level sufficient to cause clinical change, but when they do, the effects on menstruation, fertility, and sex drive are evident. However, unlike prolactinomas, these tumors do not cause galactorrhea unless they are large.

The first step in evaluating patients who have pituitary tumors producing excess hormone involves distinguishing the tumors that secrete prolactin from those that do not. Making this distinction can be difficult. Any mass within the sella turcica that sufficiently distorts the pituitary stalk interrupts the flow of dopamine from the hypothalamus to the anterior pituitary gland. Because prolactin release from the pituitary gland is tonically inhibited by dopamine, interference with the transmission of dopamine to the pituitary gland results in a moderate rise in prolactin (the "stalk effect"). Only patients with prolactin levels higher than 100 ng/mL can be safely assumed to have a true prolactinoma, and even they are occasionally found to have nontumoral causes for the high level. The most common alternative cause of an elevated prolactin level is the use of psychotropic drugs such as risperidone, about which the physician should inquire in any patient presenting with prolactin excess (Molitch, 2005). Patients who have serum prolactin levels lower than 100 ng/mL may harbor a smaller or less efficient prolactinoma but also may simply show physiologic hyperprolactinemia from impaired stalk function. The cause must be determined because tumors secreting prolactin are usually amenable to medical therapy, whereas tumors that secrete other hormones or are nonfunctional usually require surgery. Because there is a rough correlation between prolactin level and tumor size, an astute clinician can often decide this issue by comparing these 2 features, but in some patients the distinction can be made only by pathologic analysis of excised tumor tissue.

Changes in Vision

Vision can be affected in 2 ways by a pituitary tumor. Most commonly, loss of peripheral vision occurs when the tumor grows into the suprasellar cistern and compresses the optic chiasm, optic nerve, or both from below. This defect is usually bitemporal, beginning in the upper outer quadrants of the visual field and progressing to complete bitemporal hemianopia in severe cases. However, the position of the chiasm relative to the stalk is variable, so the presentation is not stereotypical. With longstanding compression of the optic apparatus comes optic atrophy visible on funduscopic examination, which results in permanent loss of visual acuity and perhaps decreased color vision. The less common disturbance of vision occurs when the tumor extends into or compresses the cavernous sinus. Such a lesion can disturb the function of the third, fourth, or sixth cranial nerve on the affected side, resulting in diplopia and, if the oculomotor nerve is affected, ptosis and pupillary dilitation.

Headache

Headache as a symptom has very poor sensitivity and specificity for the detection of intracranial disease. Many patients with pituitary tumors describe headache as part of their symptoms, and indeed it may lead to the performance of the scan that discloses the tumor. Nevertheless, headache is often simply coincidental with pituitary tumors, particularly in patients with small, noninvasive tumors. Even large tumors extending far from the sella turcica or those invading or compressing the pain-sensitive dura mater of the sella and cavernous sinus wall show little correlation between tumor size and degree of headache. At M. D. Anderson Cancer Center, we routinely tell patients that the only proof that the headache results from the pituitary tumor comes when surgical cure of the tumor resolves the headache. However, in many patients, an excellent resection is obtained but the headache persists and requires treatment by medical means.

Sudden severe headache suggests a sudden increase in the size and composition of a preexisting pituitary tumor. In such patients, hemorrhage within the pituitary adenoma produces an apoplectic syndrome of acute headache and sudden neurologic decline caused by bleeding across the diaphragma sellae into the subarachnoid space, acute compression of the sellar dura mater or the adjacent cavernous sinuses, or compression of the hypothalamus or its vascular supply. These patients often have coincident acute diplopia and may have a sudden decrease in vision. Hemorrhaging tumors require urgent surgical excision to maximize the chances for recovery of visual function (Randeva et al, 1999).

Laboratory Investigation

In the standard laboratory workup of a patient with a suspected pituitary tumor, a panel of hormones is measured to provide both direct and indirect evidence of the hormone function directed from the tumor and from the normal pituitary gland. At M. D. Anderson, new patients are routinely assessed for levels of prolactin, TSH, FSH, LH, IGF-I, testosterone (in men), estradiol (in women), and cortisol. Interpretation of these hormone values can be somewhat complex, since normal values vary with age (e.g., IGF-I) or time of day (e.g., cortisol), depend on the phase of the menstrual cycle (e.g., FSH and LH), or require measurement of a second messenger hormone for proper interpretation (e.g., TSH levels cannot be interpreted properly unless L-thyroxine [T_4] and sometimes α subunit are measured as well to allow differentiation of pituitary hypersecretion from the elevation of TSH caused by primary thyroid insufficiency). In women, the estradiol level is a fairly sensitive index of gonadal failure, but it cannot be interpreted in the absence of concomitant levels of FSH and LH. The ACTH level is not usually measured directly because it is normal in many patients with Cushing's disease. In addition, assays of ACTH tend to be inaccurate because proteases in plasma degrade the sample unless inhibitors are added and the tube is kept chilled (which is rarely done in practice). The activity of the pituitary-adrenal axis is better assessed by measuring levels of cortisol, which is one of the main adrenal hormones produced in response to adrenocorticotropic stimulation. Because both cortisol and ACTH are produced according to a diurnal rhythm, standard measurement of serum cortisol levels is performed at 8:00 a.m., when these levels are relatively high. Occasionally, dynamic testing is necessary to determine the pituitary hormone reserve from the normal gland. This testing is largely confined to after surgery and to patients undergoing a workup for Cushing's disease, for whom the results may allow the source of excess ACTH to be pinpointed.

After a suitable interval following surgical excision of a pituitary tumor, baseline hormone values are remeasured. Early testing of cortisol function on the first postoperative day has been advocated, but in general there is no standard point at which to take such measurements. In Cushing's disease in particular, gradual restoration of normal hormone levels may take up to 3 months; thus, some patients can appear to have persistent disease at first when in fact the disease ultimately goes into remission (Pereira et al, 2003). If a hormone deficit exists before surgery, restoration to at least a partial degree will occur in 50% of patients, but 15% of patients will show new deficits in anterior pituitary function (Webb et al, 1999).

The function of the posterior lobe is initially assessed by taking a careful patient history of urinary frequency and thirst pattern and measuring serum glucose and sodium levels. A normal blood glucose level (ideally in the fasting state) rules out diabetes mellitus, and patients with normal sodium levels have a normal vasopressin level or have compensated for its lack by increasing fluid intake. Diabetes insipidus exists in very few patients seen in consultation for suspected pituitary tumor, but it occurs much more frequently after surgery, when about 15% to 20% of patients show the phenomenon transiently and about 0.5% permanently. By contrast, at least half of patients with metastatic cancer involving the pituitary gland present with diabetes insipidus. These patients do not recover posterior lobe function with surgical decompression and require lifelong hormone replacement with desmopressin, which is a synthetic analog of vasopressin administered by nasal spray or as a pill.

RADIOLOGIC EVALUATION

The best method of imaging the pituitary fossa and adjacent structures is MRI. The advantages of such imaging over older forms (e.g., computed tomography, skull radiography, and angiography) are so great that it does not make sense to initiate evaluation of a patient today by any other technique. Improvements in MRI sensitivity now allow detection of tumors as small as 2 mm in diameter. A pituitary adenoma is typically seen on contrast scans as hypointense or isointense relative to brain tissue, whereas normal gland is slightly hyperintense due to the absence of the blood-brain barrier in its vasculature. The best delineation of tumor from normal gland occurs in scans performed 2 to 5 minutes after the intravenous injection of gadolinium. However, even tumors larger than 2 to 3 mm in diameter sometimes escape detection on scans if they produce a signal that is truly isointense to that of normal gland, and some patients with microadenomas at surgery show no abnormality on preoperative MR images. The latter phenomenon occurs primarily in Cushing's disease; in patients with this disease, no tumor may be visible on MR images even though biochemical testing can pinpoint a tumor to the sella turcica in a patient with profound clinical evidence of the disease, which can be caused by even small disturbances in the rhythm or level of ACTH secretion from a minute tumor. Thus, MRI is most useful in declaring the presence of a pituitary tumor, but it is not required for that diagnosis. MRI also assists in delineating the extent of the tumor and the structure of the sphenoid sinus, the knowledge of which is very helpful in conducting surgery safely.

TREATMENT

Why Treat Pituitary Tumors?

The clinical significance of small, nonfunctional pituitary adenomas is hotly debated. It is likely that such tumors can be left alone and watched on scans performed at intervals. Most will not grow or cause problems for the patient. On the other hand, hormonally active tumors, even small ones, usually require treatment to prevent the long-term sequelae of hypersecretion. Patients with Cushing's disease or acromegaly rarely reach normal life expectancy because of the diseases' untoward effects on a variety of organ systems, particularly the cardiovascular system. Acromegaly also imposes a 3-fold excess risk of carcinoma of the colon, and patients with uncontrolled GH excess require ongoing screening for polyps by colonoscopy. Patients with prolactinomas may require treatment to correct the infertility that such tumors impose and to prevent accelerated osteoporosis. TSH-secreting tumors are quite disruptive and also adversely affect the heart. Finally, any pituitary tumor, functional or nonfunctional, that reaches the optic chiasm can endanger vision, and an increasing field cut is an absolute indication for surgical intervention, no matter what hormone the tumor secretes. As a whole, patients with pituitary tumors are twice as likely to die in any given year than is the population at large (Nilsson et al, 2000).

Treatment of pituitary tumors aims at eliminating hormone excess, preventing optic nerve dysfunction, restoring or preserving normal pituitary function, avoiding complications from therapy, and preventing tumor regrowth. These aims apply to any treatment—medical, surgical, or radiologic—used to control or cure pituitary neoplasms.

Overview of Surgical Treatment of Pituitary Tumors

Transsphenoidal surgery allows entry into the sella turcica in the safest possible way in any patient with a small pituitary tumor and no or moderate extrasellar extension. In this approach, the surgeon does not enter the intracranial compartment and uses a midline trajectory that avoids cranial nerves and carotid arteries to either side of the gland. The incision in such surgery can be placed along the mucosa on the inner surface of the upper lip or along the mucoperichondrium overlying the nasal septum within the nasal cavity. These routes are referred to as the sublabial and endonasal approaches, respectively. In the former, numbness of the upper front teeth persists for 6 to 8 weeks after surgery. In the latter, nasal ache may occur but is transient. Both approaches lead to the same corridor of access to the sella turcica, and ideally a surgeon should be adept at both.

Transsphenoidal approaches are used for tumors confined to the sella turcica, but they can also be valuable in debulking tumors with extrasellar extension. Tumors with suprasellar extension causing optic nerve compression may be completely removable through transsphenoidal surgery, but tumors with lateral extension may require craniotomy. Some patients with complex tumors require a staged approach that starts with a transsphenoidal operation to remove midline components of the tumor and ends with craniotomy to complete the decompression of the optic apparatus (Figure 10–1). Tumors that extend into the cavernous sinus usually elude complete surgical excision, and at M. D. Anderson, these extensions are typically removed only when the tumor growth is relentless in that area, endangers optic nerve function, or has already shut down function in cranial nerves traversing the cavernous sinus (i.e., by creating ptosis and loss of eye movements).

Endoscopy has become increasingly popular in pituitary surgery in the past 5 years. As endoscopic instrumentation has developed with better optics and differently angled scopes, it has been applied as an adjunct to open surgery to allow visualization of the tumor laterally placed in the sella turcica or superiorly placed over the tuberculum sellae or as the primary tool for visualization (replacing the operative microscope). Although endoscopy certainly can be used to extend the surgeon's reach, no randomized study comparing endoscopic versus classic open removal of pituitary tumors has been performed. As in transsphenoidal surgery, the surgical outcome of endoscopy is highly dependent on the surgeon's experience. At M. D. Anderson, endoscopy is currently used

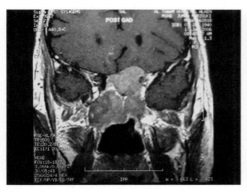 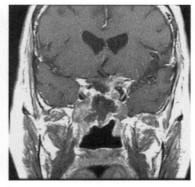

A   B

Figure 10–1. A 65-year-old man underwent transsphenoidal surgery to remove a clinically nonfunctional pituitary macroadenoma and then sellar radiotherapy. Ten years later, after he developed a homonymous hemianopia, coronal, postcontrast MR images showed a large recurrence filling the sphenoid sinus, sella turcica, and suprasellar cistern with obscuration of the bony outlines of the sella turcica and compression of the optic apparatus (A). This tumor was incompletely (90%) removed by a second transsphenoidal surgery, and a craniotomy was performed to resect residual suprasellar tumor encasing the left optic nerve (B). This combination of approaches restored the patient's vision and achieved gross total removal of the tumor. The patient remains at high risk for recurrence but cannot undergo radiotherapy again for fear of inducing an optic neuropathy.

to examine areas within the sella turcica or sphenoid sinus that cannot be directly seen; the most common of these areas is the medial wall of the cavernous sinus.

Additional adjuncts useful in surgery include computer-assisted navigation and intraoperative MRI. In the former, the surgeon uses an optically tracked pointer to overlay the tumor location in a virtual 3-dimensional space on the multiplanar MR images captured preoperatively. This technology is useful in skull base surgery, but for most pituitary tumors confined to the immediate environs of the sella turcica, it is a relatively expensive and not necessarily superior alternative to fluoroscopy, which defines the surgical trajectory in a sagittal plane just as well as more complicated equipment does. Intraoperative MRI is available at only a few centers, but it provides a valuable means of identifying residual tumor that may escape the notice of the surgeon within the difficult anatomy of the sellar region (Bohinski et al, 2001). However, as with most new technologies, it remains debatable whether these new tools in the hands of an inexperienced surgeon confer facility equal to that of a seasoned surgeon with extensive transsphenoidal experience using established techniques.

Specific Tumor Types

Prolactin-Secreting Adenomas

Although 30% of pituitary adenomas secrete prolactin, such tumors represent a minority in surgical practice because they are generally treated medically before surgery is considered. The current medical therapy of choice is the dopamine agonist cabergoline, which inhibits prolactin release (Verhelst et al, 1999). A positive response to this drug (i.e., normalization of prolactin levels and cessation of tumor growth) occurs in up to 90% of patients taking it. However, the adverse effects, which include nausea, vomiting, orthostatic hypotension, and occasional psychotic reactions, occur in 10% to 15% of patients and therefore limit its use. Older drugs such as bromocriptine are still used but are less convenient for patients. One reason is that bromocriptine is given several times a day, whereas cabergoline is administered twice weekly; therefore, use of the latter drug increases compliance and thus drug efficacy. Another reason is that because cabergoline is a D_2 receptor-specific agonist, it tends to provoke fewer adverse effects than bromocriptine, which affects both D_1 and D_2 receptors. Patients who cannot tolerate bromocriptine can often tolerate cabergoline. Typically, prolactin levels are normalized in 80% to 90% of patients treated with a dopamine agonist, but tumor shrinkage occurs in two thirds or less.

The response to medical therapy in patients with prolactinomas depends on the tumor size and the prolactin level. Patients with smaller tumors and lower prolactin levels respond best. If the prolactin level before treatment is higher than 1,000 ng/mL (the normal level is less than 25 ng/mL), the level usually decreases with medical therapy but does not normalize. Most prolactinomas cause hormone elevation in the range of 50 to 250 ng/mL, and 80% to 90% of patients with this level of prolactin show normalization of the hormone level, tumor reduction, or both in response to dopamine agonist therapy.

Many patients with prolactinomas receive dopamine agonist therapy year after year. It is, however, entirely appropriate to stop treatment in patients who have received it for at least 2 years to determine whether high prolactin levels recur after long-term suppression. After cabergoline is withdrawn, 10% of patients whose tumors have completely regressed show no recrudescence of their prolactin excess (Biswas et al, 2005). For this reason, we recommend stopping drug therapy at biennial or triennial intervals and monitoring hormone levels and scans for any sign of tumor recurrence.

Surgery for prolactinomas is used when medical treatment fails or is not completely successful or if a patient cannot tolerate the adverse effects of dopamine agonists (Hamilton et al, 2005). These drugs induce some fibrosis within the tumor and may make tumor excision more difficult and tumor delineation from normal gland more problematic. As a result, it is best to decide no later than 6 to 12 months after initiating medical therapy whether surgery will be used.

Surgical excision is most successful for microadenomas and tumors showing prolactin levels in the lower end of the abnormal range (i.e., 50 to 100 ng/mL). Most smaller tumors (85% to 90%) can be completely resected, but patients with larger tumors and tumors that express higher prolactin levels (which correspond to larger tumors) are less readily cured. For instance, 90% of patients with microadenomas and 40% of patients with tumors producing more than 200 ng/mL prolactin, but only 6% of patients with tumors producing more than 1,000 ng/mL prolactin, will go into remission after surgery (Tyrrell et al, 1999). Fifteen years after surgery, 15% of patients who experience initial remission will have relapsed to hyperprolactinemia.

Radiotherapy is generally reserved for patients in whom regrowth has occurred and who do not wish to pursue further surgery. It is also used when a complete excision cannot be achieved because of tumor infiltration into the adjacent dura mater or into the cavernous sinus. In external beam radiotherapy, a fractionated dose of 45 to 50 Gy is given over 4 to 6 weeks by a limited-field technique that excludes structures outside a 4-cm window centered on the sella turcica. This technique is quite effective in controlling most residual prolactinomas. However, the proximity of most irradiated tumors to normal gland and parapituitary structures can lead to gradual onset of hypopituitarism (typically over 5 years and occurring in 50% of patients) or optic neuropathy (rare, but showing a similar time course). Radiotherapy works better on small tumors than on large ones, and it may take several years after completion of treatment for the prolactin level to go as low as it ever will.

To focus the beam of radiation on the tumor target and exclude non-neoplastic tissue, techniques for stereotactic localization and delivery have been developed (Brada et al, 2004). These techniques usually involve attachment of a stereotactic ring to the patient's head with fiducial markers that can be used to transform the 2-dimensional space of the images into a composite 3-dimensional space. Although in theory stereotactic techniques such as the linear accelerator or the Gamma Knife reduce the risk of radiation damage to normal structures, the pituitary gland is still typically within the field and thus hypopituitarism is not always prevented. Radiation damage to the medial temporal lobe is also occasionally seen, but this damage is usually asymptomatic and clears with time. When the cavernous sinuses are included in the radiation field, 10% to 15% of patients develop cranial neuropathy within 3 years of stereotactic radiotherapy (Tischler et al, 1993). The practical limitation in applying radiosurgical techniques is simply a question of distance. For the safe delivery of a concentrated dose of radiation to a pituitary tumor, the edge of the tumor must be 5 mm or more from the nearest edge of the optic apparatus. Thus, most patients with macroadenomas do not qualify for radiosurgery. At M. D. Anderson, in many instances we debulk a tumor by transsphenoidal surgery to remove all of the tumor except the portion within the cavernous sinus, which is more safely treated with radiosurgery.

In current practice at M. D. Anderson, patients with prolactinomas are first offered cabergoline. If they cannot tolerate its adverse effects, they then typically undergo surgery. Those with progressive visual loss due to a macroadenoma are treated with surgery if their vision is quite tenuous, but a minor field cut still permits the use of cabergoline instead of surgery, and this vision deficit often clears as the tumor shrinks over the ensuing several months. Radiotherapy is reserved for those few patients in whom tumors regrow after surgery or whose tumors cannot be completely excised, as determined using radiographic or biochemical criteria.

GH-Secreting Adenomas

The mainstay of treatment for GH-secreting tumors is surgery. These tumors are usually relatively small when found, since even small tumors can elevate GH levels significantly. Although there has been some enthusiasm for preoperative treatment with octreotide, a short-acting somatostatin analog, we have not found this agent to be particularly helpful and it is not routinely used at M. D. Anderson. Octreotide can shrink tumors by 10% to 20%, which is not enough to make surgery easier or to warrant the inconvenience and delay imposed by such therapy.

Drugs used against GH-secreting tumors include both short-acting and long-acting somatostatin analogs. The latter have become more popular for obvious reasons. The short-acting analogs require injection as often as 3 times daily, whereas the long-acting versions (e.g., octreotide LA) can be given monthly. In some patients, somatostatin analogs cause gastrointestinal upset or gallstones, which may limit the use of these drugs. Dopamine agonists have also been used against GH-producing tumors, but they work for only 10% to 20% of patients, which compares poorly with octreotide, which reduces GH levels in 70% to 80% of patients. Bromocriptine has limited use in managing acromegaly, whereas cabergoline works almost as well as the somatostatin analogs in some patients. Because cabergoline is an oral medication and is significantly cheaper than octreotide, it may be a reasonable alternative. Other drugs, including radionuclide-labeled preparations, that target somatostatin receptors are now being studied and will likely become part of the menu of therapy for acromegaly (Oberg, 2004).

Maximal resection via a transsphenoidal approach is the first step in managing GH-secreting tumors (Figure 10–2). If GH and IGF-I levels are still high after surgery, drug therapy is instituted. Radiotherapy is quite effective, but it puts the long-term integrity of normal gland in jeopardy, so we reserve this modality for patients whose tumors are refractory to medical therapy and for patients who prefer to avoid lifelong injections.

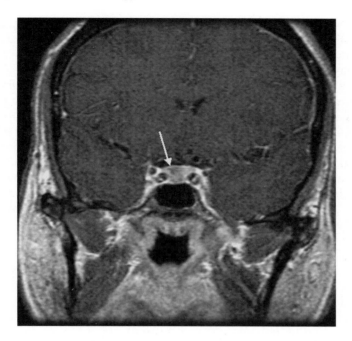

Figure 10–2. A 54-year-old woman presented with a multinodular goiter; during thyroidectomy, a follicular adenoma on a hyperplastic background was found. Workup revealed an elevated IGF-I level, and acromegaly was noted on physical examination. Coronal, postcontrast MR images of the sella turcica showed a focal area of hypointensity consistent with pituitary adenoma (arrow), which was resected by transsphenoidal surgery. The acromegaly regressed, and IGF-I levels decreased significantly but did not normalize. The patient was offered octreotide LA or pegvisomant, but she declined medical therapy. Sellar radiotherapy induced a slow decrease of the IGF-I level to normal over the next 18 months. Because GH and IGF-I are growth factors for some tumors, it is interesting to speculate on the role that this patient's longstanding acromegaly had in promoting the initiation or growth of the thyroid neoplasm.

The most recent addition to the medical menu for treating acromegaly is the GH receptor antagonist pegvisomant, which eliminates clinical acromegaly without directly affecting tumor growth (Trainer et al, 2000). Pegvisomant is a relatively new drug, so its value in long-term use has not been established. There is some concern, however, that pegvisomant may allow unchecked tumor growth over time and thereby endanger vision and anterior pituitary function, since its mechanism of action decreases the potential negative feedback by IGF-I at the level of the pituitary gland. Thus far, such fears have not been realized, but follow-up over at least 10 years is needed before any conclusion can be drawn.

The physiologic changes that accompany acromegaly make surgery on GH-secreting tumors challenging and more technically difficult than in any other type of pituitary tumor except ACTH-secreting tumors. Anesthetic considerations include the potential for difficult intubation due to macroglossia and soft tissue hypertrophy around the larynx, the possibility of cardiomyopathy in longstanding cases, and the presence of arterial hypertension and diabetes mellitus in many patients. From the neurosurgeon's perspective, difficulty of access can arise due to the narrowed nasal passage imposed by osseous hypertrophy of the midface, particularly the occasional presence of a tortuous carotid artery wandering as far as the midline, where it may sit directly along the trajectory of the surgical approach and may be a potentially fatal trap. GH-secreting tumors also tend to infiltrate the sellar dura mater more than other tumors do, such that a complete macroscopic and radiographic resection may still be associated with ongoing GH excess, albeit at a lower level than before surgery. In patients with GH-secreting tumors, the hormone excess is usually controlled relatively easily by somatostatin analogs but frustrates the surgeon and causes further inconvenience to the patient. Surgical success has been defined differently by different authors, but the most vigorous modern definition of "remission" requires a GH level of 2.3 ng/mL or less. Although IGF-I levels are theoretically more reliable measures of ongoing hormonal status, they have not been used as extensively in reporting patient outcomes. Overall, about 85% of patients with microadenomas and 40% to 50% of patients with macroadenomas achieve postsurgical remission. This remission is sustained in 60% to 80% of patients overall (Nomikos et al, 2005).

Treatment failure is usually due to residual pituitary adenoma in the sella turcica or invading through the dura mater of the cavernous sinus wall. Rarely, treatment failure is due to a primary hypothalamic gangliocytoma secreting GH or GH-releasing hormone or to an ectopic site, usually the pancreas, secreting GH-releasing hormone. Such cases can be identified by measuring the plasma level of GH-releasing hormone: if it is higher than 300 ng/mL, an ectopic source is likely.

Radiotherapy can be applied to GH-secreting adenomas. Its success rate is similar to that for other secretory tumor types, although truly rigorous biochemical definitions of remission, including normalization of both GH and IGF-I levels, are generally absent in reported series. When radiotherapy is used, GH and IGF-I levels normalize an average of 1.4 years after radiosurgery, but after conventional fractioned radiotherapy, the mean time to normalization is 7.1 years (Landolt et al, 1998). Regardless, the relative risk of radiosurgery versus fractionated radiotherapy is not well understood. For example, a patient treated at M. D. Anderson had a GH-secreting adenoma that transformed to a sarcoma. We believe this conversion was fostered by the radiotherapy used to treat the postsurgical tumor residue (Prabhu et al, 2003). A review of the literature suggests that sarcomatous transformation is more common in irradiated GH-secreting tumors than in other irradiated pituitary tumor types. Thus, caution should be exercised by administering such treatment only to patients who truly need it.

ACTH-Secreting Adenomas

By definition, patients with ACTH-secreting pituitary tumors have Cushing's disease. Hypercortisolism from an unspecified extrapituitary source is denoted as Cushing's syndrome, and 70% of patients with true hypercortisolism do indeed have a pituitary tumor. The remaining 30% have a variety of underlying causes, such as an adrenal adenoma or hyperplasia, an ectopic ACTH-secreting carcinoma of the lung, or even exogenous steroid administration. The endocrine workup for a patient with suspected Cushing's disease is much more complicated than that for a patient with any other pituitary tumor; please refer to Nieman and Ilias (2005) for a full description of that workup. The basic purposes of the workup are to confirm that hypercortisolism is indeed present and to identify the source of the hypercortisolism. Diagnosis can be difficult because even the sensitive MRI of today fails to show a tumor in 20% to 30% of patients with pituitary-based Cushing's syndrome. Biochemical evaluation of patients with Cushing's disease must take into account the normal diurnal variation in the levels of ACTH and cortisol. Such episodic secretion still occurs when an adenoma is present, but neoplastic corticotrophs are relatively insensitive to negative feedback from glucocorticoids of any source. Such tumors are therefore relatively autonomous, and only a third show evidence of sensitivity to hypothalamic control. Cortisol excess is recognized by determining whether the blood levels are appropriate to the time of day that the samples were collected, and even more effectively, by collecting urine over 24 hours to eliminate diurnal variation. Salivary sampling, which is now available in many centers, adds a measure of convenience to cortisol determination. When confusion persists after several rounds of blood and urine collection, provocative tests are used to clarify the presence of true hypercortisolism and to establish its etiology. The most popular is the dexamethasone suppression test, which is available in several variations and is 90% accurate. Stimulation tests using corticotrophin-releasing factor, which causes a normal or excessive increase in ACTH level in patients with Cushing's disease, are also used, but they induce little response in patients with tumors at other sites. This test is also 90% accurate.

Much has been published about the utility of bilateral sampling of the inferior petrosal sinus. This technique compares ACTH levels in blood collected from the petrosal sinus through a transvenous catheter with ACTH levels in peripheral blood. In theory, this method should detect a central-to-peripheral gradient that confirms the presence of a pituitary tumor, and it may also lateralize an occult tumor to the right or left side of the gland. In practice, the test is useful for confirming a suspicion of a pituitary tumor, but intermixing of blood between the 2 cavernous sinuses frequently leads to inaccurate lateralization. The rate of false lateralization approaches 45%, so we do not use this test for lateralizing at M. D. Anderson. Adding stimulation by corticotrophin-releasing factor increases the accuracy of this method to almost 100% when a central-to-peripheral gradient of ACTH less than 3.0 is used as the criterion for a positive diagnosis.

Almost all patients with Cushing's disease undergo transsphenoidal surgery as first-line treatment. Most ACTH-secreting pituitary tumors are microadenomas, and as such, the transsphenoidal approach is appropriate and achieves a cure rate of 80% to 90% in skilled hands. Surgery is always more fraught with technical difficulty and potential complications in patients with Cushing's disease than in patients with other pituitary tumor types. Because of the poor medical condition often seen in patients with chronic cortisol excess, presurgical planning requires a good understanding of the patient's baseline cardiac status. Patients with Cushing's disease have vascular fragility and bleed more easily during surgery. In addition, the typically small size of ACTH-secreting adenomas has 2 implications. (1) The dura mater of the sellar floor is not thinned by pressure from the adjacent tumor and thus venous channels present in normal patients do not disappear. For this reason, it may be difficult to control bleeding from this site, which can obscure the intrasellar contents. (2) The tumor may not be immediately evident, and careful exploration may be necessary to discover it. MR images can be useful in guiding the surgeon to the appropriate location within the pituitary gland. However, a significant percentage of patients with Cushing's disease have subtle or occult tumors that MR images do not show well. In such cases, systematic exploration of the gland is performed using a series of vertical cuts that do not harm its secretory capacity. At M. D. Anderson, we do not rely on lateralization data from petrosal sinus sampling because these data have little better than 50% accuracy at most institutions, including ours. If the tumor cannot be found, a hemihypophysectomy can be performed to remove about 40% of the bulk of the anterior lobe on the side suspected of harboring the tumor. Although some authors advocate a complete hypophysectomy in such cases, we believe it is better to remove half the gland because treatment failure can be converted to success by subsequent use of stereotactic radiosurgery to maintain intact pituitary function for 3 to 5 years before hypopituitarism sets in. Remission of macroadenomas occurs in two thirds of patients after surgery, and the relapse rate of patients whose tumors (of any size) initially go into remission is 5% over 4 years and 10% over 10 years. Patients with macroadenomas relapse sooner and more often than do patients with smaller tumors.

On occasion, a tumor is not found during surgery or a patient does not go into remission after partial or total removal of the anterior lobe of the pituitary gland. In such cases, one must suspect a misdiagnosis of a pituitary source for Cushing's syndrome, and a renewed search should be instituted for other causes of cortisol excess. It is therefore of paramount importance that a rigorous review of endocrine data be conducted by the endocrinologist and the surgeon in concert before plans are made to resect a pituitary tumor in someone with suspected Cushing's disease, particularly if no tumor is visible on MR images.

Radiotherapy is infrequently used as the primary treatment for ACTH-secreting adenomas because these tumors are slow to respond to ionizing radiation and because this therapy puts anterior pituitary function at risk. In some centers, stereotactic radiosurgery has been used as the primary treatment for a number of patients. However, for patients who have microadenomas, radiosurgical targeting is not sufficiently precise to exclude the pituitary gland from the radiation field. The dose of radiation given in the typical single fraction is 20 Gy or more and may induce hypopituitarism. Therefore, at M. D. Anderson, we prefer to use surgery as first-line therapy, especially since it cures a significant proportion of patients without inducing hypopituitarism, and to reserve stereotactic radiosurgery as second-line therapy. Ablation of the adrenal glands has been performed in years past but carries the risk of inducing Nelson's syndrome, in which a previously quiescent adenoma of the pituitary gland converts to a more aggressive form due to loss of negative feedback from the adrenal gland. Therefore, adrenal gland ablation is a third-line treatment at our institution.

In summary, when Cushing's disease is suspected, patients are subjected to a rigorous and lengthy endocrine evaluation before any treatment is considered. The evaluation includes the repeated sampling of blood for morning cortisol measurement and the collection of 24-hour urine volumes to prove hypersecretion. Because some patients harbor tumors that secrete cortisol episodically, patients with appropriate symptoms who fail to show cortisol excess on 1 or 2 samples are repeatedly evaluated. Most go on to dexamethasone suppression testing, but petrosal sinus sampling is considered for patients in whom no radiographic abnormality can be seen on MR images of the sella turcica. At that point, surgery—typically a transsphenoidal approach with vigorous exploration of the sella turcica—is planned. The stakes for a patient with Cushing's disease are quite high in light of the significant detriment this disease has on quality of life and life expectancy. After surgery, testing is repeated over the first 2 to 3 months; should cortisol excess persist, MR imaging is repeated to detect further surgically resectable tumor. In the absence of such tumor, radiosurgery is then considered.

TSH-Secreting Adenomas

Tumors secreting TSH are the rarest class of pituitary tumors and form less than 1% of tumors in any large series. The rarity is probably exaggerated by the tendency of physicians to misdiagnose these cases as primary hyperthyroidism, which is much more common than the hyperthyroid syndrome typically produced by such pituitary tumors. The typical patient with TSH-secreting adenoma has been misdiagnosed with primary thyroid disease for years, and many have been treated with thyroid gland ablation without success. The delay, and likely the ablation, allow the tumor to enlarge, become more invasive, and to resist complete surgical removal. However, when such tumors are found early, they can be cured surgically. In the largest series of TSH-secreting adenomas to date, which was compiled in Belgium, long-term remission was achieved by a combination of surgery and radiotherapy or octreotide-based therapy in 40% to 50% of patients (Socin et al, 2003).

A detectable level of TSH in the early postoperative period indicates the possibility of incomplete resection. Radiotherapy is a common adjunct to surgery for these patients. Bromocriptine will not control these tumors, but the somatostatin analog octreotide can control excess secretion, and in some patients this drug will cause gross tumor shrinkage. The workup of patients with TSH-secreting pituitary adenomas before and after surgery should include determination of the molar ratio of α subunit to TSH. An elevated ratio implies an imbalance between the production of α and β subunits that combine to form a complete TSH molecule. This phenomenon is seen in pituitary tumors but not in normal thyrotrophs. Endocrine assessment of patients with an elevated ratio is complicated for those who have previously been treated inappropriately with thyroid gland ablation. Such patients may have hypothyroidism rather than hyperthyroidism due to end-organ failure, so obtaining a careful medical history is mandatory when a TSH-secreting adenoma is suspected.

A word of caution about a related pitfall in assessing any patient with pituitary gland enlargement: primary hypothyroidism may itself cause thyrotroph hyperplasia and lead to pituitary gland enlargement, which can mimic an adenoma. Patients with primary hypothyroidism have a symmetrically enlarged pituitary gland of homogeneous appearance. They should not undergo transsphenoidal surgery but instead should be given exogenous thyroxine, which will allow resolution of the pituitary gland enlargement as the euthyroid state is restored.

Clinically Nonfunctional Adenomas

Clinically nonfunctional adenomas include true null cell adenomas secreting no hormone of any kind, α subunit–secreting adenomas producing no active hormone, and secretory tumors producing hormone in amounts too small to cause clinical changes in endocrine function. In the last category, many tumors produce FSH, LH, or both as assessed by immunohistochemical analysis. Such gonadotropin-secreting tumors exist on a spectrum that at the lower end includes tumors previously classified as nonsecreting and at the higher end includes tumors that produce detectable elevations of gonadotropin in the peripheral blood.

About 40% of pituitary adenomas are clinically nonfunctional. These tumors produce symptoms only by compressing the pituitary gland (causing hypopituitarism) or the optic apparatus (causing visual loss). About half of such "nonfunctional" tumors stain positively for 1 or more glycoprotein hormones or their subunits (α or β). The lack of clinical activity stems from the inefficient release of hormone or from the production of hormone with low bioactivity. Treatment for these tumors is largely surgical (Figure 10–3). Medical therapy in this circumstance tends to encompass only hormone supplementation to correct deficiencies in pituitary function.

Because of the adherence of a tumor to the dura mater or its invasion of parasellar structures, surgical excision is incomplete in a significant number of cases, and some clinicians argue that residual tumor should be treated with radiotherapy to prevent regrowth. On the basis of published series and a review of our own quite extensive case series at M. D. Anderson, we believe that at least 90% of residual fragments are devascularized and do not grow over time and that further treatment should be reserved for the 10% that prove their growth potential (Park et al, 2004). For many of the tumors that do regrow, we resect again. If ongoing tumor growth is ultimately proven in a location such as the cavernous sinus, where a truly complete elimination of tumor cannot be safely achieved, we offer radiotherapy using focal stereotactic or conformal techniques and a limited field. We strive for maximal resection of pituitary tumors

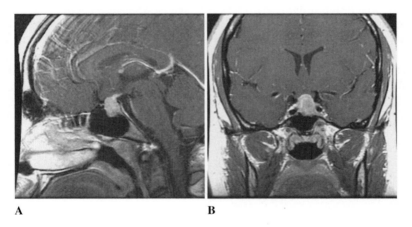

A   **B**

Figure 10–3. A 17-year-old girl with a significant history of psychosis and behavioral problems presented with intractable headache and subjective loss of vision unconfirmed by perimetry. Her serum prolactin level was normal. Postcontrast sagittal (A) and coronal (B) MR images showed a tumor extending from the sella turcica into the suprasellar cistern, where the optic chiasm is lifted slightly. During transsphenoidal surgery, the tumor was found to be a (benign) pituitary adenoma producing ACTH. Because the patient had no evidence of cortisol excess before surgery, the tumor was considered clinically nonfunctional. The patient is being monitored for recurrence with serial imaging.

and suggest annual follow-up for 5 to 7 years after resection. Typically, radiotherapy follows a second surgery only if further residual tumor still exists or if the pathologic appearance of the tumor has changed after the first resection in a way that suggests anaplasia.

Gonadotropin-secreting tumors are treated in a similar way as true null cell adenomas are. The main reason to distinguish between them is the possibility of treating the former medically. Because dopamine suppresses gonadotropin secretion in the normal pituitary gland, bromocriptine or cabergoline is occasionally used to manage FSH- or LH-secreting adenomas. Efforts at securing consistently effective medical therapy for such tumors are ongoing. Current interest is centered on strategies to manipulate gonadotropin-releasing hormone, the hypothalamic factor that controls FSH and LH release by normal pituitary cells.

Pituitary Tumors Needing No Treatment

In the MRI era, patients frequently consult us after a pituitary tumor has been found on a scan that was performed to investigate unrelated complaints such as persistent headache or dizziness. At M. D. Anderson, these patients receive an endocrine workup to search for pituitary hyperfunction. If the workup results are negative, the tumors are called "incidentalomas" and are followed conservatively without active treatment. The chance of such a small tumor showing growth over time is unknown. Although macroadenomas typically need treatment, microadenomas must be analyzed carefully from a hormonal standpoint before any decisions about therapy are made. Even the secretory microadenomas can sometimes be managed conservatively, although only prolactinomas are ever treated this way. Prolactinomas may spontaneously involute, or their ability to oversecrete may strengthen with time. In a study of 30 patients with small prolactinomas who were not treated at all, 14 showed no change in prolactin level over time, 6 showed a gradual increase, and 10 showed a decrease (Schlechte et al, 1989). For female patients with small nonfunctional tumors or with prolactin-secreting microadenomas, we often suggest monitoring of those who have some menstrual cycles and of those who do not wish to bear children and reserving intervention until tumor growth or increased secretory activity occurs.

MALIGNANT PITUITARY TUMORS

Truly malignant pituitary tumors are unusual. These tumors tend to be invasive, proliferate rapidly, or metastasize to distant sites. Invasion means, first and foremost, dural invasion. The dura mater sits immediately adjacent to the pituitary gland, as it lines the sides and floor of the sella turcica. Thus, it is interposed between the pituitary tumor and several of the anatomic compartments into which the tumor may extend (i.e., the sphenoid sinus and cavernous sinuses). The incidence of dural invasion was reported by the Mayo Clinic to be 40% by gross description, but this rate climbed to 85% with microscopic verification (Selman et al, 1986). Like meningiomas, pituitary tumors can invade the dura mater and adjacent bone but typically do not invade the brain. Thus, it is clear that many "benign" adenomas with an indolent clinical course can invade, so invasion is not a perfect criterion for pituitary tumor malignancy.

Microinvasion of normal gland by tumor occurs frequently along the pseudocapsule that such tumors typically form around themselves. Failure to recognize such invasion during surgery is one of the leading causes of tumor recurrence. Tumors that tend to be invasive include those that secrete TSH, large prolactinomas associated with very high serum prolactin levels, and tumors that secrete GH and so cause acromegaly. Invasion usually affects the floor of the sella turcica, which can be thinned and eroded. Tumor enlargement also extends the tumor into the suprasellar cistern by stretching the diaphragma sellae, an arachnoid layer that separates the subarachnoid space above from the intrasellar space below. In some patients, a dumbbell-like extension of the pituitary tumor reaches through the small opening provided in the diaphragma for the pituitary stalk. A truly large pituitary tumor pushing up into the third ventricle may ultimately cause hydrocephalus if it reaches the foramina of Monro. The most common sequela of suprasellar extension is compression of the optic chiasm or optic nerves, leading to loss of the temporal portions of the visual field. In patients with lateral extension into the cavernous sinuses, which occurs less frequently, the dura mater is physically breached by the tumor, which then fills the sinusoidal spaces within the sinus and encases the carotid artery and cranial nerves. The cavernous sinus typically expands as its dural boundaries are stretched by the tumor. Cranial nerve dysfunction occurs only in later stages of the disease. However, cranial nerve malfunction (typically oculomotor paresis) can occur due to compression of the cavernous sinus rather than frank invasion. Cavernous sinus compression can be relieved by surgery, and the associated cranial neuropathies will improve over 3 to 6 months. Patients with encasement of the cranial nerves by the tumor within the cavernous sinus have a much worse prognosis for neurologic improvement. The internal carotid artery is quite sturdy and resists narrowing from tumor compression, but arterial narrowing can occur and may be devastating to patients with poor collateral flow through an anatomically incomplete circle of Willis.

The histologic hallmarks of malignancy are often absent in patients with invasive pituitary adenomas. Pathologic factors such as *p53* status, apoptosis, epidermal growth factor receptor expression, and especially tumor cell proliferation (measured by using, for example, the MIB-1 labeling index) all correlate well with the degree of invasiveness and are most pronounced in frankly metastatic pituitary tumors. These factors may be used as loose predictors of the likelihood of recurrence after surgical excision.

Metastases from pituitary tumors are very rare and are the hallmark of the true pituitary carcinoma (Scheithauer et al, 2005). Although most patients with such metastases have clinically nonfunctional tumors, all functional adenoma types have been reported in the literature on pituitary carcinomas. In half of patients with these metastases, the tumors disseminate within the neuraxis, and most show cytologic features of malignancy, including pleomorphism, nuclear atypia, and mitotic figures. Occasionally, a patient will show leptomeningeal dissemination and have positive cytologic results for malignant cells within the spinal fluid. Of those patients with metastases to extraneural sites, half have an ACTH-secreting tumor. About half of pituitary carcinomas metastasize to the liver; lesser proportions metastasize to the bone, lung, and lymph nodes. Overall, pituitary carcinomas are nonfunctional in half the cases and secrete ACTH in 22% of cases, GH in 13%, and prolactin in 11% (Mountcastle et al, 1989). Although it appears that nonfunctional adenomas are somewhat overrepresented, in the absence of immunohistochemical staining on all tumors, some of these cases may actually represent gonadotropin-secreting tumors.

Pituitary carcinomas can be indolent or aggressive. The patient survival duration ranges from 1 month to 10 years or more. Most of these tumors start as slowly growing adenomas and progress over years to become more aggressive tumors. Radiotherapy can cause sarcomatous transformation of adenomas (many of which are GH-secreting tumors, which seem to be more sensitive to such transformation), but more than half of patients with pituitary carcinomas have not been exposed previously to sellar radiotherapy. Thus, the role of radiotherapy as a transforming agent remains unclear.

Treatment protocols are difficult to devise consistently for pituitary neoplasms. Even aggressive treatment confers a relatively short survival benefit. The classic oncologic approach—maximal resection of the primary site and surgically accessible metastatic sites followed by radiotherapy and finally cytotoxic chemotherapy—is rarely applied to pituitary tumors because of anatomic constraints. In addition, no chemotherapy protocols have been devised. Chemotherapy has typically been provided ad hoc, and only the occasional patient has shown a response, which is usually temporary. In a study by Kaltsas et al (1998), lomustine and 5-fluorouracil were given to 7 patients with aggressive tumors, 4 of whom had frank carcinomas. The tumors shrank temporarily, but all 7 patients died of their disease 3 to 65 months after the treatment was started. At M. D. Anderson, we usually initiate a sarcoma regimen (often including ifosfamide) for these lesions, but we too have had limited success in controlling their growth.

Although the development of skull base approaches over the past 20 years has made surgery feasible within the cavernous sinus, these approaches are not free of risk. We have attempted to use such approaches in selected patients who have aggressive intracavernous disease that is expanding actively and is threatening the integrity of the optic apparatus. Both cavernous sinus exenteration and partial cleanout of the cavernous sinus with preservation of the neurovascular structures have been tried. In frankly malignant tumors, neither approach has ultimately succeeded, although some palliation has been obtained. In light of the dismal natural history of this disease, patients with pituitary carcinomas should generally undergo as aggressive a resection as anatomic and technical factors permit.

METASTASES TO THE PITUITARY GLAND FROM SYSTEMIC CANCER

Because pituitary adenomas are common in the population at large, oncologists often assume that a sellar tumor in a patient with systemic cancer is a pituitary adenoma. Although this assumption is often correct, enough patients present with metastases to the pituitary gland or to its sellar enclosure that consideration must be given to true metastatic disease (Figures 10–4 and 10–5). Making this distinction is important because the surgical and medical treatments are very different for benign disease and malignant disease.

Between 1% and 4% of pituitary neoplasms are metastases arising from distant primary sites. Carcinomas of the breast constitute 50% of such tumors, and carcinomas of the lung constitute 20% (Komninos et al, 2004). Less common primary tumors include gastrointestinal cancer (6%), prostate cancer (6%), and melanoma (2%). Pituitary metastases are diagnosed first by clinical suspicion, second by the presence of diabetes insipidus (which is seen in up to 70% of patients with symptomatic pituitary metastases but in fewer than 1% of patients with pituitary adenomas at presentation), and finally by MRI findings. Although not a particularly reliable symptom in elucidating sellar pathology, headache is present in two thirds of patients with metastases, probably because of the more active irritation of the sellar dura mater with such rapidly growing tumors. MR images must be checked for the concomitant presence of cerebral metastases.

Many pituitary metastases produce no symptoms, but metastatic deposits are found at autopsy in the pituitary glands of up to 5% of patients with systemic cancer. Antemortem diagnosis typically follows the development of hypopituitarism, visual loss, or diplopia from cavernous sinus involvement, but diagnosis can be difficult because the constitutional symptoms of systemic cancer can mimic those of anterior pituitary dysfunction. Diabetes insipidus is seen at presentation in 45% to 70% of these patients; other patients develop it later in the course of the disease. Distinguishing an adenoma from a metastasis is often difficult because both can invade the cavernous sinus, sphenoid bone, or clivus.

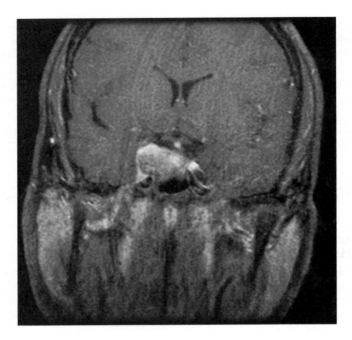

Figure 10–4. A 35-year-old woman had epithelioid sarcoma of the axilla and chest wall and multiple recurrences necessitating a forequarter (i.e., intrascapulothoracic) amputation. The patient underwent MRI after the onset of headache, lactation, and diplopia from a right abducens palsy. The image showed a sellar mass invading or compressing the right cavernous sinus. Because a metastatic sarcoma was suspected, the tumor was resected by transsphenoidal surgery. The tumor was somewhat hemorrhagic, indicating a degree of apoplexy. Pathologic analysis revealed a null cell pituitary adenoma, and the symptoms cleared soon after surgery. This case illustrates the principle that a history of malignant tumor does not exclude the concomitant presence of a more benign (albeit, in this case, invasive) pituitary tumor.

However, on MR images, pituitary adenoma appears as an area of focal hypointensity relative to normal gland (Figure 10–4), whereas metastases are typically enhanced by contrast and appear as relatively diffuse enhancements within the sella turcica. There is little to distinguish metastases from normal gland (Figure 10–5). In some cases, the metastases may also show a heterogeneous enhancement pattern that lacks the focality necessary to demonstrate an adenoma.

At M. D. Anderson, as long as the clinical and radiographic scenario is classic for this condition, the asymptomatic patient with incidentally discovered pituitary metastasis is usually treated with radiotherapy. If there is any uncertainty about the diagnosis, the patient may undergo excisional biopsy of the tumor or may simply be monitored and rescanned in

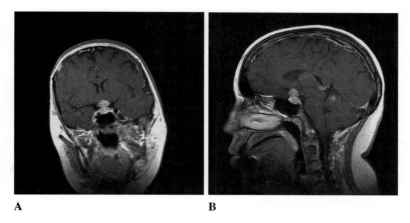

A **B**

Figure 10–5. A 23-year-old woman with multiple endocrine neoplasia (type IIB) was being actively treated for medullary thyroid carcinoma metastatic to lung, bone, and subcutis at multiple sites. She admitted to worsening headache and then loss of peripheral vision. She also experienced polyuria and polydipsia consistent with diabetes insipidus. MR images showed a dumbbell-shaped sellar and suprasellar tumor with diffuse pituitary gland involvement and chiasmatic compression (A), which is the classic appearance for metastases; parenchymal metastases were also seen in the cerebellum (B). The patient underwent transsphenoidal surgery, and subtotal resection allowed decompression of the optic apparatus and restoration of vision. The patient underwent whole-brain radiotherapy but died 2 months later from progression of the brain metastases.

6 to 8 weeks, assuming that optic compression is not already present. The patient who presents with optic nerve dysfunction typically undergoes transsphenoidal resection, which is likely to be subtotal. The tumor residue is then treated with limited-field external beam radiotherapy or with conformal radiotherapeutic techniques that protect the optic chiasm. Local control of these tumors using this scheme is achieved in 80% of patients, most of whom have coincidental metastases to other sites and are therefore treated with chemotherapy. The relative contributions of site-directed therapy and systemic therapy are difficult to tease out, but both types of therapy result in good palliation and good preservation of vision in most patients.

SPECIAL SITUATIONS

Cystic Lesions of the Sella Turcica

A differential diagnosis of a cystic mass centered on the sella turcica includes cystic pituitary adenoma, Rathke's cleft cyst, pars intermedia cyst, and craniopharyngioma. These 4 entities cover more than 95% of such lesions. Metastasis to the pituitary gland is very rarely seen in a cystic form.

Cystic Pituitary Adenomas

The treatment of a cystic pituitary adenoma is transsphenoidal resection of the tumor sustaining the cyst and emptying of the cyst during the surgery. Many such tumors are multiloculated and require aggressive exploration to break the fenestrations within the cyst to ensure complete emptying. Most cystic adenomas are nonfunctional, and as long as the cyst is well opened and the tumor well removed, they ultimately respond to surgical excision as well as their noncystic counterparts do.

Rathke's Cleft Cysts

Rathke's cleft cysts are congenital lesions arising from the remnants of Rathke's pouch, a dorsal invagination of the stomodeal ectoderm. They are not neoplastic lesions but rather true cysts lined with a ciliated epithelium, which is their pathologic hallmark under light microscopy. Although relatively common at autopsy, most of these cysts remain asymptomatic. They may cause symptoms by enlarging enough to compress the anterior lobe of the pituitary gland and thereby cause hormone deficits or to produce visual loss by compressing the optic chiasm. Treatment of Rathke's cleft cysts is restricted to those cysts that compress or endanger the optic chiasm or when diagnostic confusion arises. Usually a transsphenoidal approach with fenestration and marsupialization of the cyst prevent recurrence. At M. D. Anderson, we do not attempt to strip the lining of the cyst from within the sella turcica because this procedure will damage the pituitary gland and cause cerebrospinal fluid to leak.

Pars Intermedia Cysts

Pars intermedia cysts are benign congenital lesions that arise in the cleft between the anterior and posterior lobes of the pituitary gland. They are rarely symptomatic, but with increasingly sensitive scanning techniques, they are now occasionally identified. A symptomatic pars intermedia cyst is rarely seen and thus rarely requires transsphenoidal resection; when it is removed, though, it tends to separate nicely from the adjacent glandular tissue and thus can be "cured."

Craniopharyngiomas

Craniopharyngiomas are cystic tumors that are almost always benign (see chapter 4). Such tumors are usually identifiable on MR images by their contrast-enhanced pattern and signal characteristics, which are distinct from those of cystic pituitary adenomas. In addition, these tumors tend to adhere firmly to the structure from which they arise, are more often suprasellar than intrasellar, and are in close apposition to the pituitary stalk. Large craniopharyngiomas may reach the hypothalamus and adhere to its inferior surface. Thus, the risk of injury to the hypothalamus, the pituitary stalk, or the pituitary gland itself is relatively high when resection is undertaken, and a fine balance must be struck between the imperatives to cure and to preserve function. Surgery for craniopharyngioma is one of the more difficult undertakings in surgery aimed at the sella turcica, and it is best performed aggressively by a skillful surgeon with much experience with this tumor type. When surgical resection is subtotal, craniopharyngiomas readily recur, forming complex multiloculated cysts that become even more difficult to remove safely in subsequent operations. Radiotherapy is often used as an adjunct to surgery and occasionally is used as the primary treatment. However, in light of the diagnostic difficulties inherent in determining the etiology of a cystic sellar lesion, it may be prudent to establish a diagnosis histologically before exposing the patient to the potential adverse effects of radiotherapy.

Pituitary Tumors Associated with Tumor Syndromes

Pituitary adenomas may be a manifestation of multiple endocrine neoplasia type 1 (MEN1). MEN1 is uncommon, and most pituitary tumors seen in clinical practice have no link with it. Nonetheless, the reported prevalence of pituitary tumors in patients with a defective *MEN1* tumor-suppressor gene (located on chromosome 11p) ranges from 10% to 65%. These patients also tend to have parathyroid adenomas (which cause hyperparathyroidism and thus hypercalcemia) and pancreatic islet cell neoplasms (which cause peptic ulcers and other digestive difficulties as well as hypoglycemia from insulin excess). Because parathyroid tumors are seen in more than 95% of patients with MEN1, clinicians can most easily screen patients with pituitary tumors for this genetic syndrome by assessing serum calcium and albumin levels and interpreting the results appropriately.

Pituitary tumors are the initial manifestation of MEN1 in 17% of patients with the disease (Verges et al, 2002). Although such adenomas are by repute more aggressive and difficult to cure than sporadic tumors are, we have found no such distinction at M. D. Anderson and have achieved similar cure rates for tumors, regardless of whether they are associated with a defective *MEN1* gene. About 60% of these adenomas with a defective *MEN1* gene are prolactinomas, and only 15% are nonfunctional; thus, these types are overrepresented and underrepresented, respectively, compared with sporadic tumors. GH-secreting adenomas are occasionally seen, and on rare occasions patients present with a pancreatic tumor that secretes GH-releasing factor and with clinical acromegaly from hyperplasia of the pituitary somatotrophs rather than a true adenoma. Macroadenomas are 3 times more likely than microadenomas in the context of MEN1, which is a reversal from the usual distribution of tumor size. The criteria directing surgical or other treatment for pituitary tumors with a defective *MEN1* gene are similar to those applied to patients without a genetic mutation.

The only other genetic syndromes clinically associated with pituitary tumorigenesis are the McCune-Albright syndrome and Carney's complex. Diagnosing McCune-Albright syndrome requires the presence of at least 2 of the following features: polyostotic fibrous dysplasia, café au lait spots, and autonomous endocrine hyperfunction. The endocrine disruption most commonly arises outside the pituitary gland (as in gonadotropin-independent precocious puberty) but sometimes from an

KEY PRACTICE POINTS

- Any patient harboring a tumor that occupies the sella turcica should undergo rigorous hormonal evaluation and be examined for pituitary hypofunction (indicating compression of the normal gland) and hyperfunction (indicating a pituitary tumor secreting excess hormone).

- Not all sellar tumors are pituitary tumors. Careful radiologic evaluation using MRI is essential for determining the appropriate differential diagnosis for such lesions.

- A homogeneously enhancing, symmetrically enlarged pituitary gland may represent a case of pituitary hyperplasia due to thyrotroph hyperplasia. Any such case should be examined clinically and biochemically for evidence of hypothyroidism, which if corrected would prevent inappropriate surgery.

- If a pituitary tumor secretes prolactin, it can likely be treated successfully with a dopamine agonist. However, it is not appropriate to treat patients medically who have relatively large pituitary tumors with modestly elevated levels of prolactin (25 to 75 ng/mL) because these tumors are typically nonfunctional adenomas that are unresponsive to such drugs and are better treated with surgery.

- In general, patients requiring surgery for a pituitary tumor are treated most safely and effectively with a transsphenoidal approach. Craniotomy is reserved for patients who have tumors with suprasellar or lateral extensions that are inaccessible via the transsphenoidal approach.

- Patients with systemic cancer who show a sellar tumor on MR images may harbor metastases to the pituitary gland instead of a pituitary adenoma. Metastases to the pituitary gland are seen most commonly in persons with carcinomas of the lung or breast. The hallmark is diabetes insipidus, which pituitary adenomas rarely cause. Patients with a sellar tumor and diabetes insipidus are presumed to have a metastatic deposit in the sella turcica unless proven otherwise.

- Metastases to the sella turcica can be treated effectively with surgery and radiotherapy and possibly chemotherapy, depending on the source of the tumor. Such treatment should be undertaken to preserve the patient's vision.

associated pituitary adenoma, which typically causes acromegaly. Carney's complex arises from disruption of the gene encoding a regulatory subunit of protein kinase A. This syndrome induces cardiac, cutaneous, and mammary myxomas; skin pigmentation; melanotic schwannomas; and endocrine hyperfunction manifested usually as primary adrenocortical nodular hyperplasia or as pituitary adenoma. All pituitary tumors reported in patients with Carney's complex have been GH positive, and most are associated with clinical acromegaly (Watson et al, 2000). Thus, a patient with this syndrome who shows signs of Cushing's disease is more likely to have an extrapituitary source of ACTH excess. In addition, a person who shows increasing levels of IGF-I over time may benefit from surgical exploration of the sella turcica, even in the absence of a tumor on MR images.

SUGGESTED READINGS

Asa SL. *Tumors of the Pituitary Gland*. Washington, DC: Armed Forces Institute of Pathology; 1998.

Biswas M, Smith J, Jadon D, et al. Long-term remission following withdrawal of dopamine agonist therapy in subjects with microprolactinomas. *Clin Endocrinol* 2005;63:26–31.

Bohinski RJ, Warnick RE, Gaskill-Shipley MF, et al. Intraoperative magnetic resonance imaging to determine the extent of resection of pituitary macroadenomas during transsphenoidal microsurgery. *Neurosurgery* 2001;49:1133–1143.

Brada M, Ajithkumar TV, Minniti G. Radiosurgery for pituitary adenomas. *Clin Endocrinol* 2004;61:531–543.

Ezzat S, Asa SL, Couldwell WT, et al. The prevalence of pituitary adenomas: a systematic review. *Cancer* 2004;101:613–619.

Hamilton DK, Vance ML, Boulos PT, Laws ER. Surgical outcomes in hyporesponsive prolactinomas: analysis of patients with resistance or intolerance to dopamine agonists. *Pituitary* 2005;8:53–60.

Hardy J. Transsphenoidal microsurgery of the normal and pathological pituitary. *Clin Neurosurg* 1969;16:185–217.

Holdaway IM, Rajasoorya C. Epidemiology of acromegaly. *Pituitary* 1999;2:29–41.

Jenkins PJ, Mukherjee A, Shalet SM. Does growth hormone cause cancer? *Clin Endocrinol* 2006;64:115–121.

Kaltsas GA, Mukherjee JJ, Plowman PN, Monson JP, Grossman AB, Besser GM. The role of cytotoxic chemotherapy in the management of aggressive and malignant pituitary tumors. *J Clin Endocrinol Metab* 1998;83:4233–4238.

Komninos J, Vlassopoulou V, Protopapa D, et al. Tumors metastatic to the pituitary gland: case report and literature review. *J Clin Endocrinol Metab* 2004;89: 574–589.

Landolt AM, Haller D, Lomax N, et al. Stereotactic radiosurgery for recurrent surgically treated acromegaly: comparison with fractionated radiotherapy. *J Neurosurg* 1998;88:1002–1008.

Molitch ME. Medication-induced hyperprolactinemia. *Mayo Clin Proc* 2005; 80:1050–1057.

Mountcastle RB, Roof BS, Mayfield RK, et al. Pituitary adenocarcinoma in an acromegalic patient: response to bromocriptine and pituitary testing: a review of the literature on 36 cases of pituitary carcinoma. *Am J Med Sci* 1989;298: 109–118.

Nieman LK, Ilias I. Evaluation and treatment of Cushing's syndrome. *Am J Med* 2005;118:1340–1346.

Nilsson B, Gustavasson-Kadaka E, Bengtsson BA, Jonsson B. Pituitary adenomas in Sweden between 1958 and 1991: incidence, survival, and mortality. *J Clin Endocrinol Metab* 2000;85:1420–1425.

Nomikos P, Buchfelder M, Fahlbusch R. The outcome of surgery in 668 patients with acromegaly using current criteria of biochemical 'cure.' *Eur J Endocrinol* 2005;152:379–387.

Oberg K. Future aspects of somatostatin receptor-mediated therapy. *Neuroendocrinology* 2004;80:57–61.

Park P, Chandler WF, Barkan AL, et al. The role of radiation therapy after surgical resection of nonfunctional pituitary macroadenomas. *Neurosurgery* 2004;55: 100–106.

Pereira AM, van Alken MO, van Dulken H, et al. Long-term predictive value of postsurgical cortisol concentrations for cure and risk of recurrence in Cushing's disease. *J Clin Endocrinol Metab* 2003;88:5858–5864.

Prabhu SS, Aldape KD, Gagel RF, Benjamin RS, Trent JC, McCutcheon IE. Sarcomatous change in a growth hormone-secreting pituitary adenoma: possible influence by IGF-I. *Can J Neurol Sci* 2003;30:378–383.

Randeva HS, Schoebel J, Byrne J, Esiri M, Adams CB, Wass JA. Classical pituitary apoplexy: clinical features, management and outcome. *Clin Endocrinol* 1999;51: 181–188.

Scheithauer BW, Kurtkaya-Yapicier O, Kovacs KT, Young WF Jr, Lloyd RV. Pituitary carcinoma: a clinicopathological review. *Neurosurgery* 2005;56: 1066–1074.

Schlechte J, Dolan K, Sherman B, Chapler F, Luciano A. The natural history of untreated hyperprolactinemia: a prospective analysis. *J Clin Endocrinol Metab* 1989;68:412–418.

Selman W, Laws ER, Scheithauer BW, Carpenter SM. The occurrence of dural invasion in pituitary adenomas. *J Neurosurg* 1986;64:402–407.

Socin HV, Chanson P, Delemer B, et al. The changing spectrum of TSH-secreting pituitary adenomas: diagnosis and management in 43 patients. *Eur J Endocrinol* 2003;148:433–442.

Tischler RB, Loeffler JS, Lunsford LD, et al. Tolerance of cranial nerves of the cavernous sinus to radiosurgery. *Int J Radiat Oncol Biol Phys* 1993;27:215–221.

Toogood A. Safety and efficacy of growth hormone replacement therapy in adults. *Expert Opin Drug Saf* 2005;4:1069–1082.

Trainer PJ, Drake WM, Katznelson L, et al. Treatment of acromegaly with the growth hormone receptor antagonist pegvisomant. *N Engl J Med* 2000;342: 1171–1177.

Tyrrell JB, Lamborn KR, Hannegan LT, et al. Transsphenoidal microsurgical therapy of prolactinomas: initial outcomes and long-term results. *Neurosurgery* 1999;44:254–261.

Verges B, Boureille F, Goudet P, et al. Pituitary disease in MEN type 1 (MEN1): data from the France-Belgium MEN1 Multicenter Study. *J Clin Endocrinol Metab* 2002;87:457–465.

Verhelst J, Abs R, Maiter D, et al. Cabergoline in the treatment of hyperprolactine-mia: a study in 455 patients. *J Clin Endocrinol Metab* 1999;84:2518–2522.

Watson JC, Stratakis CA, Bryant-Greenwood PK, et al. Neurosurgical implications of Carney complex. *J Neurosurg* 2000;92:413–418.

Webb SM, Rigla M, Wagner A, Oliver B, Bartumeus F. Recovery of hypopitu-itarism after neurosurgical treatment of pituitary adenomas. *J Clin Endocrinol Metab* 1999;84:3696–3700.

11 MANAGEMENT OF LUNG CANCER, BREAST CANCER, AND MELANOMA METASTATIC TO THE BRAIN

Jeffrey S. Weinberg

Chapter Overview 225
Introduction 226
Decision Analysis 227
   Clinical Assessment 227
   Brain Tumor Characteristics and Treatment Alternatives 228
      Imaging Characteristics 228
      Treatment Options Based on Tumor Characteristics 229
Lung Cancer Brain Metastases 232
   Epidemiology 232
   Brain Metastases from Lung Cancer 232
   Treatment of Metastatic Lung Cancer to the Brain 232
Breast Cancer Brain Metastases 235
   Epidemiology 235
   Brain Metastases from Breast Cancer 236
   Treatment of Metastatic Breast Cancer to the Brain 237
Malignant Melanoma Brain Metastases 238
   Epidemiology 238
   Brain Metastases from Malignant Melanoma 238
   Treatment of Metastatic Melanoma to the Brain 239
Conclusion 241
Key Practice Points 241
Suggested Readings 241

CHAPTER OVERVIEW

Lung cancer, breast cancer, and melanoma metastasize to the brain more frequently than other cancers do. These cancers can present incidentally (i.e., on magnetic resonance images performed for staging purposes) or can cause seizures or symptoms due to mass effect on the surrounding brain. A careful assessment of the stage of the cancer, the patient's medical condition, and the imaging characteristics must be performed. Treatment for brain metastases can involve surgical resection, stereotactic radiosurgery (SRS), whole-brain radiotherapy, or any combination of the 3 modalities. As a general rule, whole-brain radiotherapy is used for radiosensitive tumors, for multiple lesions, or prophylactically in patients with small cell lung cancer. It can also be used after surgical resection or SRS. Surgery is reserved for lesions that are larger than 3 cm (larger than 2 cm for melanomas). SRS can be used for single or multiple small lesions. Communication with all members of the treatment team must take place for the most comprehensive and patient-specific treatment plan to be devised.

INTRODUCTION

The management of metastatic tumors to the brain has changed in the modern era as technologic advances have led to better treatment. These advances have allowed surgery to be performed more safely and radiation to be delivered more accurately. Thus, the philosophy has changed from treating the whole brain to treating individual lesions. As a result, patients who have metastatic tumors to the brain and were once thought to be end-stage with a median survival duration of 4 months (with steroid treatment only) now live for a long time and frequently die from systemic disease progression rather than intracranial disease.

Many types of systemic cancer metastasize to the brain; carcinomas of the lung, breast, and skin do so the most frequently. Twenty-five percent of patients with cancer will develop brain metastases at some point. An estimated 170,000 patients in the United States develop metastatic brain tumors each year. The primary route of entry for cancer to the brain is the bloodstream (i.e., hematogenous). The lymphatic system is not present in the brain, so spread via this route is impossible. Single lesions in the brain are more frequent than multiple lesions. The sensitivity of magnetic resonance imaging (MRI) and the longer survival duration of patients due to better systemic treatments have resulted in an increasing number of patients being diagnosed with lesions earlier in their treatment and with multiple brain metastases.

The most common modalities used to treat brain metastases are whole-brain radiotherapy (WBRT), surgery, and stereotactic radiosurgery (SRS). Steroids are frequently used when there is edema and the patient is symptomatic from the edema, but they are not directly therapeutic. WBRT involves treating the entire brain with radiation, regardless of the tumor location within the brain. This modality is frequently used when there are multiple brain tumors or extremely radiosensitive lesions. Surgery is used for single or multiple metastases, especially when the targeted lesion is large (i.e., larger than 3 cm) or is causing mass effect on the surrounding tissue and symptoms. Surgery for biopsy or resection is needed if the histologic type is in question (e.g., in a patient with multiple systemic malignancies or an unknown primary tumor). SRS is a treatment option for patients with single or multiple small lesions (3 cm or smaller is the general rule) or for patients with similarly sized lesions who are medically unable to undergo craniotomy.

This chapter reviews the decision analysis behind the treatment recommendations for patients with metastatic brain tumors from the lung, breast, or skin. The process involves evaluating the patient for the state of the systemic disease, prognosis, and medical condition. More important, the characteristics of the brain lesions themselves must be critically analyzed with respect to the treatment options available to determine the optimal treatment regimen.

DECISION ANALYSIS

Many common features enter into the decision analysis before a specific treatment for a patient can be recommended. These features are outlined next. The unique features of the primary cancers (lung, breast, and skin) will be discussed in the remainder of the chapter.

Clinical Assessment

The prognosis of a patient who has had all intracranial tumors resected is equivalent to the prognosis of a patient without brain disease who has an otherwise similar stage of systemic cancer. Several studies have suggested that aggressive treatment of single or multiple brain lesions (via surgical resection or SRS) with or without radiotherapy results in excellent outcomes (Patchell et al, 1990; Bindal et al, 1993). Patients who receive treatment for a limited number of brain metastases will usually succumb to systemic disease progression rather than progression of their brain disease.

The status of the disease is usually determined by computed tomography (CT) scans of the chest, abdomen, and pelvis and also by positron emission tomography (PET) scans or combined PET-CT scans. In patients with a long history of disease, the most recent imaging studies should be compared with those from prior studies. A sense of the disease response to the current systemic treatment and of how rapidly the disease is responding or progressing can be developed by this comparison. Frequently, an estimation of life expectancy can be obtained from the patient's medical oncologist. At M. D. Anderson Cancer Center, patients with a life expectancy of less than 3 or 4 months are rarely offered surgical intervention unless palliative surgery can be performed with acceptable morbidity.

The overall medical condition of the patient plays a large role in determining which treatments may be offered. Patients with cardiorespiratory difficulties due to age, premorbid conditions, or side effects of other therapies (e.g., immunosuppression) need to be assessed before surgical intervention can be recommended. Medical optimization should take place before surgery is performed in such patients. Patients with comorbid medical conditions are referred to an internist, cardiologist, and frequently an anesthesiologist to determine their risk before surgery is scheduled.

The patient's functional condition is assessed by using the Karnofsky performance scale (KPS). This system is based on a patient's neurologic function and symptomatology. For therapeutic evaluation, the KPS score ranges from 10 (death imminent) to 100 (normal, without complaints); 70 is the cutoff for functional independence. A second prognostication system that is frequently used is the Radiation Therapy Oncology Group's recursive partitioning analysis. This system groups patients into 3 categories: Class I (patients who are younger than 65 years old, have a KPS score of 70 or higher, and have a controlled primary tumor with no extracranial metastases), Class III (patients with a KPS score of less than 70), and Class II (all other patients). Class I patients have a much better prognosis than Class II or III patients. A third method of categorizing patients uses a score index for SRS. This score, which ranges from 0 to 2, is determined from patient age, KPS score, extracranial disease status, number of brain lesions, and largest brain lesion volume. Patients with a score index of 0 for SRS have the worst prognosis.

Patients frequently present with headache or focal neurologic deficit. Because many metastatic tumors are located in the cerebellum, headache can be due to perilesional edema or obstructive hydrocephalus. Neurologic deficit can be caused by direct involvement of the part of the brain subserving that function, or it may be due to edema and compression on eloquent parts of the brain. Steroid use should be initiated when the patient is symptomatic. Subsequent improvement in neurologic function indicates that the eloquent brain is affected by edema and that the tissue can still function. Thus, improvement is a good prognostic factor for functional outcome.

Brain Tumor Characteristics and Treatment Alternatives

Imaging Characteristics

The best method for determining the characteristics of a brain tumor is MRI with and without contrast. T1- and T2-weighted images, diffusion-weighted images, and fluid-attenuated inversion recovery (FLAIR) sequences should be performed. At M. D. Anderson, T1-weighted imaging series with gadolinium enhancement are routinely performed in the axial, coronal, and sagittal planes to provide the best assessment of the tumor's location as well as the normal anatomic landmarks for delineating the eloquent brain (Figure 11–1). These series are also the best means of characterizing the

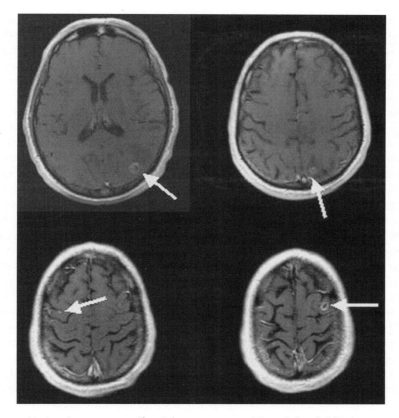

Figure 11–1. A sequence of axial postcontrast T1-weighted MR images of a patient with metastatic renal cell carcinoma. The arrows point to 4 separate metastases. The 2 lesions in the top row are associated with peritumoral edema seen as areas of hypointensity surrounding the metastases, which are enhanced after gadolinium administration.

lesion, and they aide the clinician in developing a differential diagnosis. Furthermore, these imaging sequences provide a framework for determining optimal treatment. The location, size, and number of lesions must be determined before a treatment course can be recommended.

Treatment Options Based on Tumor Characteristics

Determining the tumor's location is a critical step in choosing the optimal approach to treatment. Tumors in a superficial location are generally considered surgically accessible and therefore easily removed, but even tumors in the eloquent brain or in deep locations, including the thalamus and brainstem, can be reached with modern surgical approaches and techniques. In that sense, all tumors are operable. However, one must weigh the risk of surgery (i.e., the possible complications) with the risk of not removing the lesion in a patient who may have a limited life span. SRS is a minimally invasive technique that is potentially less expensive and less invasive than surgery and can be performed as an outpatient procedure. On the other hand, SRS does not protect against hemorrhage immediately after treatment, and there is the possibility of delayed radiation necrosis, a need for steroids, and neurologic deficit; thus, surgery may be a more viable alternative for some patients. In addition, because approximately 10% of patients who have systemic cancer can have a brain lesion unrelated to their malignancy, SRS may not be a viable treatment alternative if tissue confirmation for diagnostic purposes is warranted.

Single lesions larger than 3 cm in the largest diameter are traditionally removed surgically. Lesions 1 cm or smaller are routinely treated with SRS because even with the technologic advances in stereotactic localization and ultrasonography, smaller lesions are frequently difficult to identify at the time of surgery. As a rule of thumb, SRS cannot be used for tumors larger than 3 cm, but this rule needs to be evaluated in the context of the histologic characteristics of the tumor being treated. For example, at M. D. Anderson, the use of SRS for melanoma tumors larger than 2 cm^3 has been ineffective.

No prospective randomized trial has determined whether surgery or SRS is superior for treating single brain metastases. In published retrospective clinical series, both treatments have been touted as being better than the other. Until recently, patients at M. D. Anderson who had single lesions were offered the chance to participate in a randomized controlled trial comparing surgery and SRS for lesions thought to be surgically accessible and that fit the criteria for SRS. Accrual is completed, and the data are being analyzed.

Regardless of the type of study, published data must be screened carefully. The definition of local control in patients treated with SRS is no growth or shrinkage of the lesion. Few articles discuss the development of radiation necrosis and the need for steroids. Future studies will need to assess steroid use, quality-of-life issues, and neurocognitive outcomes related to complications of any and all treatments for brain metastases.

WBRT is used for patients with multiple or radiosensitive lesions. WBRT was the standard of care before the development of SRS and safe surgical techniques. Theoretically, WBRT treats lesions visible on MR images as well as lesions that are too small to be visualized. With a small number of lesions (which can be treated with surgery or SRS), delaying the use of WBRT may be beneficial. It can be used later if more lesions develop or if the tumor recurs after surgery or SRS.

The most important part of treatment discussions with the patient is a balanced presentation of the alternatives. At M. D. Anderson, patients are counseled on the advantages and disadvantages of surgery and SRS. The advantages of surgical resection are that tissue is obtained for histologic confirmation, mass effect is relieved and frequently results in weaning off of steroids, the entire gross lesion can usually be removed, and the likelihood of morbidity or neurologic deficit is recognized immediately after the operation and rehabilitation can begin immediately. The disadvantages of surgical resection are that it is invasive, the risk of neurologic deficit is acute, it is more costly than SRS, and an inpatient hospital stay is required. In contrast, the benefits of SRS are that it is noninvasive and avoids the risks of open surgical intervention, it is less expensive than surgical resection, and it is an outpatient procedure. The disadvantages of SRS are that no tissue is obtained, the tumor may not respond to the treatment, mass effect is not relieved, edema may not be relieved and may even be exacerbated and require chronic steroid use, protection against the risk of hemorrhage from tumors that tend to bleed (e.g., melanomas and renal cell carcinomas) is not immediate, and radiation necrosis may develop 3 months or later after treatment and cause neurologic symptoms and necessitate steroid treatment or surgical resection.

The number of lesions in the brain needs to be defined before a treatment course can be recommended. This information, the status of the patient's systemic disease, and the patient's neurologic status are used to determine the best course of treatment. Even for patients with many metastatic brain lesions, resection of a single large, symptomatic tumor can relieve mass effect, improve symptoms, and provide time to initiate other therapies. Data from M. D. Anderson have suggested that resection of 2 or 3 brain metastases can be performed with the same morbidity or mortality rates as resection of a single brain metastasis and that the prognosis is the same (Bindal et al, 1993). Thus, resection of multiple lesions in their entirety may be as effective as resection of a single lesion. This is not to suggest that resection of all lesions should be undertaken in all patients with multiple lesions; this intervention needs to be evaluated in the context of the other patient characteristics. For patients with multiple lesions, a combination of therapies (e.g., resection for larger lesions plus SRS for remaining smaller lesions) may be the best option.

Analysis of the literature reveals a number of problems that make determining the "best" treatment or describing the "standard of care" impossible. Besides a few articles that have described prospective, randomized controlled studies that examined the use of WBRT after resection of single brain metastases, almost all of the information that is available to aid in the decision-making process is based on retrospective data. The other issue is that very few, if any, of the studies are analyzed according to the histologic type of the metastases. For this reason, it is hard to determine whether similar treatment algorithms should be followed for metastatic lung cancer, breast cancer, melanoma, and other cancers. The hope for the future is that well-designed prospective, randomized controlled trials can be performed and that these questions will be answered for each histologic type.

The purpose of this section was to discuss decision making for patients with metastatic tumors to the brain. Specific surgical techniques that enhance the safety of surgery are not included, but an article by Weinberg et al (2001) provides further reading on that subject.

LUNG CANCER BRAIN METASTASES

Epidemiology

Lung cancer is the most frequently diagnosed cancer in the world and the second most frequently diagnosed cancer in the United States. In the United States, an estimated 172,570 people were diagnosed with lung cancer in 2005, and 163,510 people died from this disease. The incidence of brain metastases in lung cancer patients has been estimated to range from 18% to 65%. In autopsy studies, the incidence of brain metastases approaches 50% in both patients with non-small cell lung carcinoma (NSCLC) and patients with small cell lung carcinoma (SCLC) (Frazier et al, 2004). Brain metastases in lung cancer patients are a considerable cause of morbidity and mortality, and the neurosurgeon is frequently called on to provide treatment for the metastasis before therapy for the systemic disease is introduced. In addition, at M. D. Anderson, untreated brain metastasis is often an exclusion criterion for clinical trials; thus, brain metastasis treatment may take precedence over systemic therapy.

Lung cancer is most frequently diagnosed initially by radiography of the chest and confirmed with a CT scan of the chest. Staging is routinely performed using a CT scan of the abdomen to search for hepatic and adrenal metastases and a PET scan to look for metabolically active lesions that are too small to be visualized on CT scans. The workup continues with percutaneous biopsy or open surgical resection of the primary lesion if clinically indicated.

Brain Metastases from Lung Cancer

More and more frequently, lung cancer patients are being staged with MRI of the brain to determine whether brain metastases are present. Brain metastases from lung cancer are usually single or solitary. Brain metastases may occur in as many as 40% of patients with no neurologic symptoms and in up to 17.5% of patients with stage III NSCLC (Salbeck et al, 1990). In light of these statistics, MRI of the brain is indicated for patients with neurologic symptoms. For asymptomatic patients, brain imaging is generally suggested for staging of SCLC and for patients with advanced stage NSCLC.

Treatment of Metastatic Lung Cancer to the Brain

In general, treatment options consist of surgery, SRS, and WBRT. Steroids are initiated for patients with neurologic symptoms due to the tumor.

Surgical resection is indicated to obtain a histologic diagnosis if the diagnosis is uncertain or if the lesion is large and causing mass effect, hydrocephalus, or herniation

Patients with SCLC usually have a poor prognosis, yet the brain metastases are considered radiosensitive. A mainstay of treatment for patients with SCLC is prophylactic cranial irradiation (PCI). Early clinical evidence suggested that PCI was associated with increased survival duration, but it was not until 1999, when the Prophylactic Cranial Irradiation Overview Collaborative Group published their results (Auperin et al, 1999), that this practice was solidified. In that study, compared with untreated SCLC patients, SCLC patients treated with PCI had a higher 3-year survival rate (15.3% vs 20.7%) and a lower incidence of brain metastases (58.5% vs 33.3%). If brain lesions are present at diagnosis or develop before PCI, WBRT is frequently the treatment of choice. A response rate of 50% to WBRT is possible, as is improved neurologic function. One study used hyperfractionated PCI (for a total of 36 Gy) to decrease the risk of brain metastasis recurrence without affecting the neurocognitive outcome (Wolfson et al, 2001). In a prospective randomized trial that examined 505 SCLC patients, the brain as the first site of relapse was 20% for patients treated with PCI and 37% for untreated patients ($P < 0.001$), but survival rates did not change significantly (Arriagada et al, 2002). In summary, SCLC metastases in the brain are generally radiosensitive lesions. Therefore, if a patient is symptomatic from even a single large lesion, steroid treatment is initiated. If the symptoms resolve, WBRT or SRS may be initiated with the hope of avoiding surgery even for large (i.e., 3- to 4.5-cm) lesions. Because of this radiosensitivity, the fact that many patients have multiple brain lesions, and the utility of PCI, neurosurgeons are not usually consulted for patients with SCLC metastatic to the brain.

SCLC metastases to the brain may also be treated successfully with chemotherapy. A 1992 meta-analysis indicated a 76% response rate in patients with brain metastases at cancer diagnosis who were treated with etoposide or teniposide along with either cisplatin or carboplatin (Kristensen et al, 1992). More recent data suggest that SCLC brain metastases respond to topotecan and that the response of the primary lesion to this agent may be indicative of the response of the metastatic lesions as well (Korfel et al, 2002). Currently, the use of chemotherapy to manage brain metastases in patients with SCLC is undergoing evaluation, and it is not considered the primary treatment option.

In patients with NSCLC (e.g., adenocarcinoma or squamous cell carcinoma), the decision analysis is more complicated. Before the development and refinement of SRS techniques, WBRT was the mainstay of treatment and the standard of care. Now with earlier detection due to MRI and better prognosis due to improved systemic therapy, more brain metastatic lesions are being discovered. Furthermore, because of earlier detection, the lesions are frequently asymptomatic and small. Evidence is convincing that patients with the brain as the only site of extrapulmonary disease at presentation should receive aggressive treatment. Data from M. D. Anderson suggest that NSCLC patients with American Joint Committee on Cancer thoracic stage I and solitary brain metastases treated with either surgical resection or SRS have a comparable outcome as patients with similar stage disease and no brain metastases. In this cohort, resection of both the primary tumor and the brain lesion vastly improved the 1-year survival rate compared with no resection or resection at just 1 site (50% vs 0% to 2%) (Read et al, 1989).

Surgery may not be an option for NSCLC patients if the brain lesion is small. If there is a single lesion smaller than 2 or 3 mm, we will frequently delay treatment and obtain a new MR image in 6 to 8 weeks. This deliberate delay allows the lesion to grow and thus makes for easier and more accurate targeting with SRS and, more important, allows time for the growth of other radiographically occult lesions and hence their detection. We are frequently concerned that there is more than 1 lesion but that they are too small to be seen on the MR images. This concern applies to lesions from breast cancer and melanoma as well.

Direct treatment (e.g., surgery or SRS) of the brain lesion at the time of relapse is beneficial. Surgery for brain metastasis at M. D. Anderson is frequently performed as a palliative procedure because of the improvement that can be gained by relief of mass effect in the case of large lesions. Both surgery and SRS are associated with increased patient survival and improved local control. The utility of WBRT after surgical resection of the brain lesion was demonstrated in a prospective randomized trial of patients with multiple histologic types of tumor to improve local and distant control but not to prolong survival time (Patchell et al, 1998). Although that trial did not include lung cancer patients specifically, another prospective randomized trial suggested that resection of a single brain metastasis is superior to WBRT alone (Patchell et al, 1990; Vecht et al, 1993).

Recent data also suggest that SRS is a useful method for treating NSCLC brain metastases, particularly for patients with advanced systemic disease, small lesions (3 cm or smaller), or up to 5 lesions or who are medically unfit to undergo craniotomy. Even though a trial comparing surgical resection and SRS has not been performed, the trend at M. D. Anderson is to use SRS to treat patients with up to 3 brain lesions who are diagnosed with brain metastases at presentation. SRS with or without WBRT is associated with improved long-term survival compared with WBRT alone. A median survival duration of 10 months and an 84% local control rate are achieved by Gamma Knife SRS treatment of NSCLC brain metastases (Kim et al, 1997). Improved survival is associated with a higher KPS score, female gender, adenocarcinoma, a longer time from diagnosis of the lung cancer to development of the brain lesions, smaller lesion size, and limited systemic disease. The addition of WBRT has been associated with improved local and distant control but not with improved survival. Future trials will determine the benefit of multimodality treatments using surgical resection and SRS with or without WBRT.

At M. D. Anderson, for patients with brain metastases from lung cancer, the trend is to be very aggressive with treatment at the time of diagnosis of the brain lesions. If the lesions are 2 cm or smaller and fewer than 4 are present, SRS is frequently used. We recommend surgery for single or multiple large lesions and then SRS for any untreated lesions. WBRT is usually recommended for patients who have more than 3 brain lesions at first presentation of the lesions under the assumption that since there is significant tumor burden, WBRT will confer improved local and distant control. In addition, other radiographically imperceptible lesions may be present and treated with this modality. Patients undergo MRI of the brain 1 month after completion of WBRT and up to every 3 months if the disease remains stable. At recurrence, the decision analysis is repeated.

BREAST CANCER BRAIN METASTASES

Epidemiology

Breast cancer is the most common cancer and the second-leading cause of cancer deaths among females. An estimated 211,240 women in the United States and 1.2 million women worldwide were expected to be diagnosed in 2005, and 40,410 women were expected to die secondary to breast cancer. The incidence of this disease has increased over time, whereas survival and mortality rates have improved as a result of earlier detection (due to public awareness of the need for self-examination and mammography) and improved treatment. Risk factors for breast cancer include a family history of the disease, genetic predisposition (e.g., *BRCA1* and *BRCA2* mutations), Caucasian race, late age at first full-term pregnancy, early menarche, late menopause, and use of hormones after menopause (American Cancer Society, 2005). Mutations in *BRCA1* and *BRCA2* are responsible for a large proportion of inherited breast cancer. These mutations are associated with young age at diagnosis, bilateral disease, ovarian cancer, a family history of breast and ovarian cancer, family members under 50 years old with breast cancer, and family members with breast cancer who are Ashkenazi Jews. The effects these gene mutations have on the prognosis of patients with breast cancer are unclear, although cancer in the contralateral breast in patients after breast conservation therapy is more likely when there is a *BRCA* mutation (Pierce et al, 2000).

In reported series of breast cancer, the most frequent types of invasive disease are infiltrating ductal carcinoma (65% to 80% of cases) and infiltrating lobular carcinoma (5% to 10% of cases). For patients with infiltrating ductal carcinoma, poor survival is associated with a high tumor grade, a large tumor size, and the presence of lymph node metastases. For patients with certain subtypes of infiltrating lobular carcinoma, the prognosis is similar. Both cancer types present with palpable breast masses, although the latter can present with multiple lesions within the ipsilateral breast. Staging is performed using the tumor, node, metastases (TNM) schema created by the American Joint Committee on Cancer. The presence of estrogen and progesterone receptors as well as the epidermal growth factor receptor HER2 is associated with improved survival because of better responses to hormonal therapy and trastuzumab, respectively. Predictive factors of a worse outcome include a lack of these receptors, the presence of lymphatic or vascular invasion, and a high mitotic rate.

Patients with metastatic disease obviously have a worse prognosis than patients without metastasis. Multiple metastatic sites, a short interval to presentation of metastases, and a lack of estrogen and progesterone receptors or HER2 are associated with a poorer prognosis. Brain metastases from breast cancer are the second most common metastatic lesions in women (behind brain metastases from lung cancer) and are more likely to occur before rather than after or during menopause. Autopsy studies of women with breast cancer have revealed that as many as 22% of women have brain metastases and that during the course of their illness, 10% will develop clinical manifestations of central nervous system involvement. Lung as the first site of breast cancer recurrence, a negative receptor status, and a high lactate dehydrogenase level before treatment may predict the development of brain metastases.

Brain Metastases from Breast Cancer

Intracranial metastases can take the form of intraparenchymal, dural-based, or leptomeningeal lesions. Many patients with metastatic breast cancer lesions to the brain present with single intraparenchymal lesions, although more than half of patients have multiple brain lesions. The lesions can be incidental (i.e., found on staging workup), or patients can be symptomatic and present with headache, focal neurologic deficit, seizure, or increased intracranial pressure. Dural-based lesions can be confused with meningiomas if they are single or solitary. Meningioma is less likely to be in the differential diagnosis when there are multiple lesions. Leptomeningeal disease can occur as a result of direct seeding of the cerebrospinal fluid by cancer cells or as a complication of surgery for the brain lesion.

Because of the inherent radiosensitivity of breast cancer metastases, the management of brain lesions secondary to breast cancer is slightly more complicated than the management of lung cancer metastasized to the brain. Even large lesions can be temporized with steroids and be treated successfully with radiotherapy. Unlike lung cancer metastases, there is no evidence to support the idea that any type of breast cancer is more susceptible than another to a particular type of treatment once it has metastasized to the brain. New biologic chemotherapeutic agents that can be targeted directly to receptors have been used with mild success. Breast tumors that have HER2 respond to the anti-HER2 chemotherapeutic agent trastuzumab. However, because this drug cannot penetrate the blood-brain barrier, patients treated with trastuzumab may develop brain metastases despite the extracranial disease showing a response. This situation indicates an affinity of HER2-positive tumor cells for the central nervous system, poor trastuzumab penetration into the central nervous system, or late tumor development in patients who are living longer (Bendell et al, 2003).

Treatment of Metastatic Breast Cancer to the Brain

The main modalities used to treat metastatic breast cancer to the brain are WBRT, surgery, and SRS. Evaluation of the patient should include the extra-cerebral and intracerebral tumor burden and the patient's medical condition, performance status, and symptomatology. Typically, tumors larger than 3 cm are surgically removed because they can cause mass effect or increased intracranial pressure (due to edema, hydrocephalus, etc.). In an M. D. Anderson study of patients treated with surgical resection, the median survival duration was 16 months, and WBRT after surgical resection was found in a multivariate analysis to reduce mortality by 60% (Pieper et al, 1997). Because breast cancer is extremely radiosensitive, patients with even large lesions or multiple lesions may respond to WBRT. Data from this article as well as data from a prospective randomized trial by Patchell and associates (1998) that examined the use of WBRT after resection in patients with different malignancies confirm the benefit of WBRT on both local and distant control. However, Patchell and colleagues found no effect on survival. Unfortunately, there are no data describing the quality of life or neurocognitive deficits in patients who undergo WBRT and survive long after. Therefore, the medical condition and prognosis of breast cancer patients must be critically analyzed before global brain therapy (i.e., WBRT) can be recommended over a targeted one (i.e., surgery or SRS).

Direct treatment of single or multiple lesions by SRS has proven efficacy. In a recent study, patients treated with SRS had a median overall time to progression of 10 months (Goyal et al, 2005). The authors were unable to assess the effect of WBRT added to the SRS on local control or patient survival. A second series of patients with large tumor volumes and multiple lesions (some patients had more than 6) resulted in a median overall time to progression of 7.5 months (Lederman et al, 2001). Because of the paucity of articles specifically addressing surgery and SRS for a pure breast cancer brain metastasis population and because no prospective randomized trial has been performed, it is difficult to compare the treatment modalities and determine which are superior.

For this reason, when a patient at M. D. Anderson with breast cancer is diagnosed with brain metastases, a referral to a neurosurgeon is usually initiated. Frequently, SRS is recommended for 1 to 3 lesions that are 3 cm or smaller. WBRT may or may not be recommended for these patients.

If there is widely metastatic disease, multiple brain lesions, or both at the time of diagnosis, WBRT is used with or without SRS. The success of newly developed targeted therapies has improved the prognosis of patients with breast cancer, thus warranting this aggressive multimodality approach. Surgery is reserved for lesions that are large, are symptomatic, or do not respond to primary treatment in patients who have otherwise stable or slowly progressive disease and who are medically able to tolerate the surgery.

MALIGNANT MELANOMA BRAIN METASTASES

Epidemiology

Malignant melanoma was diagnosed in an estimated 59,580 people in the United States in 2005 and was responsible for approximately 7,700 deaths that year. Malignant melanoma accounts for 79% of deaths due to skin cancer, and the annual death rate is 2.3 per 100,000 population (Liu and Herlyn, 2005). Because of early detection, 83% of cases are diagnosed while the cancer is localized. Eleven percent are diagnosed after the cancer has spread to regional lymph nodes, and only 3% are diagnosed after the cancer has already metastasized. For the remaining cases, the staging information at diagnosis is unknown. The 5-year relative survival rates are 98.3% for patients with localized disease, 63.8% for patients with regional lymph node metastases, 16.0% for patients with distant metastases, and 80.9% for patients with unstaged disease (Liu and Herlyn, 2005). Because of the referral pattern at M. D. Anderson, patients are frequently referred to us with either locoregional metastases or more distant spread of disease.

Exposure to ultraviolet light has been identified as the greatest environmental risk factor (even in childhood) for melanoma and is thought to effect malignant transformation through its interaction with the retinoblastoma gene (*Rb*), hepatocyte factor/scatter factor, or both. Other risk factors for melanoma include a large number of moles, congenital nevi, a prior history of melanoma, a family history of melanoma, fair complexion, older age, and a tendency to burn during sun exposure. Characteristics of the primary lesion, such as tumor thickness, ulceration, and Clark level of invasion, have been associated with poor outcome. At more advanced stages of the disease, the number of involved lymph nodes, the tumor burden, satellite or in-transit metastatic lesions, ulceration, and tumors thicker than 3 mm may be predictive of distant metastases and forebode a worse outcome.

Brain Metastases from Malignant Melanoma

Brain metastases from melanoma are the third most common metastatic brain lesions, behind lung and breast cancer brain metastases. The most common route of entry into the central nervous system is hematogenous spread. At M. D. Anderson, most patients with stage III or IV disease are screened with MRI of the brain before treatment is initiated. Because of this procedure, many patients are diagnosed with asymptomatic brain metastases. In patients who present with symptoms, headache, focal neurologic deficit, and seizure are the most frequent complaints. The tumors can be single or multiple. The tumors are frequently located in the cerebrum, but they can also be found in the cerebellum and brainstem.

The characteristics of melanoma brain metastases on MR images can be confusing because these tumors tend to hemorrhage. This hemorrhage may be silent and found incidentally on routine brain imaging. Hemorrhage is clinically relevant if it occurs in the eloquent brain, causes seizure, or creates a clot large enough to cause headache or obstructive hydrocephalus. Melanoma lesions can be hyperintense on T1-weighted images as a result of acute hemorrhage or the degree of melanin in the lesion. These lesions are brightly enhanced after the administration of intravenous contrast (e.g., gadolinium) (Figure 11–2). Image analysis for treatment decision making is critical, as a hemorrhage may obscure the actual melanotic lesion. The actual contrast-enhanced tumor may not be apparent on an MR image amid the bright signal from the acute hematoma.

Treatment of Metastatic Melanoma to the Brain

The treatment of these lesions is guided by the principles described at the outset of this chapter (see section on Decision Analysis). In patients

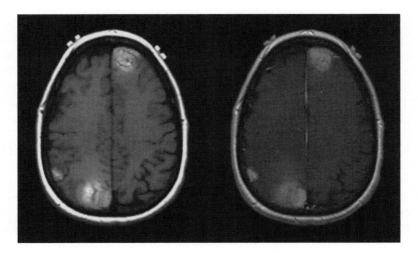

Figure 11–2. Axial precontrast (*left*) and postcontrast (*right*) T1-weighted MR images of a patient with metastatic melanoma. The 2 larger metastases were associated with hemorrhage (subsequently confirmed at the time of surgery). The smaller lesion was deeply melanotic but was without hemorrhage (also confirmed at the time of surgery).

with a single or solitary brain lesion who have limited extracranial disease, direct therapy with either surgery or SRS is frequently recommended. Recent data from M. D. Anderson have demonstrated that in contrast to lung and breast cancer metastases that are 2 to 3 cm, which can be successfully treated with SRS, melanoma lesions with a volume greater than 2 cm^3 do not respond well to SRS (Selek et al, 2004). The trend now is to offer surgery for patients with single or solitary melanoma lesions that are greater than 2 cm^3 regardless of whether symptoms are present. For incidentally found small metastatic lesions, SRS is usually recommended.

For patients with multiple lesions, multidisciplinary treatment is frequently needed. Surgery is usually recommended for large hemorrhagic or symptomatic lesions. In general, if the patient has 1, 2, or 3 lesions, SRS is used as a primary treatment. At M. D. Anderson, a 75% local control rate with SRS was realized for such patients (Selek et al, 2004). Other study series have documented similar results. From those articles, it is apparent that limited systemic disease, a high KPS score, and an intracranial tumor volume of 3 cm^3 or less are associated with a better response to SRS. None of these articles could confirm a benefit from adding WBRT to the treatment regimen.

The utility of WBRT after surgery for brain metastases resection has been verified in a prospective randomized trial (Patchell et al, 1998). However, as specifically related to melanoma, the data are controversial. Whereas the data from the radiosurgery articles mentioned in the previous paragraph could not confirm the utility of WBRT, other data contradict those results. Data from M. D. Anderson have suggested that WBRT after resection of solitary melanoma brain metastases results in improved brain control (by decreasing the rate of recurrence) and a longer median patient survival time (18 vs 6 months; $P = 0.002$) (Skibber et al, 1996). The median survival time was 25 weeks among patients who received WBRT alone, 45 weeks among patients who received WBRT and underwent surgical resection, and 54 weeks in patients with no extracranial disease (Ellerhorst et al, 2001).

Recent data suggest that new chemotherapeutic agents are effective against melanoma brain metastases. Temozolomide is now being used alone or in combination with WBRT for melanoma metastatic to the brain. In 1 study, 12 of 34 patients treated with temozolomide had stable disease, partial remission, or complete remission (Hofmann et al, 2006). The median survival duration was 8 months, and when the treatment was combined with SRS, the duration increased to 9 months. At M. D. Anderson, the use of chemotherapy as a primary treatment for brain metastases is being undertaken only for asymptomatic patients with small lesions. These patients are followed closely, and neurosurgical consultation is obtained when the lesions fail to respond to treatment and grow, hemorrhage, or become symptomatic.

CONCLUSION

Brain metastases from lung cancer, breast cancer, and melanoma are a significant cause of morbidity and mortality among cancer patients. The need for therapy and the type of therapy to be recommended can be determined only after a thorough patient examination, including assessment of the extent of extracranial disease, KPS score, anticipated radiosensitivity of the lesion, and analysis of brain imaging studies to identify the number and size of the lesions. Further studies are needed to confirm the utility of chemotherapy. Multidisciplinary treatment is usually needed. Communication among the patients' caregivers is of paramount importance in determining the combination of modalities that would be most effective.

KEY PRACTICE POINTS

- Lung cancer, breast cancer, and melanoma are the cancers that metastasize to the brain most frequently.
- Metastatic lesions to the brain can be single, solitary, or multiple.
- A careful patient history and physical examination must be performed as well as analysis of all brain imaging studies to assess the extent of disease.
- Before an appropriate treatment can be recommended, the characteristics of the brain lesion must be understood.
- WBRT can be recommended prophylactically for patients with SCLC or multiple brain lesions or after surgical resection.
- Radiosurgery can be recommended for single or multiple lesions that are 3 cm or smaller in the largest diameter (2 cm or smaller for melanomas).
- Surgical resection is warranted for patients with limited systemic disease, for patients with brain tumors larger than 3 cm, and for patients who are medically fit to tolerate surgical intervention.
- The optimal management of brain metastases involves a multidisciplinary approach.

SUGGESTED READINGS

American Cancer Society. *Breast Cancer Facts & Figures, 2005–2006*. Atlanta, GA: American Cancer Society; 2005.

Arriagada R, Le Chevalier T, Riviere A, et al. Patterns of failure after prophylactic cranial irradiation in small-cell lung cancer: analysis of 505 randomized patients. *Ann Oncol* 2002;13:748–754.

Auperin A, Arriagada R, Pignon JP, et al. Prophylactic cranial irradiation for patients with small-cell lung cancer in complete remission. Prophylactic Cranial Irradiation Overview Collaborative Group. *N Engl J Med* 1999;341:476–484.

Bendell JC, Domchek SM, Burstein HJ, et al. Central nervous system metastases in women who receive trastuzumab-based therapy for metastatic breast carcinoma. *Cancer* 2003;97:2972–2977.

Bindal RK, Sawaya R, Leavens ME, Lee JJ. Surgical treatment of multiple brain metastases. *J Neurosurg* 1993;79:210–216.

Ellerhorst J, Strom E, Nardone E, McCutcheon I. Whole brain irradiation for patients with metastatic melanoma: a review of 87 cases. *Int J Radiat Oncol Biol Phys* 2001;49:93–97.

Frazier JL, Garonzik IM, Rhines LD. Metastatic lung cancer. In: Sawaya E, ed. *Intracranial Metastases: Current Management Strategies.* Houston, TX: Blackwell Futura; 2004:199–220.

Goyal S, Prasad D, Harrell F Jr, Matsumoto J, Rich T, Steiner L. Gamma knife surgery for the treatment of intracranial metastases from breast cancer. *J Neurosurg* 2005;103:218–223.

Hofmann M, Kiecker F, Wurm R, et al. Temozolomide with or without radiotherapy in melanoma with unresectable brain metastases. *J Neurooncol* 2006;76: 59–64.

Kim YS, Kondziolka D, Flickinger JC, Lunsford LD. Stereotactic radiosurgery for patients with nonsmall cell lung carcinoma metastatic to the brain. *Cancer* 1997;80:2075–2083.

Korfel A, Oehm C, von Pawel J, et al. Response to topotecan of symptomatic brain metastases of small-cell lung cancer also after whole-brain irradiation. A multicentre phase II study. *Eur J Cancer* 2002;38:1724–1729.

Kristensen CA, Kristjansen PE, Hansen HH. Systemic chemotherapy of brain metastases from small-cell lung cancer: a review. *J Clin Oncol* 1992;10: 1498–1502.

Lederman G, Wronski M, Fine M. Fractionated radiosurgery for brain metastases in 43 patients with breast carcinoma. *Breast Cancer Res Treat* 2001;65:145–154.

Liu ZJ, Herlyn M. Molecular biology of cutaneous melanoma. In: Vincent J, DeVita T, Hellman S, Rosenberg SA, eds. *Cancer: Principles and Practice of Oncology.* Philadelphia, PA: Lippincott Williams & Wilkins; 2005:1745–1753.

Patchell RA, Tibbs PA, Regine RF, et al. Postoperative radiotherapy in the treatment of single metastases to the brain: a randomized trial. *JAMA* 1998;280: 1485–1489.

Patchell RA, Tibbs PA, Walsh JW, et al. A randomized trial of surgery in the treatment of single metastases to the brain [see comment]. *N Engl J Med* 1990;322: 494–500.

Pieper DR, Hess KR, Sawaya RE. Role of surgery in the treatment of brain metastases in patients with breast cancer. *Ann Surg Oncol* 1997;4:481–490.

Pierce LJ, Strawderman M, Narod SA, et al. Effect of radiotherapy after breast-conserving treatment in women with breast cancer and germline *BRCA1/2* mutations. *J Clin Oncol* 2000;18:3360–3369.

Read RC, Boop WC, Yoder G, Schaefer R. Management of nonsmall cell lung carcinoma with solitary brain metastasis. *J Thorac Cardiovasc Surg* 1989;98(5 Pt 2): 884–890; discussion 890–891.

Salbeck R, Grau HC, Artmann H. Cerebral tumor staging in patients with bronchial carcinoma by computed tomography. *Cancer* 1990;66:2007–2011.

Selek U, Chang EL, Hassenbusch SJ 3rd, et al. Stereotactic radiosurgical treatment in 103 patients for 153 cerebral melanoma metastases. *Int J Radiat Oncol Biol Phys* 2004;59:1097–1106.

Skibber JM, Soong SJ, Austin L, Balch CM, Sawaya RE. Cranial irradiation after surgical excision of brain metastases in melanoma patients. *Ann Surg Oncol* 1996;3:118–123.

Vecht CJ, Haaxma-Reiche H, Noordijk EM, et al. Treatment of single brain metastasis: radiotherapy alone or combined with neurosurgery? *Ann Neurol* 1993;33: 583–590.

Weinberg JS, Lang FF, Sawaya R. Surgical management of brain metastases. *Curr Oncol Rep* 2001;3:476–483.

Wolfson AH, Bains Y, Lu J, et al. Twice-daily prophylactic cranial irradiation for patients with limited disease small-cell lung cancer with complete response to chemotherapy and consolidative radiotherapy: report of a single institutional phase II trial. *Am J Clin Oncol* 2001;24:290–295.

12 NEOPLASTIC MENINGITIS

Morris D. Groves

Chapter Overview 245
Introduction 246
Epidemiology 246
Pathophysiology 247
Diagnosis 247
    Symptoms and Signs 247
    Diagnostic Studies 250
        Cerebrospinal Fluid Analysis 250
        Neuroimaging 251
        Cerebrospinal Fluid Flow Studies 252
        When Cerebrospinal Fluid Analytic Results and
        Neuroimaging Results Disagree 252
Disease Management 253
    External Beam Radiotherapy 254
    Intrathecal Chemotherapy 255
        Route of Administration of Intrathecal Chemotherapy 255
        Commonly Used Intrathecal Chemotherapies 255
        Experimental Intrathecal Treatments for Neoplastic Meningitis 256
    Systemic Chemotherapy 257
    Adverse Effects of Therapy 257
Prognosis 258
The Future of Neoplastic Meningitis Treatment 259
Key Practice Points 260
Suggested Readings 260

CHAPTER OVERVIEW

Leptomeningeal dissemination of systemic cancer, which is also known as neoplastic meningitis, occurs in roughly 5% to 8% of cancer patients. Because of the increasing survival of cancer patients and the use of new drugs that inadequately penetrate the brain and cerebrospinal fluid, this percentage may increase. Neoplastic meningitis is usually diagnosed late in a patient's disease course and carries a poor prognosis. Symptoms are related to the cerebral hemispheres, cranial nerves, and spinal nerves. Treatment of neoplastic meningitis is multidisciplinary and is targeted toward palliation, preservation of neurologic function, and prolongation of life. Radiotherapy, intrathecal chemotherapy, systemic chemotherapy, and surgical procedures to provide easy cerebrospinal fluid access or diversion are used. Current interventions provide modest benefit, and newer therapies are needed to extend patient survival beyond the current average of 4 to 6 months.

INTRODUCTION

Neoplastic meningitis (NM) refers to the dissemination of cancer to the pia mater, subarachnoid space, cerebrospinal fluid (CSF), and arachnoid membrane. NM can be a metastatic manifestation of many different malignancies, especially adenocarcinomas, and it carries a poor prognosis. Treating patients with NM requires the expertise of neuro-oncologists, medical oncologists, neurosurgeons, and radiation oncologists. The goals of treatment are primarily palliation and the prevention of neurologic deficits. Because of improvements in treatment for many other cancers, NM is likely to become a more frequently encountered clinical problem. This chapter focuses on NM secondary to solid tumors, but many of the concepts are relevant to the diagnosis and treatment of leptomeningeal involvement of leukemia and lymphoma (see chapter 13).

EPIDEMIOLOGY

On the basis of the total number of cancers diagnosed per year, roughly 60,000 to 70,000 individuals in the United States will develop NM each year, and probably 30% to 50% of them will have the condition confirmed with CSF analysis. Most patients with NM have disseminated cancer at the time of diagnosis, although 20% to 35% of patients may not have identifiably active malignant disease outside the nervous system. Between 6% and 38% of patients have no history of known malignant disease (Olson et al, 1974; Wasserstrom et al 1982). Approximately one third of patients with NM will have evidence of metastatic spread to other areas of the central nervous system (CNS), such as the brain or spine parenchyma or the epidural space (Wasserstrom et al, 1982; Balm and Hammack, 1996). According to an autopsy study, up to 19% of patients with cancer who have neurologic symptoms will have evidence of leptomeningeal involvement of their cancer (Glass et al, 1979).

The incidence of NM varies depending on the histologic characteristics of the primary cancer. Approximately 2% to 5% of patients with breast cancer, 6% to 25% of patients with small cell lung cancer, and 1% to 5% of patients with non-small cell cancer eventually develop NM (Hitchins et al, 1987; Balm and Hammack, 1996). Melanoma patients can have up to a 23% risk of developing NM. Lymphoma and leukemia may involve the leptomeninges in up to 6.3% and 10% of cases, respectively. Other malignancies, including gliomas, some genitourinary cancers, gastrointestinal cancers, and sarcomas, can also metastasize to the leptomeninges. Because of improvements in cancer treatments, the increasing sensitivity of modern diagnostic tests, and the relative sanctuary of the CNS and CSF from large-molecule systemic therapies, the number of persons diagnosed with NM each year will likely increase.

PATHOPHYSIOLOGY

Once malignant cells gain access to the spinal fluid pathways, the cells can be dispersed throughout the CNS by direct extension along the leptomeninges, or they can exfoliate and be carried to other parts of the CNS by CSF flow. New metastatic deposits invade the subpial parenchyma, penetrate spinal nerve roots, and produce subarachnoid masses. The blood-brain barrier, which prevents large, hydrophilic chemotherapeutic agents from entering the CNS, creates a sanctuary for malignant cells and may predispose cancer patients to the development of NM and other CNS metastases.

Malignant cells can gain access to CSF pathways by the routes depicted in Figure 12–1. These routes include direct extension from parenchymal or epidural metastases (synchronous intraparenchymal brain metastases occur in 28% to 75% of patients with NM [Glass et al, 1979; Wasserstrom et al, 1982; Balm and Hammack, 1996]); perineural spread along cranial or spinal nerves; hematogenous spread through arachnoid vessels, the choroid plexus, or the internal spinal venous (Batson's) plexus; or perivenous spread from bone marrow metastases. Intraoperative spread is possible, especially during surgery for posterior fossa metastases. The proximity of tumors to CSF pathways may play a part in their propensity to enter the CSF, as demonstrated by the fact that primary brain tumors such as ependymomas, pineoblastomas, and medulloblastomas are more often associated with NM than are the more common intraparenchymal primary brain tumors.

DIAGNOSIS

Symptoms and Signs

Symptoms and signs of NM are referable to the specific neural structures involved with the tumor. Symptoms and signs are organized into 3 neuroanatomic groups: cerebral, cranial nerve, and spinal. The most common symptoms and signs of NM and their incidence at the time of presentation are listed in Table 12–1. Headache, mental status change, diplopia, back or neck pain, and leg weakness or numbness are the most common complaints. Headache can be due to elevated intracranial pressure from

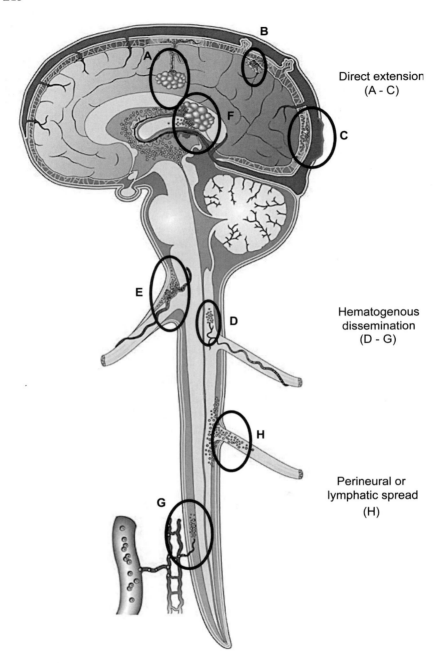

Figure 12–1. The CNS and potential sites of entry of malignant cells resulting in NM. Direct extension of malignant cells into the subarachnoid space can occur from parenchymal brain metastases via the Virchow-Robin spaces (A), by migration through the brain parenchyma (B), or from adjacent dural structures (C).

Table 12–1.   Most Common Symptoms and Signs of NM at Time of Presentation

Neuraxis Level	Incidence of Symptoms		Incidence of Signs	
	Symptom	%	Sign	%
Cerebral				
	Headache	51–66	Mental status changes	27–62
	Mental status changes	26–33	Seizure or syncope	11–18
	Gait difficulty	27	Papilledema	11
	Nausea or vomiting	22–34	Diabetes insipidus	4
	Incoordination	20	Hemiparesis	2
	Loss of consciousness	4	Cerebellar signs	15
	Dizziness	4		
Cranial nerve	Diplopia	20–36	III, IV, or VI	5–36
	Vision loss	9–10	II	6–19
	Facial numbness	10	V	6–10
	Tinnitus or hearing loss	10–14	VII	10–30
	Hypogeusia	4	VIII	7–18
	Dysphonia or dysphagia	2–7	IX or X	2–6
	Vertigo	2	XII	5–10
Spinal				
	Lower motor neuron weakness	34–46	Nuchal rigidity	9–13
	Paresthesia	33–42	Leg or arm weakness	73
	Radicular pain	26–37	Any sensory loss	32
	Back or neck pain	31–37	Straight leg raise test, positive result	15
	Bowel or bladder dysfunction	16–18	Anal sphincter dysfunction	5–14

Adapted from Groves MD. Leptomeningeal carcinomatosis: diagnosis and management. In: Sawaya R, ed. *Intracranial Metastases: Current Management Strategies.* Malden, MA: Blackwell Publishing; 2004:309–330 with permission.

Figure 12–1. *(continued)* Hematogenous tumor dissemination can occur through the radicular arteries (D) or veins (E), the choroid plexus (F), or the vena cava and the valveless venous plexus (G). Malignant cells can also enter the nervous system through direct extension from the nerves (H) or lymphatics. Adapted from Groves MD. The pathogenesis of neoplastic meningitis. *Curr Oncol Rep* 2003;5:15–23 with permission from Current Science, Inc.

obstruction of CSF flow at the level of the arachnoid granulations or the ventricular foramina with resulting communicating or noncommunicating hydrocephalus. Cognitive change resulting from NM can include memory loss, lethargy, extreme somnolence, and even loss of consciousness. Seizure occurs in up to 18% of patients with NM. Cancer cells near the surface of the brain may cause impairment due to brain invasion or possibly due to a metabolic steal phenomenon in which the malignant cells use glucose that would otherwise be available for nearby neurons. Symptoms referable to involvement of the cranial nerves and lumbosacral roots are common because of the frequent accumulation of malignant cells around the gravitationally dependent skull base and lumbosacral regions.

Diagnostic Studies

Cerebrospinal Fluid Analysis

When NM is considered a diagnostic possibility and lumbar puncture is safe, CSF must be evaluated for malignant cells. Cytologic examination to identify malignant cells is the *sine qua non* of diagnosis in NM, but the sensitivity of a single CSF cytologic examination can be as low as 45% (Olson et al, 1974). Several physician-dependent actions have been shown to minimize false-negative CSF results, including (1) withdrawing at least 10.5 mL of CSF for cytologic analysis, (2) immediately processing the CSF specimen, (3) obtaining CSF from a site adjacent to areas suspicious for NM, and (4) repeating this procedure if the initial cytologic test result is negative (Glantz et al, 1998a). The sensitivity of CSF cytologic analysis is improved to more than 77% if more than 1 CSF analysis is performed (Olson et al, 1974; Wasserstrom et al, 1982; Posner, 1995). The variability of CSF test results from the lumbar space versus those from a ventricular reservoir is high enough that lumbar CSF should be obtained, particularly for assessment of response to treatment.

The likelihood of obtaining a positive cytologic result is higher than 60% when neuroimaging findings are suggestive of NM but 25% when neuroimaging reveals no suggestion of NM. Other routine data collected at the time of lumbar puncture can assist in the diagnosis. CSF pressure is higher than 150 mm H_2O (16 cm H_2O) in 30% to 57% of patients at the time of their initial lumbar puncture (Olson et al, 1974). The CSF white blood cell count is elevated in more than 50% of patients with NM and is usually comprised of lymphocytes or polymorphonuclear leukocytes (Olson et al, 1974; Wasserstrom et al, 1982), although this cell count can be normal in as many as one third of patients with a positive cytologic result. A CSF protein concentration higher than 50 mg/dL is found in more than 70% of patients with NM (Olson et al, 1974). Finally, a CSF glucose concentration lower than 60 mg/dL (3.33 mmol/L) is found in up to 77% of patients with NM (Olson et al, 1974), and if infection can be excluded, this finding is highly suggestive of NM.

Neuroimaging

Imaging of the symptomatic areas of the nervous system is needed to identify changes suggestive of NM; imaging of the entire neuraxis is usually necessary for disease staging. Radiographic abnormalities suggestive of NM include leptomeningeal, subependymal, dural, and cranial nerve enhancement and communicating hydrocephalus. Typical imaging findings of NM are depicted in Figures 12–2, 12–3, and 12–4. Neuroimaging findings are more likely to be abnormal for patients with NM from solid tumors than for patients with NM from hematologic malignancies (90% vs 55%, respectively). Approximately 50% of patients with NM and spine-related symptoms will have abnormal imaging results (Wasserstrom et al, 1982).

Magnetic resonance imaging is more sensitive than computed tomography in detecting leptomeningeal enhancement, but among patients who cannot undergo magnetic resonance imaging, contrast-enhanced computed tomography or computed tomographic myelography can provide

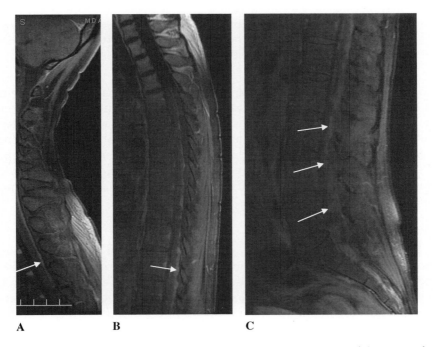

A   B   C

Figure 12–2. T1-weighted gadolinium-enhanced sagittal images of the spine of a 39-year-old woman with small cell lung carcinoma and back pain. (A) Smooth enhancement on the dorsal surface of the spinal cord. (B) Nodular enhancement mostly on the dorsal surface of the lower thoracic cord. (C) Nodular, bulky enhancement in the nerve roots of the cauda equine. Scale shows 1-cm intervals.

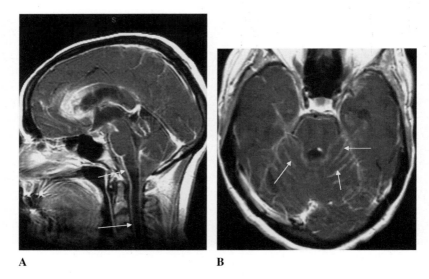

A   **B**

Figure 12–3. T1-weighted gadolinium-enhanced images of the brain of a 44-year-old woman 22 months after the diagnosis of glioblastoma multiforme, now with memory loss and confusion. (A) Sagittal image. Thick sugar-coated enhancement on the anterior and posterior of the brain stem and spinal cord (arrows). (B) Axial image. Classic pattern of enhancement of the cerebellar folia (arrows).

diagnostic information. Because areas of leptomeningeal enhancement are suggestive—but not diagnostic—of NM, one must consider other conditions that can give similar appearances, such as postcraniotomy or postlumbar puncture leptomeningeal changes, calvarial metastases causing dural engorgement, local infection, and inflammatory disease. Patients with positive CSF cytologic results and normal neuroimaging results may have a better prognosis than patients with abnormal imaging results (Glantz et al, 1999b).

Cerebrospinal Fluid Flow Studies

CSF flow is assessed by injecting a radioactive tracer (usually pentetic acid labeled with indium 111) and looking for areas of occult CSF flow obstruction or loculation. As many as 70% of patients with NM can have obstructed CSF ventricular outlets. CSF flow evaluation is usually performed after placement of an intraventricular catheter. Focal radiotherapy administered to areas of CSF flow obstruction has been shown to improve patient survival (Glantz et al, 1995; Chamberlain et al, 1999).

When Cerebrospinal Fluid Analytic Results and Neuroimaging Results Disagree

When imaging is suggestive of NM but malignant cells cannot be found in the CSF, or when only indirect indicators of NM (such as elevated protein

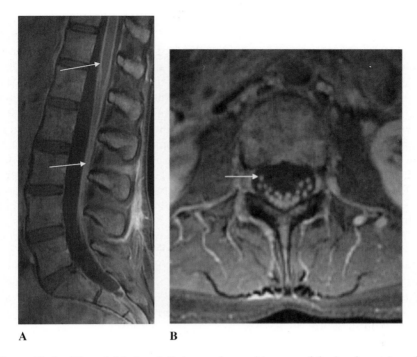

A **B**

Figure 12–4. T1-weighted gadolinium-enhanced images of the lumbar spine of a 40-year-old woman with breast cancer and back pain. (A) Sagittal image. Sugar-coated enhancement of the lower cord and nerve roots (arrows). (B) Axial image. Brightly enhanced nerve roots (arrow).

concentration or depressed glucose concentration) are found on CSF testing, additional markers such as α-fetoprotein, β-human chorionic gonadotropin, carcinoembryonic antigen, and β_2-microglobulin may be useful. Up to 3 lumbar puncture samples may increase diagnostic sensitivity; rarely, meningeal biopsy is necessary. Sampling the CSF from the cisternal area can increase the yield and should be considered when symptoms and signs are referable to the brain or cranial nerves. Time, repeat imaging, and CSF assessment usually resolve the diagnostic dilemma. Occasionally, when clinical features and neuroimaging results typical of NM are found but repeated CSF analyses are nondiagnostic, a presumptive diagnosis can be declared and treatment instituted without cytologic confirmation.

DISEASE MANAGEMENT

The management of NM is controversial because of the lack of strong evidence of the efficacy of current treatment, the poor overall prognosis, and the risk of toxicity from treatment. Fixed neurologic deficits rarely improve and patients do not survive long, although early diagnosis and treatment before the development of significant neurologic disabilities may improve quality of life and prevent neurologic death. The survival of patients with NM is poor and treatment is considered palliative, but aggressive treatment (radiotherapy and intrathecal [IT] chemotherapy) directed at the leptomeningeal disease may increase the survival duration by 3 weeks to 3 months (Balm and Hammack, 1996). The goals of treatment for patients with NM are to improve or stabilize neurologic deficits and to prolong survival. With no therapy, the median survival duration is 4 to 6 weeks and death most often results from progressive neurologic decline. Therapy for NM can provide effective local control such that most patients eventually succumb to systemic disease rather than the neurologic complications of their cancer (Wasserstrom et al, 1982).

Treatment of NM should target the entire neuraxis because tumor cells are generally thought to disseminate throughout the CSF. Both bulky disease and malignant cells floating in the CSF must be addressed; therefore, both focal and more systemic treatments are needed. Proper management of the patient's underlying systemic malignancy should accompany any treatment directed to the CSF. Patients who may derive the most benefit from treatment are those whose underlying tumor is quiescent or is known to be responsive to the available treatments. Guidelines recently published by the National Comprehensive Cancer Network (2006) suggest stratifying patients as having either poor risk or good risk of survival to determine whether aggressive treatment should be instituted. These guidelines define poor-risk patients as those with (1) a low Karnofsky performance scale score, (2) multiple, serious, fixed neurologic deficits, and (3) extensive systemic disease with few treatment options. Supportive care and radiotherapy to symptomatic sites of disease are suggested for poor-risk patients. The guidelines define good-risk patients as those with (1) a high Karnofsky performance scale score, (2) no fixed neurologic deficits, (3) minimal systemic disease, and (4) reasonable systemic treatment options, if needed.

Patients with NM can be physically or cognitively impaired and may require more assistance than the immediate family can provide. For practicality and safety, modifications of the home and special means of transportation may be necessary. Addressing the psychologic burden of NM on patients and their caregivers is also an integral part of the care of each patient.

External Beam Radiotherapy

External beam radiotherapy can be useful in several clinical scenarios for patients with NM. Treatment should be considered to areas of CSF flow obstruction or where bulky disease is identified. Typical radiation doses are 30 Gy given in 10 fractions; patients with breast cancer, leukemia, and lymphoma are considered the best candidates for this therapy. Craniospinal radiotherapy is rarely used because of the significant myelosuppressive and gastrointestinal toxicities with which it is associated. Palliative radiotherapy to areas of symptomatic disease may be given to patients who are good candidates for more aggressive approaches.

Intrathecal Chemotherapy

IT chemotherapy is used to treat subclinical leptomeningeal deposits and tumor cells suspended in the CSF and to prevent further seeding of the leptomeninges. The use of IT chemotherapy versus systemic chemotherapy is debatable. At least 1 report has suggested that IT chemotherapy increases toxicity without added benefit over radiotherapy and systemic chemotherapy (Bokstein et al, 1998). Another study showed a better survival outcome for patients treated with systemic methotrexate (MTX) rather than IT MTX (Glantz et al, 1998b).

Route of Administration of Intrathecal Chemotherapy

For patient comfort and better CSF distribution of chemotherapeutic drugs, most patients have a ventricular reservoir placed for drug delivery. Intralumbar delivery of chemotherapeutic drugs may result in drug placement outside the thecal sac and increased variability of ventricular drug concentrations. For patients with CNS leukemia, drug delivery via an Ommaya reservoir appears to improve the durability of remission compared with intralumbar drug delivery (Bleyer and Poplack, 1979). The reservoir is usually well tolerated, but complications such as misplacement, catheter tip occlusion, and infection can occur in as many as 5% of patients.

Commonly Used Intrathecal Chemotherapies

IT chemotherapies commonly used to treat NM include MTX, cytarabine (Ara-C), and thiotepa (triethylenethiophosphoramide). Very few randomized trials have compared the efficacy of these drugs. In a study comparing IT MTX and IT thiotepa in 59 patients with solid tumors, there was no significant difference in the median survival duration between the 2 treatment groups (Grossman et al, 1993). Another study comparing IT MTX alone or with IT Ara-C found no significant difference in outcomes for 44 patients with meningeal carcinomatosis (Hitchins et al, 1987).

MTX is the most commonly used IT drug for treating NM. It is a cell cycle phase–specific antimetabolite that acts primarily during the S phase. Typical dosing schemes use MTX (10 to 12 mg) mixed with preservative-free normal saline and delivered intrathecally twice a week for 8 doses. If a response is noted with clearing of malignant cells from the CSF, the treatment is decreased to once a week for 4 doses, then twice monthly for 4 doses, and then monthly for a variable time. Intraventricular injections of

MTX result in therapeutic concentrations (greater than 1 μM) that persist for 48 hours. With the use of MTX, along with radiotherapy as needed, up to 50% of patients with NM can be clinically stabilized or improved (Wasserstrom et al, 1982; Hitchins et al, 1987). MTX toxicities such as myelo-suppression and mucositis can be prevented by using folinic acid, which does not enter the CNS and leaves the MTX within the CNS unantagonized.

Ara-C is a synthetic pyrimidine analog that is relatively specific to the S phase of the cell cycle. It is used most commonly in patients with menin-geal leukemia or lymphoma. A new method of delivery for Ara-C was recently approved for lymphomatous meningitis: DepoCyt is an injectable sustained-release formulation of Ara-C that extends the terminal half-life of free Ara-C in the CSF from 3.4 to 140 hours, allowing for treatment twice monthly instead of twice weekly. Measurable Ara-C concentrations can be maintained in the lumbar and ventricular CSF for up to 2 weeks after a sin-gle dose of DepoCyt. A randomized trial demonstrated the superiority of DepoCyt over standard Ara-C in treating lymphomatous meningitis (Glantz et al, 1999b). That study of 28 patients demonstrated a number of improvements with DepoCyt over standard Ara-C: a higher response rate (71% vs 15%), a longer median time to neurologic progression (78.5 vs 42 days), and a longer median overall survival duration (99.5 vs 63 days). The most common adverse events with DepoCyt were headache, arach-noiditis, nausea, vomiting, and fever. DepoCyt has also been studied in patients with breast cancer and other solid tumors but has not been found to offer significant improvement over IT MTX (Glantz et al, 1999a).

Thiotepa is an alkylating agent that has induced tumor responses in some patients. It is usually administered in 10- to 15-mg IT doses on a similar schedule as IT MTX. IT thiotepa was prospectively compared with IT MTX in patients with NM, but no significant difference in efficacy was noted between the 2 drugs, although thiotepa was more myelosuppres-sive (Grossman et al, 1993).

Even though combination chemotherapy improves outcomes in many systemic cancers, improvement has not been seen in studies of IT combi-nation chemotherapy for NM. Studies of the IT combinations of MTX and thiotepa; MTX and Ara-C; MTX, thiotepa, and Ara-C; and MTX, thiotepa, Ara-C, and hydrocortisone have failed to demonstrate improved response rates or survival rates compared with single-drug regimens (Hitchins et al, 1987; Stewart et al, 1987), although they have demonstrated increased myelosuppression and neurotoxicity (Stewart et al, 1987).

Experimental Intrathecal Treatments for Neoplastic Meningitis

Numerous IT strategies have been and are being tested for use in patients with NM. These strategies include the use of alkylating agents such as temozolomide, mafosfamide, diaziquone, and ACNU (the abbreviation of the chemical name of nimustine) and the topoisomerase inhibitor topote-can. No IT cytotoxic treatment has yet been shown to be superior to the standard available agents. Laboratory and clinical studies continue to evaluate other IT strategies using immunotherapy (including interleukin-2), radiolabeled monoclonal antibodies, free radionuclides, and gene therapy.

Systemic Chemotherapy

Even though it is not well studied in NM, systemic chemotherapy may have a role in treating this disease. Retrospective evidence indicates that systemic chemotherapy with or without IT chemotherapy may increase patient survival duration (Boogerd et al, 1991). Therapeutic CSF concentrations of most drugs are not generally considered to be achievable, although there is strong evidence that cytotoxic MTX concentrations (1 µM and higher) can be achieved after high-dose administration (Glantz et al, 1998b). Intravenous systemic therapies directed toward NM may be less toxic than IT chemotherapy but no less efficacious (Bokstein et al, 1998). Hormonal therapy in conjunction with IT therapy may result in better overall survival for patients with NM (Boogerd et al, 1991), and there are case reports of hormonally responsive NM from breast cancer. At M. D. Anderson Cancer Center, unless contraindicated, we usually prefer that patients remain on effective antitumor therapy for their systemic disease while being treated for NM.

Adverse Effects of Therapy

Major toxicities can result from delivery of IT chemotherapy or radiotherapy to the CNS (Chamberlain et al, 1997). IT Ara-C–associated neuropathy or myeloneuropathy can occur. IT MTX can cause acute arachnoiditis, nausea, vomiting, and mental status change, and high CSF concentrations of IT MTX may be associated with seizure (Bleyer et al, 1973). IT MTX can also cause mucositis and myelosuppression if not followed by systemic administration of folinic acid. The toxicity of IT thiotepa is similar to that of IT MTX but may cause more hematologic toxicity (Grossman et al, 1993). Radiotherapy may worsen myelosuppression in patients heavily pretreated with chemotherapeutic drugs and may increase the likelihood of neurotoxicity from IT chemotherapy (Bleyer et al, 1973). Necrotizing leukoencephalopathy associated with IT MTX, especially when MTX is administered after radiotherapy, is a feared complication in patients with NM. A less fulminate leukoencephalopathy, manifested by dementia, seizure, progressive tetraparesis, and change in white matter, may be more likely to occur in patients undergoing IT chemotherapy than in patients undergoing systemic chemotherapy (Bokstein et al, 1998).

Chronic arachnoiditis, or CSF flow obstruction due to arachnoid granulation blockade by cellular debris, can cause symptoms of cerebral hypoperfusion, usually due to a relative increase in intracranial pressure compared with systemic blood pressure. This condition is frequently misdiagnosed as seizure activity. Resolution of symptoms with simple CSF drainage via the Ommaya reservoir or lumbar puncture can help alleviate the patient's symptoms and avoid inappropriate use of anticonvulsants. Long-term management of this problem can be accomplished with frequent CSF draws, CSF diversion with a ventriculoperitoneal shunt, or administration of acetazolamide or steroids.

PROGNOSIS

Treating NM from solid tumors will stabilize or improve neurologic symptoms in about 45% of patients (Wasserstrom et al, 1982). Without therapy, patients with NM have a very poor prognosis; survival duration is about 3 to 6 weeks, and progressive neurologic dysfunction is often the cause of death (Wasserstrom et al, 1982; Balm and Hammack, 1996). A number of factors have been identified that may be predictive of longer patient survival or greater tumor response, although there is not complete agreement in the literature on the implications of all factors. Table 12–2 lists some

Table 12–2. Patient- and Treatment-Related Factors That May Be Predictive of Patient Survival or Tumor Response

Factor	Effect on Survival or Response*
CSF cleared of cells with IT chemotherapy	+ + +
No CSF block, or CSF block cleared	+ +
Controlled systemic disease	+
History of intraparenchymal tumor	+
Karnofsky performance scale score ≥70	+
Longer duration of neurologic symptoms	+
Concomitant systemic and IT chemotherapy	+
Treatment with IT chemotherapy	+
Female sex	+
Negative neuroimaging results	+
Longer pretreatment duration of CSF disease	+
Spinal involvement	+
Long delay from diagnosis to neurologic symptoms	+
Low CSF protein concentration	+
High CSF protein concentration	+ 0 – –
Low CSF glucose concentration	0 –
Cerebral involvement or encephalopathy	– – –
Eastern Cooperative Oncology Group score >3	–
Cranial nerve deficit	–
Progressive systemic disease at study entry	–

* Each symbol in this column represents a result from 1 published study. +, Positive effect; 0, no effect; –, negative effect.
Adapted from Groves MD. Leptomeningeal carcinomatosis: diagnosis and management. In: Sawaya R, ed. *Intracranial Metastases: Current Management Strategies*. Malden, MA: Blackwell Publishing; 2004:309–330 with permission.

Table 12–3. Average Median Survival Duration of Patients with NM, by Histologic Type

Histologic Type	Number of Studies	Median Survival Duration (Weeks) of Relevant Studies	
		Average	Range
Breast	13	16.5	5–38
Lung	3	15	8–22
Small cell lung cancer	4	8.6	4–15.5
Non-small cell lung cancer	3	13	9–20
Lymphoma	9	16	8.8–32
Gastrointestinal	1	7	

Adapted from Groves MD. Leptomeningeal carcinomatosis: diagnosis and management. In: Sawaya R, ed. *Intracranial Metastases: Current Management Strategies.* Malden, MA: Blackwell Publishing; 2004:309–330 with permission.

patient- and treatment-related factors that may affect survival and response. In particular, treatment that clears malignant cells from the CSF appears to correspond with an improved overall survival (Hitchins et al, 1987; Boogerd et al, 1991; Glantz et al, 1999b). Glantz and colleagues (1999b) found evidence that those patients who responded to IT chemotherapy had improvements in quality-of-life measures. Table 12–3 provides the averages of the median survival durations of patients from a number of studies in which specific primary histologic types and outcomes for each group could be ascertained. Recent studies have reported time to neurologic progression after the initiation of treatment, which may be a more useful tool than survival in assessing treatment efficacy in NM.

THE FUTURE OF NEOPLASTIC MENINGITIS TREATMENT

Patients with NM require the expertise of neurosurgeons, radiation oncologists, medical oncologists, and neuro-oncologists. Despite the collective expertise, the effect of treatment on patients' outcomes has been unimpressive. Relatively few therapeutic agents have been tested for NM. One goal for the future is to test novel agents in this setting. Regimens that combine cytotoxic and noncytotoxic treatments that target tumor cell invasion, migration, and angiogenesis may have a role in the treatment of NM. Future clinical trials will need to group patients with the same underlying histologic types to better determine the efficacy of targeted therapies in specific disease states. To achieve meaningful outcomes from clinical trials, the cooperation of multiple centers will be necessary. Ultimately, significant improvement in outcomes for patients with NM will stem from a better understanding of the molecular factors that promote metastasis and from the application of that understanding toward the development of novel treatments for patients with this serious metastatic complication.

KEY PRACTICE POINTS

- The incidence of NM will likely increase as patients with cancer live longer.
- Clinical symptoms or signs localized to multiple regions of the nervous system should raise the diagnostic suspicion of NM.
- Finding malignant cells in the CSF is the *sine qua non* of diagnosis, but strong clinical and imaging evidence of disease may occasionally be enough to initiate treatment.
- Patients with a low Karnofsky performance scale score and patients who present with encephalopathy or fixed cranial nerve deficits may be better served with palliative care.
- Ventricular access devices allow for better distribution of intrathecally administered drugs.
- CSF flow study results shown to be normal are needed to help minimize the toxicity of intrathecally delivered drugs by preventing loculation of the administered drugs and prolonged high drug concentrations adjacent to nervous system tissue.
- External beam radiotherapy can be useful in relieving obstructed CSF flow and in treating nodular disease.
- IT MTX given concurrently with or after radiotherapy increases the risk of CNS toxicity.
- Symptoms of cerebral hypoperfusion with syncope or near-syncope can be due to elevated CSF pressure from obstructed CSF outflow or from arachnoiditis. High CSF pressure should be treated with CSF diversion, acetazolamide, or steroids.

SUGGESTED READINGS

Balm M, Hammack J. Leptomeningeal carcinomatosis. Presenting features and prognostic factors. *Arch Neurol* 1996;53:626–632.

Bleyer WA, Drake JC, Chabner BA. Neurotoxicity and elevated cerebrospinal-fluid methotrexate concentration in meningeal leukemia. *N Engl J Med* 1973;289: 770–773.

Bleyer WA, Poplack DG. Intraventricular versus intralumbar methotrexate for central-nervous-system leukemia: prolonged remission with the Ommaya reservoir. *Med Pediatr Oncol* 1979;6:207–213.

Bokstein F, Lossos A, Siegal T. Leptomeningeal metastases from solid tumors: a comparison of two prospective series treated with and without intra-cerebrospinal fluid chemotherapy. *Cancer* 1998;82:1756–1763.

Boogerd W, Hart AA, van der Sande JJ, Engelsman E. Meningeal carcinomatosis in breast cancer. Prognostic factors and influence of treatment. *Cancer* 1991;67: 1685–1695.

Chamberlain MC, Kormanik PA, Barba D. Complications associated with intra-ventricular chemotherapy in patients with leptomeningeal metastases. *J Neurosurg* 1997;87:694–699.

Chamberlain MC, Kormanik P, Jaeckle KA, Glantz M. [111]Indium-diethylenetri-amine pentaacetic acid CSF flow studies predict distribution of intrathecally administered chemotherapy and outcome in patients with leptomeningeal metastases. *Neurology* 1999;52:216–217.

Fizazi K, Asselain B, Vincent-Salomon A, et al. Meningeal carcinomatosis in patients with breast carcinoma. Clinical features, prognostic factors, and results of a high-dose intrathecal methotrexate regimen. *Cancer* 1996;77:1315–1323.

Glantz MJ, Cole BF, Glantz LK, et al. Cerebrospinal fluid cytology in patients with cancer: minimizing false-negative results. *Cancer* 1998a;82:733–739.

Glantz MJ, Cole BF, Recht L, et al. High-dose intravenous methotrexate for patients with nonleukemic leptomeningeal cancer: is intrathecal chemotherapy necessary? *J Clin Oncol* 1998b;16:1561–1567.

Glantz MJ, Hall WA, Cole BF, et al. Diagnosis, management, and survival of patients with leptomeningeal cancer based on cerebrospinal fluid-flow status. *Cancer* 1995;75:2919–2931.

Glantz MJ, Jaeckle KA, Chamberlain MC, et al. A randomized controlled trial comparing intrathecal sustained-release cytarabine (DepoCyt) to intrathecal methotrexate in patients with neoplastic meningitis from solid tumors. *Clin Cancer Res* 1999a;5:3394–3402.

Glantz MJ, LaFollette S, Jaeckle KA, et al. Randomized trial of a slow-release versus a standard formulation of cytarabine for the intrathecal treatment of lymphomatous meningitis. *J Clin Oncol* 1999b;17:3110–3116.

Glass JP, Melamed M, Chernik NL, Posner JB. Malignant cells in cerebrospinal fluid (CSF): the meaning of a positive CSF cytology. *Neurology* 1979;29:1369–1375.

Grossman SA, Finkelstein DM, Ruckdeschel JC, Trump DL, Moynihan T, Ettinger DS. Randomized prospective comparison of intraventricular methotrexate and thiotepa in patients with previously untreated neoplastic meningitis. Eastern Cooperative Oncology Group. *J Clin Oncol* 1993;11:561–569.

Hitchins RN, Bell DR, Woods RL, Levi JA, A prospective randomized trial of single-agent versus combination chemotherapy in meningeal carcinomatosis. *J Clin Oncol* 1987;5:1655–1662.

National Comprehensive Cancer Network. *NCCN Clinical Practice Guidelines in Oncology, Version 2.2006. Central Nervous System Cancers*. National Comprehensive Cancer Network; 2006.

Olson ME, Chernik NL, Posner JB. Infiltration of the leptomeninges by systemic cancer. A clinical and pathologic study. *Arch Neurol* 1974;30:122–137.

Pfeffer MR, Wygoda M, Siegal T. Leptomeningeal metastases—treatment results in 98 consecutive patients. *Isr J Med Sci* 1988;24:611–618.

Posner JB. Leptomeningeal metastases. In: Posner JB, ed. *Neurologic Complications of Cancer*. Philadelphia, PA: F.A. Davis; 1995:143–171.

Stewart DJ, Maroun JA, Hugenholtz H, et al. Combined intraommaya methotrexate, cytosine arabinoside, hydrocortisone and thio-TEPA for meningeal involvement by malignancies. *J Neurooncol* 1987;5:315–322.

Wasserstrom WR, Glass JP, Posner JB. Diagnosis and treatment of leptomeningeal metastases from solid tumors: experience with 90 patients. *Cancer* 1982;49:759–772.

13   Lymphoma Affecting the Central Nervous System

Barbara Pro

Chapter Overview 263
Introduction 263
Diagnosis and Staging 264
Treatment 266
    Radiotherapy 266
    Methotrexate-Based Chemotherapy 267
    Neurotoxic Effects of Treatment 268
    Other Adverse Effects of Treatment 269
    Intrathecal Chemotherapy 270
Salvage Treatment 270
Key Practice Points 271
Suggested Readings 271

CHAPTER OVERVIEW

Primary central nervous system lymphoma (PCNSL) is defined as extra-nodal lymphoma that arises in the central nervous system. Symptomatic therapy alone results in a median survival duration of only 2 to 3 months. Radiotherapy often produces complete remission, but the response is transient and the median survival duration of patients is 12 to 18 months. First-generation chemotherapy (e.g., the combination of cyclophosphamide, doxorubicin, vincristine, and prednisone and similar regimens) commonly used to treat systemic non-Hodgkin's lymphoma is ineffective in treating PCNSL, partly because of the blood-brain barrier. The addition of methotrexate-based chemotherapy to radiotherapy significantly improves the outcome of patients with PCNSL. However, neurotoxicity is a significant and severe complication, particularly for patients over the age of 60 years.

INTRODUCTION

Primary central nervous system lymphoma (PCNSL) is defined as non-Hodgkin's lymphoma that at the time of diagnosis is confined to the central nervous system. This disease typically involves the brain and less commonly the eyes, leptomeninges, and spinal cord. PCNSL accounts for approximately 4% to 7% of primary brain tumors and occurs more frequently in patients who are immunocompromised, particularly those with AIDS. However, in contrast to the incidence of PCNSL in immunocompetent patients, the incidence of AIDS-related PCNSL has decreased significantly in the last decade, after the introduction of highly active antiretroviral therapy. The etiology of the disease is still poorly understood. The Epstein-Barr virus appears to have a role in the pathogenesis of this disease in immunocompromised patients but not in immunocompetent patients (Auperin et al, 1994). A pathogenetic role of other viruses such as human herpesvirus 8 has been suggested but needs to be confirmed (Corboy et al, 1998).

DIAGNOSIS AND STAGING

PCNSL can affect all age groups, but the peak incidence occurs during the fifth to seventh decades of life in immunocompetent individuals. The most common presenting symptoms and signs are focal neurologic deficits (70% of cases) and behavioral and cognitive changes (43% of cases) (Bataille et al, 2000). Seizures occur in 15% to 20% of cases. The prevalence of ocular involvement at diagnosis has varied from 5% to 20% in the literature; the most common visual complaints are floaters and blurred vision. The initial evaluation for the diagnosis of suspected PCNSL should include cranial magnetic resonance imaging (MRI; preferred), computed tomography (CT), or both. MRI and CT can provide results that are suggestive of but not conclusive for PCNSL. Typically, PCNSL appears as isodense or hyperdense lesions on CT scans, and lesions show homogeneous enhancement after the administration of intravenous contrast. On T1-weighted MR images, the lesions are isodense or hypodense and typically show homogeneous enhancement after administration of gadolinium. PCNSL commonly involves the subcortical white matter; the lesions are adjacent to the ventricles and are solitary in most cases.

The diagnostic procedure of choice for PCNSL is stereotactic needle biopsy. Surgical resection does not improve survival and is indicated only in cases with signs of herniation. To help with the decision of the best diagnostic approach, a neurosurgical consultation should be obtained as soon as a diagnosis of PCNSL is suspected. Patients treated with steroids can have false-negative biopsy results, so steroids should be withheld until the biopsy is performed. Lumbar puncture for cerebral spinal fluid (CSF) studies is an important test for the diagnostic workup, but it should be avoided in patients with large posterior fossa lesions or evidence of a midline shift. CSF evaluation should include basic studies such as cell count, protein concentration, and glucose concentration; lactate dehydrogenase and β_2-microglobulin levels; cytology and flow cytometry; and polymerase chain reaction for clonal immunoglobulin gene rearrangements. Most patients have elevated levels of CSF proteins, whereas positive cytology findings are reported to be between 26% and 31% among immunocompetent patients (Fine and Mayer, 1993). An elevated lactate dehydrogenase or β_2-microglobulin level is suggestive of lymphomatous involvement. Figure 13–1 shows the diagnostic workup for suspected PCNSL and the procedures used to stage the disease.

Most PCNSLs exhibit a B-cell immunophenotype. Accordingly, the tumor cells express B-cell antigens such as CD19 and CD20. T-cell lymphomas are extremely rare; they represent approximately 2% of all PCNSL cases. In immunocompetent patients, the most common histologic subtype of PCNSL is diffuse large cell lymphoma, whereas in AIDS-related PCNSL, the tumor cells are more often immunoblastic, Burkitt's lymphoma-like, or large atypical. The mitotic activity for all cases of PCNSL is generally high, indicating a very aggressive tumor. Microscopically, PCNSL infiltrates are typically patchy, poorly demarcated, and angiocentric. The last characteristic is a key histologic feature of lymphoma (Figure 13–2).

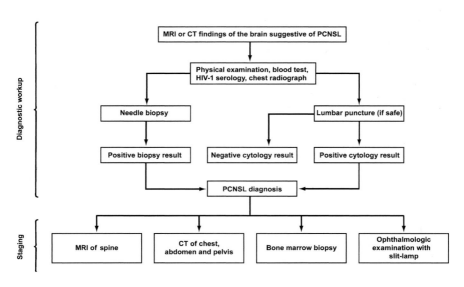

Figure 13–1. Diagnostic workup for suspected PCNSL and staging of the diagnosed disease. In light of the rarity of spinal cord involvement, MRI of the spine is indicated only when the clinical suspicion of spinal cord tumor is high.

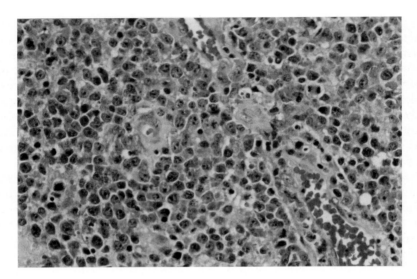

Figure 13–2. PCNSL infiltrates are typically patchy, poorly demarcated, and angiocentric. A characteristic feature is perivascular infiltration. Courtesy of Dr. John T. Manning, M. D. Anderson Cancer Center, Houston, TX.

TREATMENT

PCNSL is a highly aggressive tumor, and the median survival duration is only 2 to 3 months for untreated patients. Because of the rarity of this disease and the need to improve patient outcome, we encourage patients with PCNSL to participate in prospective trials.

Radiotherapy

In the past, whole-brain radiotherapy (WBRT) was the conventional treatment for patients with PCNSL. As primary therapy, radiotherapy is associated with an initial response in up to 80% of patients, but this response is short lived. In a Radiation Therapy Oncology Group prospective study, patients were given 40-Gy WBRT plus a focal boost of 20 Gy to the tumor site (Nelson et al, 1992). The reported local control rate was 39%, and 79% of recurrences occurred in the boosted fields. The median survival time was 11.6 months. Patients over 60 years of age did significantly worse: their median survival time was 7.6 months.

Subsequently, to improve patient survival, several studies have explored the combination of chemotherapy and radiotherapy. Lachance and colleagues (1994) were the first to report on the use of the combination of cyclophosphamide, doxorubicin, vincristine, and prednisone plus WBRT in the initial treatment of PCNSL. Despite a significant initial radiographic response, the duration of remission was brief and the median survival time was only 8.5 months. This lack of efficacy may be partially attributable to the poor penetration of the blood-brain barrier by these chemotherapeutic agents. The Radiation Therapy Oncology Group reported similarly disappointing results a few years later (Schultz et al, 1996). Fifty-four immunocompetent patients with newly diagnosed PCNSL were treated with 3 cycles of cyclophosphamide, doxorubicin, vincristine, and dexamethasone (CHOD) followed by WBRT (41.4 Gy) plus a tumor boost of 18 Gy. This regimen did not significantly improve the outcome over radiotherapy alone: the median survival duration was 16 months, and the 2-year survival rate was 42%. From these early studies it emerged that (1) radiotherapy alone is insufficient to treat PCNSL and there is no clear dose-response relationship because of the persistently high rate of local recurrence and that (2) conventional chemotherapy regimens commonly used in systemic lymphoma are ineffective in PCNSL.

Methotrexate-Based Chemotherapy

Following the first initial reports on the efficacy of high-dose methotrexate (MTX) for patients with recurrent central nervous system lymphoma, many studies have shown that high-dose MTX with leucovorin rescue is the most effective agent for treating PCNSL and should be used as the initial therapy. The addition of high-dose MTX-based chemotherapy to radiotherapy substantially extends the survival duration over radiotherapy alone. For example, Glass and colleagues (1994) reported on 25 patients treated with high-dose intravenous MTX ($3.5 \ g/m^2$) before radiotherapy. The response rate to MTX before radiotherapy was 88%, and the median duration of response was 32 months. The median patient survival duration was 33 months for the whole group and 42.5 months for those whose disease responded to the chemoradiotherapy regimen. Concerning the optimal dose of MTX to deliver, consensus is that a dose of $3 \ g/m^2$ or higher ("high dose") in a 4- to 6-hour infusion is recommended.

Although MTX is the chemotherapeutic agent with the most proven activity against PCNSL, a major question relates to the value of adding other cytotoxic drugs to MTX. In a prospective combined-modality trial, DeAngelis and colleagues (1992) treated 31 patients with intravenous MTX ($1 \ g/m^2$) given weekly for 2 weeks along with 6 doses of intrathecal MTX (12 mg per dose). This regimen was followed by WBRT and subsequent high-dose systemic cytarabine. The response rate to MTX alone was 64%, the median disease-free survival time was 41 months, and the median overall survival time was 42.5 months. More recently, the same group reported the results of preradiotherapy MTX ($3.5 \ g/m^2$) with procarbazine and vincristine followed by WBRT and high-dose cytarabine. The median survival rate was 60%, and the 5-year survival rate was 50% (Abrey et al, 2000). The results from these 2 studies suggest that other cytotoxic agents can be used with high-dose MTX to improve treatment for PCNSL, although the best combination remains to be defined. Several studies are currently investigating the role of other chemotherapeutic agents (e.g., temozolomide and topotecan) and monoclonal antibodies (e.g., rituximab) in MTX-based chemotherapy regimens as primary treatment for PCNSL.

Neurotoxic Effects of Treatment

Unfortunately, in a significant percentage of patients, the benefits of treatment are overshadowed by neurotoxicity. Delayed neurologic toxicity resulting from the combined effects of high-dose MTX and WBRT has become an increasingly recognized complication, and the risk increases with patient age. In patients older than 60 years, virtually all the long-term survivors will develop severe delayed neurotoxicity after combined treatment, as characterized by attention deficit, memory impairment, ataxia, urinary incontinence, and eventually dementia. Among younger patients, cognitive dysfunctions due to treatment are usually less severe. Hence, the role of radiotherapy as consolidation treatment for patients who have achieved complete remission after chemotherapy is controversial and should be evaluated in a phase III trial. Certainly, WBRT after MTX-based chemotherapy should be avoided in patients older than 60 years. Our current approach at M. D. Anderson Cancer Center is to use high-dose MTX-based chemotherapy for all PCNSL patients and to use WBRT in patients younger than 60 years of age but avoid or defer WBRT in older patients (Figure 13–3).

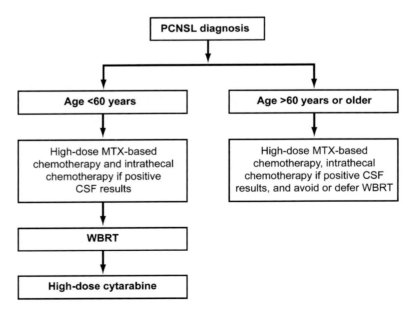

Figure 13–3. Treatment algorithm used at M. D. Anderson for patients with newly diagnosed PCNSL.

Different approaches are being taken in an effort to minimize late neurotoxicity, including the use of chemotherapy alone and the use of autologous bone marrow transplantation. Results from recent trials suggest that high-dose MTX-based chemotherapy with deferred radiotherapy produces results comparable to those achieved with concurrent chemotherapy and radiotherapy but with less neurotoxicity. In 1 series, all 31 patients initially treated with high-dose intravenous MTX without radiotherapy achieved a complete response (n = 20; 65%) or a partial response (n = 11; 35%) and were then given maintenance MTX at 3.5 g/m^2 for 3 cycles at monthly intervals and then an indefinite number of cycles at 3-month intervals (Guha-Thakurta et al, 1999). There were no cases of neutropenic fever or infection; acute renal failure was observed in 3 cycles and was reversible. The median survival time was 30 months. Among the patients who had achieved a complete response, the 2-year survival rate was 90%. After a median follow-up of 31 months, there was no evidence of encephalopathy (Guha-Thakurta et al, 1999). In another study, 52 patients were treated with high-dose MTX, procarbazine, and vincristine (Abrey et al, 2000). Twenty-two older patients in whom radiotherapy was deferred were compared with 12 older patients who received radiotherapy. The median survival duration was similar for both patient groups (33 vs 32 months), but significant delayed neurotoxicity was observed in those patients who were irradiated.

The value of intensive chemotherapy with autologous stem cell transplantation as first-line treatment is questionable as there are only limited data. In 1 study, 28 patients with newly diagnosed PCNSL were treated with 3.5 g/m^2 MTX and high-dose cytarabine as induction therapy (Abrey et al, 2003). Fourteen patients responded and were subsequently treated with carmustine, etoposide, cytarabine, and melphalan and with autologous stem cell rescue. The event-free survival time was 5.6 months for patients who had a partial response and 9.3 months for patients who had a complete response; thus, this therapy was no better than conventional chemotherapy treatment. A small study by Cheng and colleagues (2003) evaluated 7 patients with PCNSL who were treated with high-dose MTX-based chemotherapy followed by thiotepa, busulfan, and cyclophosphamide as well as autologous stem cell transplantation. Five patients had no relapse 5 to 42 months from the time of diagnosis.

Other Adverse Effects of Treatment

In our experience at M. D. Anderson, high-dose MTX does not produce significant myelosuppression, and it is well tolerated even in elderly patients. However, mucositis and hepatic, renal, and hematologic toxicities are side effects commonly seen in patients treated with high-dose MTX. We use vigorous intravenous hydration, alkalinization of the urine, and leucovorin rescue to minimize toxicity, and patients receive treatment in the inpatient setting for better monitoring. Serum MTX levels are obtained daily beginning

24 hours after MTX administration to monitor drug clearance, and the dose of leucovorin is changed depending on the serum MTX level.

Intrathecal Chemotherapy

Because it is believed that the leptomeninges and CSF are predominant sites of relapse, intrathecal chemotherapy is commonly recommended as part of the first-line therapy for patients with PCNSL. However, recent retrospective studies have failed to show a benefit by adding intrathecal chemotherapy to high-dose intravenous chemotherapy. A therapeutic concentration of MTX (10 µM) can be achieved in the CSF by using intravenous doses of 3 g/m^2 or higher. Thus, intrathecal chemotherapy can probably be avoided for most patients provided that adequate doses of intravenous MTX are used, and it should be reserved for only those patients with evidence of CSF involvement at the time of diagnosis.

SALVAGE TREATMENT

More than half of patients with PCNSL who achieve a first remission eventually suffer a relapse. The time to relapse is the most important prognostic factor of the median survival duration after relapse, which is 14 months for patients who receive second-line therapy. High-dose chemotherapy with autologous stem cell transplantation has been shown to be a feasible and active approach. In a single-institution pilot study, 20 patients with relapsed and refractory PCNSL were treated with an induction combination of cytarabine and etoposide followed by high-dose chemotherapy with thiotepa, busulfan, and cyclophosphamide and then autologous stem cell rescue (Soussain et al, 2001). The remission rate was 72%, and the 3-year estimated overall survival rate was 64%.

The regimen of procarbazine, lomustine, and vincristine (Herrlinger et al, 2000) and MTX reinduction have been shown to be effective in treating patients with recurrent disease after treatment with MTX-based chemotherapy. Additional options for salvage therapy include temozolomide, topotecan, high-dose cytarabine, and the monoclonal antibody rituximab.

Because most cases of PCNSL are B-cell neoplasms expressing the CD20 surface antigen, a potential and appealing therapeutic agent is the chimeric anti-CD20 monoclonal antibody rituximab. Schultz and colleagues (2004) treated 6 patients who had recurrent PCNSL ($n = 4$) or systemic lymphoma and central nervous system involvement ($n = 2$) with intravenous and intrathecal or intraventricular rituximab. All 4 patients with leptomeningeal disease achieved an objective response, whereas of the 2 patients with parenchymal disease, only 1 minor response was observed. Wong and colleagues (2004) investigated a combination of intravenous rituximab with the chemotherapeutic agent temozolomide in 7 patients with recurrent central nervous system lymphomas; this combination was well tolerated, and all patients achieved an objective response. Enting and colleagues (2004) reported on their study of temozolomide and rituximab in relapsed PCNSL. Fifteen patients with a median age of 69 years had a 53% objective response rate, and the median progression-free survival time of responding patients was 7.7 months.

In patients with relapse after chemotherapy alone, radiotherapy can be used. Nguyen and colleagues (2005) reported on 27 consecutive patients who failed initial high-dose MTX treatment and underwent salvage WBRT (median dose, 36 Gy). Ten patients (37%) achieved a complete response as seen on radiography, and 10 patients (37%) achieved a partial response, for a 74% overall response rate. The estimated median survival time was 10.9 months. Age less than 60 years and response to WBRT were associated with longer survival times.

KEY PRACTICE POINTS

- Stereotactic needle biopsy is the diagnostic procedure of choice for suspected PCNSL.
- When possible, the use of steroids should be withheld until the diagnosis is confirmed.
- Patients with PCNSL should be encouraged to participate in clinical trials.
- High-dose MTX-based chemotherapy followed by radiotherapy should be regarded as the standard first-line therapy for PCNSL patients younger than 60 years.
- Intrathecal chemotherapy should be used only for patients with evidence of leptomeningeal involvement.

SUGGESTED READINGS

Abrey LE, Moskowitz CH, Mason WP, et al. Intensive methotrexate and cytarabine followed by high-dose chemotherapy with autologous stem-cell rescue in patients with newly diagnosed primary CNS lymphoma: an intent-to-treat analysis. *J Clin Oncol* 2003;21:4151–4156.

Abrey LE, Yahalom J, DeAngelis LM. Treatment for primary CNS lymphoma: the next step. *J Clin Oncol* 2000;18:3144–3150.

Auperin J, Mikolt J, Oksenhendler E, et al. Primary central nervous system malignant non-Hodgkin's lymphomas from HIV-infected and non-infected patients: expression of cellular surface proteins and Epstein-Barr viral markers. *Neuropathol Appl Neurobiol* 1994;20:243–252.

Bataille B, Delwail V, Menet E, et al. Primary intracerebral malignant lymphoma: report of 248 cases. *J Neurosurg* 2000;92:261–266.

Cheng T, Forsyth P, Chaudhry A, et al. High-dose thiotepa, busulfan, cyclophosphamide and ASCT without whole-brain radiotherapy in primary CNS lymphoma. *Bone Marrow Transplant* 2003;31:679–685.

Corboy JR, Garl PJ, Kleinschmidt-DeMasters BK. Human herpes-virus 8 DNA in CNS lymphomas from patients with and without AIDS. *Neurology* 1998;48:1333–1335.

DeAngelis LM, Yahalom J, Thaler HAT, Kher U. Combined modality therapy for primary central nervous system lymphoma. *J Clin Oncol* 1992;10:635–643.

Enting RH, Demopoulos A, DeAngelis LM, Abrey LE. Salvage therapy for primary CNS lymphoma with a combination of rituximab and temozolomide. *Neurology* 2004;63:901–903.

Fine HA, Mayer RJ. Primary central nervous system lymphoma. *Ann Intern Med* 1993;119:1093–1104.

Glass J, Gruber ML, Cher L, Hochberg F. Preirradiation methotrexate chemotherapy of primary central nervous system lymphoma: long-term outcome. *J Neurosurg* 1994;81:188–195.

Guha-Thakurta N, Damek D, Polack C, Hochberg FH. Intravenous methotrexate as initial treatment for primary central nervous system lymphoma. Response to therapy and quality of life of patients. *J Neurooncol* 1999;43:259–268.

Herrlinger U, Brugger W, Bamberg M, Kuker W, Dichgans J, Weller M. PVC salvage chemotherapy for recurrent primary CNS lymphoma. *Neurology* 2000;54: 1707–1708.

Lachance DH, Brizel DM, Gockerman JP, et al. Cyclophosphamide, doxorubicin, vincristine and prednisone for primary central nervous system lymphoma: short duration of response and multifocal intracerebral recurrence preceding radiotherapy. *Neurology* 1994;44:1721–1727.

Nelson DF, Martz KL, Bonner H, et al. Non-Hodgkin's lymphoma of the brain: can high dose, large volume radiation improve survival? Report on a prospective trial by the Radiation Therapy Oncology Group (RTOG): RTOG 8315. *Int J Radiat Oncol Biol Phys* 1992;23:9–17.

Nguyen PL, Chakravarti A, Finkelstein DM, Hochberg FH, Batchelor TT, Loeffler JS. Results of whole-brain radiation as salvage of methotrexate failure for immunocompetent patients with primary CNS lymphoma. *J Clin Oncol* 2005;23:1507–1513.

Schultz H, Pels H, Schmidt-Wolf I, Zeelen U, Germing U, Engert A. Intraventricular treatment of relapsed central nervous lymphoma with the anti-CD20 antibody rituximab. *Haematologica* 2004;89:753–754.

Schultz C, Scott C, Sherman W, et al. Preirradiation chemotherapy with cyclophosphamide, doxorubicin, vincristine, and dexamethasone for primary CNS lymphomas: initial report of Radiation Therapy Oncology Group protocol 88-06. *J Clin Oncol* 1996;14:556–564.

Soussain C, Suzan F, Hoang-Xuan K, et al. Results of intensive chemotherapy followed by hematopoietic stem-cell rescue in 22 patients with refractory or recurrent primary CNS lymphoma or intraocular lymphoma. *J Clin Oncol* 2001;19:742–749.

Wong ET, Tishler R, Barron L, Wu JK. Immunochemotherapy with rituximab and temozolomide for central nervous system lymphomas. *Cancer* 2004;101: 139–145.

14 TUMORS OF THE EXTRADURAL SPINE

Ehud Mendel

Chapter Overview 274
Introduction 274
Clinical Presentation 275
Diagnostic Tests 275
Primary Bony Spinal Lesions 277
    Hemangiomas 278
    Aneurysmal Bone Cysts 278
    Osteoblastic Lesions 279
        Osteoid Osteomas 279
        Osteoblastomas 279
    Osteochondromas 280
    Giant Cell Tumors 280
    Plasma Cell Neoplasms 281
    Chordomas 281
    Ewing's Sarcomas 282
    Osteosarcomas 282
    Chondrosarcomas 282
Metastatic Spinal Lesions 284
Indications for Surgery 287
Surgical Adjuncts 288
    Embolization 288
    Transfusion 288
    Cell Saving 288
    Electrophysiologic Monitoring 288
    Intraoperative Fluoroscopy 288
Surgical Techniques 288
    Percutaneous Vertebroplasty and Kyphoplasty 289
    Approaches to the Cervical Spine 290
    Approaches to the Thoracic Spine 290
    Approaches to the Thoracolumbar Spine 290
    Approaches to the Lumbar Spine 291
    Approaches to the Sacrum 291
Adjuvant Therapies 291
    Radiotherapy 291
    Chemotherapy 292

Postoperative Care 292
    Bracing 292
    Deep Vein Thrombosis Prophylaxis and Anticoagulation 292
Key Practice Points 292
Suggested Readings 293

CHAPTER OVERVIEW

Patients who have tumors of the extradural spine often present with pain or neurologic deficit, the types of which depend on the level of spinal cord or nerve root compression. The management of these tumors has taken on an aggressive multimodal approach as a result of the development of superior imaging techniques and improved diagnostic and treatment options. The diagnostic testing options usually include radiography, computed tomography, and magnetic resonance imaging (the gold standard). Radiography can be used to diagnose malignancy, but computed tomography and magnetic resonance imaging are needed to delineate the extent of the tumor. Specific tumor types are discussed in detail in this chapter, and a distinction is made between primary and metastatic tumors. Surgery is more likely to be performed to aid in diagnosis, palliation, and restoration of spinal stability rather than to achieve oncologic cure. A multidisciplinary approach is crucial for optimal management of extradural spinal tumors; the various surgical techniques and adjuvant options are reviewed.

INTRODUCTION

The management of extradural spinal tumors has evolved rapidly over the past 20 years as the development of high-resolution imaging techniques has allowed earlier diagnosis and improved diagnostic and treatment regimens. Furthermore, recent advances in surgical technology, particularly in spinal fixation and instrumentation, and focused radiosurgical techniques have allowed an aggressive multimodal approach to managing selected vertebral column tumors, thereby resulting in improved patient evaluation and care. Extradural spinal tumors can be primary or secondary (i.e., metastatic). Both types present diagnostic and therapeutic challenges. Whether primary or metastatic, extradural spinal tumors can abut the dura matter and affect the vertebrae, soft tissue, and vascular structures. Symptoms arise from compression or invasion of the adjacent normal tissue. A multidisciplinary approach is crucial for optimal disease management. As newer management techniques become more common and as they continue to evolve, their efficacy will be evaluated.

CLINICAL PRESENTATION

Pain and neurologic compromise are common among patients with verte-bral tumors at presentation. With the advent of earlier cancer detection and high-resolution imaging, an increasing number of patients are asympto-matic at the time of discovery of both primary and metastatic spinal lesions.

On clinical presentation, the patient's history may reveal insidious and progressive pain. However, acute neck or back pain in a patient with a history of malignancy is generally assumed to be metastatic disease until proven otherwise. Whether primary or secondary, virtually all malignant tumors of the bony spine cause localized pain. Pain may arise from periosteal expansion or pathologic collapse. Radicular pain can occur when soft tissue or bone encroaches into the foramina. Nocturnal pain and pain associated with weight bearing are symptoms of destructive lesions of the vertebral column caused by skeletal metastases or primary bone tumors. Spinal instability secondary to extensive bony destruction or pathologic fractures can cause mechanical pain. The incidence of neu-rologic deficit in bony spinal tumors is directly proportional to the length of time between the onset of pain and diagnosis. More aggressive tumors will result in a more rapid onset of neurologic symptoms.

Neurologic compromise due to compression of the spinal cord or nerve roots may manifest as myelopathy or radiculopathy. Depending on the level of compression, several clinical symptoms may emerge. Patients with disease involving the cervicothoracic region may present with weakness or even muscle atrophy of the hands with or without lower extremity weak-ness and hyperreflexia. They may also present with abnormal plantar reflexes and occasionally Brown-Séquard syndrome. For patients with dis-ease involving the thoracic spine, most signs are nonspecific. Lower extrem-ity weakness, for example, is nonspecific, although a definite sensory level may localize the lesion to a specific level. Beevor's sign suggests that the lesion is at or below vertebra T9, whereas constipation, automatic bladder, spastic sphincter, and priapism suggest the lesion is above the medullary cone. Patients with lesions of the thoracolumbar junction can present with conus medullaris syndrome (motor weakness or nerve root syndromes) or cauda equina syndrome (sensory loss in the lumbosacral dermatomes with loss of sphincter tone, saddle anesthesia, absence of knee and ankle reflexes, and loss of sensation in the rectum, vagina, and urethra).

DIAGNOSTIC TESTS

Diagnostic testing often begins with plain radiography. Anteroposterior and lateral films are easy to obtain and are inexpensive, and the results are often diagnostic of malignancy. Anteroposterior and lateral films of the entire spine are also useful in assessing spinal alignment and stability. They can also be used to predict the quality of bone strength that can be expected intraoperatively. Loss of pedicle height seen on the anteroposterior film (the "winking owl" sign is seen with extensive erosion of the pedicle), a compression fracture, or destruction of several vertebrae with preservation of discs may suggest a malignant lesion. Certain areas of sclerosis can suggest an osteoblastic lesion or bone remodeling in a very slow progressive neoplastic process. Visualization of a vertebral body defect on plain radiographic film suggests at least 50% destruction of that vertebral body. However, metastatic tumors in general infiltrate the bone marrow of a vertebral body without destroying the cortical bone. If the patient has neurologic deficits due to spinal cord compression, abnormalities on plain films are noted in up to 60% to 80% of the cases (Sundaresan et al, 1990a). Dynamic flexion/extension films are useful for detecting spinal instability, although they are rarely necessary and may put the patient at increased risk of spinal cord injury.

Magnetic resonance imaging (MRI) and computed tomography (CT) are essential in delineating the extent of a tumor. Whereas MRI offers optimal visualization of epidural compression and paraspinal soft tissue involvement, CT provides better insight into the degree of bone destruction. The detection of a vertebral lesion necessitates MRI of the entire spine, at least in the sagittal plane, to determine the presence of multiple coincident lesions, which would be suggestive of metastatic disease. In cases for which MRI is contraindicated or the images are obscured by an artifact, CT myelography can provide excellent simultaneous imaging of bone anatomy and central neural constituents. Lumbar or cervical instillation of intrathecal dye may be necessary in cases of high-grade epidural compression. CT is a more sensitive method than plain radiography for detecting pathologic characteristics but is relatively nonspecific and impractical to use as a screening test. CT-guided needle biopsy is performed when there is no known malignancy and a pathologic diagnosis is desirable. Even where there is a known primary malignancy, biopsy may be appropriate to confirm a histologic diagnosis and to help determine the appropriate therapy. Percutaneous dorsal CT-guided needle biopsy can be performed routinely below the cervical spine. Cervical lesions are less amenable to percutaneous biopsy and require more dependence on a radiographic rather than histologic diagnosis before a definitive treatment is determined. CT is also very useful for surgical planning. When spinal instrumentation is planned, bone window CT with coronal and sagittal reconstruction is superior to MRI for measuring pedicle dimensions, vertebral body height, and vertebral body width in segments above and below the primary pathologic lesion.

MRI is the gold standard for studying tumors of the spine. MRI may allow elimination of the risks of lumbar puncture, and it provides superior visualization of the pathologic area and the surrounding anatomy. Nevertheless, patients with claustrophobia, indwelling pacemakers, or other metallic implants may not be able to undergo MRI. In addition, anterior or posterior spinal instrumentation in patients often renders MRI useless. Gadolinium enhancement is often useful for distinguishing between active tumor and surrounding deformed bone or soft tissue anatomy. Fat suppression techniques are useful in delineating tumors from epidural or paraspinal fatty components. The extent and degree of spinal cord compression are readily revealed on T2-weighted images. MRI is the most sensitive and specific modality for imaging spinal metastases and for distinguishing them from osteoporotic compression fractures, which are common among patients with cancer. Osteoporotic fractures are most common in the thoracic spine and do not involve the pedicle. On T1-weighted MR images, these fractures lack signal changes. In contrast, pathologic fractures are more common in the lumbar spine, generally have a homogeneously decreased signal, and may involve the pedicle.

Positron emission tomography scanning may also help to differentiate osteoporotic and pathologic compression fractures. Osteoporotic fractures evaluated more than 3 days from the onset of symptoms are generally hypometabolic, whereas most tumors are hypermetabolic (Dehdashti et al, 1996).

Angiography alone is not often useful as a diagnostic test, but it is commonly employed in conjunction with embolization before surgery and in selected cases. Spinal angiography is performed to visualize vascular tumors (e.g., renal cell carcinomas) or to embolize feeding vessels.

Radionuclide bone scanning is a sensitive but not very specific method for detecting metastatic disease in the spine (O'Mara, 1974). Bone scans are positive for most malignant spinal tumors. The sensitivity of bone scanning is decreased with hematopoietic and lymphoreticular tumors. Bone scanning relies on osteoblastic bone deposition to detect spinal metastases, so rapidly progressive and destructive tumors may not be visualized using this technique (Algra et al, 1992; Gosfield et al, 1993). This technique is also relatively insensitive with multiple myelomas that are limited to the bone marrow (Gosfield et al, 1993). Most cases of osteomyelitis, degenerative spondylosis, hemangiomas, fractures, and other benign disorders of the spine result in increased uptake of the radionuclide (Frank et al, 1990).

PRIMARY BONY SPINAL LESIONS

Primary tumors of the spine are uncommon. In a review by Dahlin (1978) of 6,221 bone tumors, fewer than 10% of all primary tumors involved the spine. Presenting symptoms include night pain, pain at rest, and neurologic deficits. The pain can be back pain or radicular pain. There is no difference between the pain symptoms of patients with benign versus malignant disease involving the spine (Weinstein, 1989). For slowly growing primary bone tumors, the interval between the onset of symptoms and diagnosis is often prolonged. These tumors can have an insidious course of nonspecific, common complaints. Often, a plain radiograph will reveal the lesion and can be diagnostic. CT and MRI are extremely valuable in exploring the extent and location of the lesion.

Hemangiomas

Hemangiomas are vascular lesions and one of the most common benign neoplasms that arise in the spinal axis from newly formed blood vessels. The incidence is not known because most hemangiomas are chance findings in patients who may have pain from unrelated causes. They are more common in females than males and are solitary two thirds of the time. Hemangiomas tend to be located in the lower thoracic or upper lumbar spine. On plain films, hemangiomas exhibit a characteristic honeycomb appearance due to linear reactive calcification around the radiolucent vascular tissue.

Most of these hemangiomas are confined to their vertebral body and are not of clinical concern. Direct compression of the spinal cord results from extension of the vascular tumor tissue into the epidural space. Pathologic fractures or epidural hemorrhage from the tumor may lead to symptoms. Spine surgeons become involved in the treatment of hemangiomas when the lesion compresses the spinal cord. Surgery is usually not indicated for the management of pain that is not associated with neurologic involvement.

Patients with asymptomatic lesions do not require further evaluation unless pain or neurologic deficits begin to develop. Those who have painful lesions should be followed closely with periodic neurologic examinations. Patients with neurologic symptoms may require surgery. Embolization followed by decompression and tumor resection generally leads to satisfactory results. Complete resection of these lesions is often possible and is recommended because of the potential morbidity and the lack of efficacy associated with radiotherapy, which is the only other reasonable treatment modality.

Aneurysmal Bone Cysts

Aneurysmal bone cysts occur most frequently in children and are uncommon in patients older than 30 years. These cysts can occur in any part of the skeleton. In the vertebrae, which constitute the location of 16% of aneurysmal bone cysts, they involve the posterior elements 60% of the time. They are often located in the lumbar vertebrae and may affect multiple lumbar levels. Aneurysmal bone cysts are benign, proliferative, lytic, rapidly expanding, and destructive lesions of the bone that can produce significant neurologic compromise. They make up approximately 20% of lesions that appear in the spine. Plain radiography and CT are the best tools with which to reach an accurate diagnosis because they can define the degree of bone destruction and the extent of the lesion. MRI reveals the degree of spinal cord compression. Selective angiography can have both diagnostic and therapeutic value (MacCarty et al, 1952). In general, complete surgical resection is the treatment of choice. Preoperative embolization can be used to minimize hemorrhage. The recurrence rate of aneurysmal bone cysts is high when resection is incomplete; in this situation, subsequent treatment such as radiotherapy or a second resection should be considered to optimize local control.

Osteoblastic Lesions

Osteoblastic lesions are benign tumors of the spine. They occur more often in males than females at presentation. Osteoid osteomas are smaller than 1.5 cm in diameter, whereas larger lesions are called osteoblastomas. Although this size cutoff is rather arbitrary, the former have a more self-limited growth potential, whereas the latter may undergo late malignant transformation. Osteoblastic lesions should be considered in any patient younger than 40 years old with back or neck pain, painful scoliosis, or radicular pain. Both tumors are characterized by a nidus of osteoid and woven bone surrounded by vascular fibrous tissue and a cap of sclerotic bone with thickened trabeculae. Radiography usually reveals a dense sclerotic rim of reactive bone surrounding a central nidus less than 2 cm in diameter. Bone scanning is the most sensitive method for locating these lesions because they have intense radionuclide uptake. Scoliosis may be present because the spine curves away from the tumor.

Osteoid Osteomas

Osteoid osteomas tend to occur in patients under the age of 30 years. They account for 21% of surgically managed benign spinal lesions. Typically, these lesions occur in the lumbar spine. Osteoid osteomas produce arachidonic acid, the breakdown product of which may cause osteolysis, which can cause pain and secondary scoliosis (Nguyen et al, 1989). The pain can be successfully treated with nonsteroidal anti-inflammatory medications. An indication for the treatment of vertebral osteoid osteoma is pain or scoliosis; in such cases, complete surgical excision is necessary to avoid recurrence. However, osteoid osteomas have been known to spontaneously resolve.

Osteoblastomas

Osteoblastomas constitute 0.5% of primary bone tumors that are managed with surgery. They usually occur in the second or third decade of life. Osteoblastomas occur almost exclusively within the posterior elements.

As with patients with osteoid osteomas, 20% to 60% of patients with osteoblastomas develop painful scoliosis. Patients may present with radicular symptoms or myelopathy due to local mass effect. Usually a single vertebra is affected; extension into surrounding soft tissue is unusual. Plain radiography and radionuclide bone scanning are diagnostic, but CT more clearly demonstrates the well-defined, oval, hyperdense nidus surrounded by sclerotic bone. MRI is useful in illustrating the presence and severity of nerve root or thecal sac effacement. A dense sclerotic bony rim encasing a soft and vascular nidus is encountered at surgery. Complete tumor removal by en bloc resection is curative. Unlike osteoid osteomas, osteoblastomas must be surgically resected. An incomplete resection carries a high risk of recurrence.

Osteochondromas

Osteochondromas, either solitary or multiple, are the most frequently encountered benign bone lesion. They consist of cartilage-covered cortical bone with underlying medullary bone. The cartilaginous cap undergoes calcification to form the osteochondroma. These lesions most commonly present in the third decade and appear more often in males than females. The lesions affect the posterior elements or the spinous process and can involve the pedicle. Approximately half of the lesions occur in the cervical spine. The diagnostic test of choice is plain radiography or CT. Osteochondromas show increased radionuclide uptake on bone scans, although less intensely than other lesions such as osteoid osteomas do. They tend to increase in size during the rapid growth of adolescence and may continue to grow throughout adulthood. Scoliosis may be present but not as frequently as it is in osteoblastic lesions. Only 1% of osteochondromas undergo malignant transformation. Surgical excision is the treatment of choice.

Giant Cell Tumors

Giant cell tumors are rare but locally aggressive. They are composed mostly of multinucleated giant cells dispersed throughout the stroma, make up about 4% of bone tumors, and occur more often in females than males. Giant cell tumors are rarely found in the spine, where they most frequently involve the sacrum (Dahlin, 1978). They usually involve a single vertebra, and imaging reveals a destructive expansile mass within the bone. Malignant transformation occurs in 10% of cases.

Depending on the location and extent of the tumor, surgical curettage or en bloc resection should be performed. Because of their large size or inaccessible location, advanced giant cell tumors are rarely amenable to complete surgical resection. A complete resection of sacral lesions usually necessitates sacrificing bowel and bladder innervation. Sacrectomy with attempted curative wide excision is warranted if the neurologic consequences are acceptable.

Giant cell tumors may be very vascular, and preoperative tumor embolization may be beneficial. To reduce local progression, radiotherapy may be
considered after a subtotal resection (Camins and Rosenblum, 1991, 1992).

Plasma Cell Neoplasms

Plasma cell neoplasms (multiple myelomas or plasmacytomas) are the
most common of all primary malignant lesions of the adult spine (Dahlin,
1978). This disease afflicts 2 to 3 people per 100,000 in the general population. It is twice as common among blacks than whites, and it occurs
slightly more often among males than females. The malignant proliferation of plasma cells occurs in bone marrow, spleen, and all lymphoid tissues. A small number of patients are diagnosed with a solitary
plasmacytoma. Plasmacytomas are usually diagnosed in middle-aged
men, who then have a median survival duration of almost 8 years. In contrast, patients who develop multiple myelomas in their seventh and eighth
decades have a 5-year survival rate of 18% (Poor et al, 1988; Rosenblum
and Camins, 1992). Characteristics of multiple myelomas are bone marrow infiltration by plasma cells and a markedly reduced immunoglobulin level. In plasmacytomas, bone marrow is negative for plasma cell
infiltration, and serum protein electrophoresis results are normal.

The treatment of choice for solitary plasmacytomas is vertebroplasty
for pain control and possibly radiotherapy afterwards for pain and tumor
control. Because approximately 50% of solitary plasmacytomas progress
to multiple myelomas within 5 years (most commonly by 3 years),
patients need to be closely followed to rule out disease progression.
Chemotherapy may be indicated for patients with multiple myelomas,
particularly if progression is documented.

Chordomas

Chordomas constitute about 5% of malignant tumors involving the spine.
These tumors arise from notochord remnants and are indolent malignancies that tend to be locally progressive and can metastasize late in their
course. About 85% of chordomas occur in the sacrum or the clivus; the
remainder occur in other parts of the spine. Fifty percent of chordomas
are sacrococcygeal, 40% are sphenoccipital, and the remaining 10% are
found in the mobile intermediate regions of the spine. About half of
chordomas occur during the fifth to seventh decades of life. The 5-year
survival rate ranges from 50% to 77%, and the 10-year survival rate is
approximately 50%.

There is general agreement that en bloc resection is the optimal intervention for chordomas. Aggressive surgery may not always be technically
feasible in advanced cases or if the patient has medical contraindications.
Tumors involving the sacrococcygeal spine require ventral, dorsal, or
combined surgical approaches. These surgical approaches should attempt
to obtain the widest possible resection while sparing normal structures as

much as possible (Sailer et al, 1988). One retrospective study of 21 patients with spinal chordomas favored a combination of surgery and radiotherapy over surgery alone (Kaparov and Kitov, 1977). Currently, there is no evidence that supports the use of chemotherapy to manage chordomas.

Ewing's Sarcomas

Ewing's sarcomas constitute 6% of primary malignant bone tumors and 3.5% of those involving the spine (Bradway and Pritchard, 1990; Sharafuddin et al, 1992; Grubb et al, 1994). These tumors develop most commonly in the first 2 decades of life, and they occur more often in males than females (Bradway and Pritchard, 1990; Grubb et al, 1994). More than half of Ewing's sarcomas of the spine occur in the sacrum; the second most common site is the lumbar spine.

In most cases, plain radiographs reveal a lytic destructive lesion that may be surrounded by a sclerotic rim. The tissue has the gross appearance of a soft, mucinous, gray-white tumor. Patients with sacral masses may have rectal masses noted on physical examination. Preoperative embolization should be considered when surgical excision is planned (Bradway and Pritchard, 1990; Sharafuddin et al, 1992). Optimal treatment includes a combination of chemotherapy, surgery, and possibly radiotherapy (Djindjian, 1989; Mohan et al, 1989). The role of surgery in the treatment of spinal Ewing's sarcoma is controversial. Surgery is indicated for diagnosis or for decompression of the spinal canal, and an attempt at maximum resection should be undertaken (Sharafuddin et al, 1992). The presence of an extraosseous soft tissue mass augments the difficulty of surgical management. In some patients, even a subtotal resection may be difficult.

Osteosarcomas

Osteosarcomas are the most common primary bone tumors found throughout the skeleton. They occasionally arise in the spine, either as primary tumors or as metastatic deposits. Primary osteosarcomas (at any skeletal site) are usually seen in young adults, whereas secondary lesions can arise in irradiated bone in older patients. In Dahlin and Coventry's series (1967), spinal osteosarcomas developed after radiotherapy in 16 of 600 cases. Because the prognosis of patients with these tumors is poor, total spondylectomy followed by radiotherapy and aggressive chemotherapy has been advocated. Long-term survival has been reported for a few patients treated using these techniques (Sundaresan et al, 1988, 1990b; Weinstein, 1991).

Chondrosarcomas

Chondrosarcomas constitute about 10% of malignant primary tumors of the spine (Dahlin, 1978). They range from almost benign-appearing round cell tumors to very malignant spindle cell sarcomas. Most chondrosarcomas are indolent and tend to recur locally over prolonged periods before spreading distantly (Sanerkin, 1980; Shires et al, 1983). They occur more often in males than females. Although they grow slowly, these lesions carry a relatively poor overall prognosis for patients. Their resistance to chemotherapy and radiotherapy contributes to the risk of local recurrence after surgery. Complete excision—en bloc, if possible—is the goal of surgery (Figure 14–1).

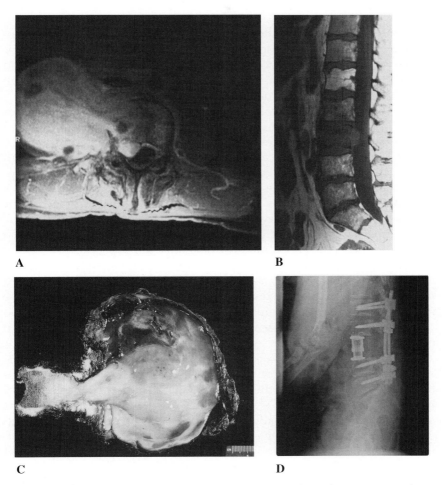

A

B

C

D

Figure 14–1. (A) Axial MR image showing a mesenchymal sarcoma involving the L3 vertebral body. (B) Sagittal MR image showing the tumor involving the entire L3 vertebral body. (C) Gross specimen of the tumor resected en bloc. The tumor is streaming into the L3 body. (D) Postoperative lateral plain radiograph showing the reconstruction. Reprinted from Mody MG, Rao G, Rhines LD. Surgical management of spinal mesenchymal tumors. *Curr Oncol Rep* 2006; 8:297–304 with permission from Current Science, Inc.

In low-grade chondrosarcomas, local control may be improved with wide resection compared with intralesional resection. Although there have been reports of longer patient survival time with multiple subtotal resections than with a debulking procedure repeated over several years, en bloc resection should be attempted when possible.

Metastatic Spinal Lesions

Between 5% and 10% of patients with all types of cancer develop symptomatic metastatic spinal disease at some point during the course of their cancer. As many as one third of these patients have spinal metastases and die with metastatic disease. In 20% of patients with vertebral column involvement, the disease progresses to spinal cord compression.

The thoracic and thoracolumbar regions constitute the locations for about 70% of all spinal metastatic deposits. The lumbar spine is involved in approximately 20% of cases and the cervical spine in 10% of cases. Breast, lung, and prostate cancers are responsible for at least half of all spinal metastatic disease. Pain is the most common presenting symptom in patients with metastatic tumors to the spine; therefore, back pain in a patient with cancer should be assumed to arise from metastatic disease until proven otherwise. Spinal instability secondary to bone destruction can cause mechanical pain, and nerve root irritation can cause radicular pain. The pain may also have a matutional component that affects patients mostly at night or in the early morning and generally abates as the day progresses. Mechanical pain tends to worsen with movement and diminish when the patient lies down. A comprehensive neurologic examination should be performed on all patients with suspected spinal metastatic disease because myelopathy can also be a sign of metastatic disease.

The primary modalities for treating metastatic disease are chemotherapy, radiotherapy, and surgery. Regardless of the treatment modality, the most important factor affecting a patient's prognosis is his or her ability to walk at the time therapy is initiated. Loss of sphincter control predicts a poor outcome and is usually irreversible. The role of surgery in metastatic spinal disease is palliative; the emphasis is on reducing pain, preserving neurologic function, and restoring mobility with maintenance of sphincter control. The relative merits of radiotherapy, surgery, or both are a matter of debate, but surgery is favored when appropriate (Patchell et al, 2003). Surgery should provide decompression of the spinal cord and nerve roots as well as stabilization of the spinal column (Figure 14–2). Cooperation between surgeons and oncologists is advisable to achieve optimal management of symptomatic spinal metastases.

The biologic properties of the primary tumor, including its growth characteristics and radiosensitivity, should determine the optimal method

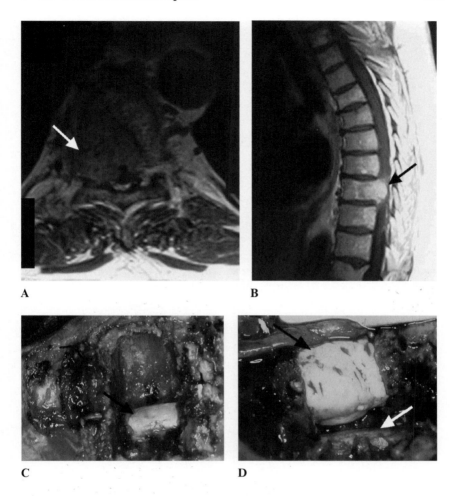

A   B

C   D

Figure 14–2. Axial (A) and sagittal (B) MR images showing compression of the thecal sac (black arrow) from a tumor originating in the vertebral body (white arrow). (C) Transthoracic vertebrectomy with removal of the diseased vertebral body. Note the decompressed thecal sac (black arrow). (D) Reconstruction with methyl methacrylate (black arrow). Note the decompressed thecal sac (white arrow).

of management of spinal metastases. The relief from pain and the preservation or restoration of neurologic function due to surgical intervention contribute to the quality of life of a cancer patient and reduce the burden of care. Radiotherapy is usually considered for metastatic tumors that are radiosensitive and cause minimal or no neurologic deficits.

Metastatic breast disease is usually radiosensitive and often responds to both hormonal and cytotoxic chemotherapy. In these cases, surgical

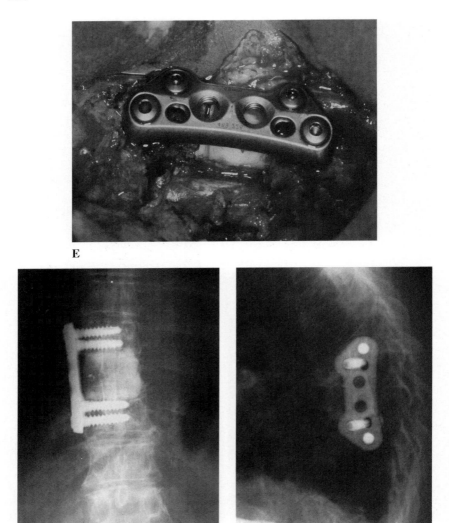

Figure 14–2. *(continued)* (E) Stabilization with titanium plate. Anteroposterior (F) and lateral (G) postoperative radiographs demonstrating the construct.

intervention may be limited. Spinal involvement from lung cancer can be a result of direct extension from a chest wall mass or a result of true hematogenous metastasis. Patients with small cell lung carcinoma in particular do not usually require surgery because these tumors are radiosensitive and rarely cause bone destruction or instability. Prostate cancer often responds to palliative nonsurgical efforts and is usually sensitive to radiotherapy, at least for a time. Prostate cancer rarely produces spinal instability until later in its course. Surgical intervention is useful if, despite radiotherapy, there is evidence of spinal instability, intractable pain due to a specific lesion, or neurologic deficits.

Squamous cell carcinoma and adenocarcinoma of the lung with spinal involvement are resistant to radiotherapy and frequently progress despite aggressive radiotherapy. Renal cell carcinoma is usually resistant to radiotherapy and is highly variable in its biologic behavior. As such, this tumor lends itself to a surgical approach. These 3 types of lesions are usually vascular and require preoperative embolization because blood loss during resection can be extensive.

INDICATIONS FOR SURGERY

Surgery of a vertebral column tumor is performed for many reasons: diagnosis, pain relief, neural decompression, restoration of spinal stability, and oncologic cure. The vast majority of vertebral column tumors are metastatic rather than primary. Because patients with vertebral column tumors typically have a limited life expectancy and may have multiple sites of disease, oncologic cure is not the usual goal of surgery. The potential benefits of surgery must be balanced against the risks of a major surgical procedure and the time needed for recuperation (typically lasting 1 to 2 months). The indications for surgery dictate the approach and goals of surgery.

Rapid neurologic deterioration due to epidural compression, especially when caused by a radioresistant tumor, is an indication for surgery. Surprisingly, there is no uniformly accepted definition of spinal instability. Thoracic kyphotic deformities greater than 20 degrees and disruption of 2 out of 3 bony columns in the thoracolumbar spine are the most commonly used definitions. Gross movement on dynamic radiographs also indicates instability. A patient's age, general well-being, and expected mobility after surgery must all be considered before surgery.

Overall, the role of surgery for patients with metastatic disease is still being defined because the goal of this intervention is palliative. Patients with widespread metastatic disease, radiosensitive tumors, a very limited life expectancy, or medical conditions that preclude surgery should first be considered for treatment using external beam radiotherapy, vertebroplasty, or steroids.

Once the decision has been made to operate on a patient with metastatic disease, there are only 2 aims for surgery: decompression of the spinal cord to improve neurologic status and stabilization of the spine to help reduce the pain caused by the underlying instability. The goal of radiotherapy either before or after surgery is to shrink the tumor. The decision to use radiotherapy and when to use it depend largely on the specific tumor and the presence of neurologic deficits.

Surgical Adjuncts

Embolization

Preoperative embolization can dramatically reduce blood loss during surgery and is generally used for vascular diseases such as metastases from renal cell carcinoma, melanoma, and thyroid carcinoma. The vascular "blush" of a tumor is usually well visualized on angiograms and guides selective embolization of the predominant vascular radicular arteries arising from the aorta. Angiography of lesions at the thoracolumbar junction also elucidates the dominant radicular artery that gives rise to spinal cord vascularization, although this information is not used to determine the side of approach or to preclude surgical resection.

Transfusion

Blood loss during surgical resection of vertebral tumors can be immense and sometimes exceeds the entire circulating blood volume. Preemptive transfusion of blood and coagulation factors must be performed to prevent hemodynamic instability or coagulopathy.

Cell Saving

Cell saving techniques generally are not used because of the concern that malignant cells may recirculate back into the bloodstream. As finer blood filtering techniques evolve, cell saving systems may find a role in vertebral tumor surgery.

Electrophysiologic Monitoring

Intraoperative somatosensory evoked potential monitoring and motor evoked potential monitoring are useful for near real-time intraoperative feedback of dorsal and ventral spinal cord function. Direct triggered electromyography stimulation of pedicle screws may also be used to assess how close these instruments are to the neural elements. Intraoperative electrophysiologic monitoring necessitates the use of nonparalyzing anesthetic techniques.

Intraoperative Fluoroscopy

Intraoperative fluoroscopy provides immediate vertebral localization when surgery begins. It also provides rough feedback on the extent of resection. Fluoroscopy is indispensable during placement of spinal instrumentation as well as during vertebroplasty and kyphoplasty.

Surgical Techniques

The surgical approach to any patient with a spinal tumor is individualized according to the goals of the procedure. A multistaged approach may be warranted for a healthy patient in whom complete cure is considered, whereas a minimally invasive palliative approach may be appropriate for a patient with diffuse systemic disease and a limited life expectancy. In general, a maximal approach necessitates a direct approach to the tumor, often regardless of anatomic obstacles. Maximal spinal tumor resection also typically requires a tailored approach to spinal reconstruction with or without an aggressive attempt at bone fusion, depending on the patient's prognosis. The following sections outline the various surgical approaches. Ventral approaches are emphasized because of the predilection of tumors to occur within the ventral spine. Laminectomy techniques alone are indicated for tumors located solely within the posterior vertebral elements.

Percutaneous Vertebroplasty and Kyphoplasty

Percutaneous needle vertebral augmentation is an effective palliative technique with which to alleviate focal midline back pain that is attributable to pathologic vertebral collapse. In these procedures, methyl methacrylate is injected into a collapsed vertebral body under direct fluoroscopic guidance (Figure 14–3). Kyphoplasty is similar to vertebroplasty but involves placement of a pressurized balloon into the collapsed vertebra before methyl methacrylate is injected. The theoretical advantages of kyphoplasty over

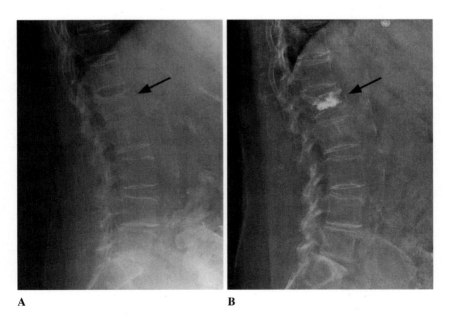

A   B

Figure 14–3. (A) Lateral radiograph of the thoracic spine showing compression of the L1 vertebral body (arrow) before vertebroplasty. (B) Lateral radiograph of the thoracic spine showing cement filling the collapsed vertebral body (arrow) after vertebroplasty.

vertebroplasty are restoration of vertebral height and more controlled injection. However, kyphoplasty is more expensive and, unlike vertebroplasty, requires general anesthesia. Both procedures appear to provide similar excellent pain relief to appropriately chosen patients.

Approaches to the Cervical Spine

High cervical (C1 and C2) vertebral body tumors may be approached directly via the transoral route with or without a transmandibular approach, depending on the degree of rostral extension of the tumor. Because this approach is destabilizing, posterior occipitocervical fusion is mandatory.

Tumors in the anterior portion of the subaxial cervical spine may be approached through the anterolateral neck. This approach is familiar to all neurosurgeons and orthopedic surgeons. Complete en bloc resections in the cervical spine are extremely challenging because of the anatomic constraints of the vertebral artery, spinal cord, and nerve roots.

Approaches to the Thoracic Spine

Tumors in the vertebral body of T1 that do not extend laterally into the paraspinal space may be approached through the low anterolateral neck. Further rostral or caudal extension of a midline ventrally placed tumor into the cervical or lower thoracic spine may be approached with the addition of anterolateral neck dissection or median sternotomy, respectively. Thoracic vertebral tumors with lateral paraspinal extension require posterolateral thoracotomy approached from the side of greatest lateral tumor extension. Tumors that circumferentially surround the thecal sac may require staged thoracotomy and posterior laminectomy. An alternative is transpedicular vertebrectomy at all thoracic levels when resection of the intralesional tumor is adequate and the risk of morbidity from thoracotomy is too high. Transpedicular vertebrectomy is facilitated by bilateral ligation of the associated nerve roots. For this reason, this technique is rarely advocated at T1 (which necessitates ligation of both T1 nerve roots) when a low anterolateral neck approach can be used instead.

Approaches to the Thoracolumbar Spine

The direct surgical approach to thoracolumbar (T10 to L1) vertebral tumors requires a thoracoabdominal approach in which a portion of the diaphragmatic crus is divided to expose the spine. The side of approach is determined by the location of the tumor within the vertebra. Tumors that extend equally on both sides are approached from the left to avoid the liver. Disrupting vital cord vascularity (by sacrificing the arteries of Adamkiewicz bilaterally at these levels) must be avoided. Vertebrectomy always requires sacrifice of at least unilateral segmental vessels at the levels involved. En bloc resection in the thoracic, thoracoabdominal, and lumbar spine is challenging and is warranted only when extralesional resection of a tumor involving no more than

270 degrees of the spinal ring will improve the oncologic prognosis compared with intralesional resection.

Approaches to the Lumbar Spine

The retroperitoneal approach is used for vertebral tumors below L1. Intralesional vertebrectomy and ipsilateral pediculectomy are possible using this approach. Transpedicular vertebrectomy is challenging because of the size of the vertebral body and the anatomic obstruction by nerve roots, which convey important lower extremity function. As for the thoracic spine, en bloc resection is a staged procedure that permits extralesional resection of tumors that involve no more than 270 degrees of the spinal ring.

Approaches to the Sacrum

Distal sacral tumors (S3 and below) may be approached solely from the back, usually without reconstruction, stabilization, or sacrifice of bowel or bladder function. Extensive high sacral tumors (S1 and S2) require complete sacrectomy. This technically challenging staged procedure requires vascular surgery, gastrointestinal surgery, and often plastic surgery support. Patients must be psychologically prepared for loss of bowel and bladder function, if they have not already been lost. There is no ideal means of reconstructing the lumbopelvic articulation, although a variety of techniques have been attempted. The transiliac rod and lumbopelvic instrumentation are the most commonly reported techniques for reconstructing.

ADJUVANT THERAPIES

Radiotherapy

The histologic characteristics of a tumor determine its sensitivity to radiotherapy. Tumors that are considered radiosensitive include plasmacytomas, multiple myelomas, and metastases due to breast cancer, prostate cancer, and small cell lung cancer. Spinal tumors of these histologic types warrant first-line radiotherapy except in cases of overt spinal cord compression and progressive neurologic deterioration. In most other cases, external beam radiotherapy after surgical resection is recommended. A recent randomized prospective trial comparing radiotherapy with surgery plus adjuvant radiotherapy to treat unifocal epidural compression due to spinal metastases demonstrated significantly better outcome in pain control, preservation of ambulation, and preservation of bowel and bladder function in the surgery plus adjuvant radiotherapy group. When used before surgery, radiotherapy predisposes up to one third of patients to infections and problems with wound healing. Newer intensity-modulated and stereotactic radiosurgical techniques may allow higher radiation doses to be delivered while limiting the doses to the thecal sac.

Chemotherapy

Chemotherapy based on the tumor's histologic type is used in appropriate circumstances. In certain instances, such as sarcomatous involvement of the spine, preoperative chemotherapy may reduce the tumor burden and facilitate surgical resection. In most other instances, malignant spinal tumors are treated with postoperative combination chemotherapy.

POSTOPERATIVE CARE

Bracing

The role of conventional spine orthoses in postoperative care remains controversial and is at the surgeon's discretion. In general, we do not routinely recommend bracing after tumor reconstructive surgery.

Deep Vein Thrombosis Prophylaxis and Anticoagulation

Deep vein thrombosis is of significant concern for patients with tumors involving the spine because of the long operating time, prolonged bed rest, and altered coagulation status. Prophylaxis against deep vein thrombosis includes passive range of motion, early ambulation, pneumatic compression boots or sequential compression devices, TED stockings, rotating beds, and anticoagulation medication if necessary. If anticoagulation medication is contraindicated, the placement of a vena caval filter can be considered.

KEY PRACTICE POINTS

- Recent advances in surgical technology, particularly in spinal fixation and instrumentation, and focused radiosurgical techniques have allowed an aggressive approach for managing selected vertebral column tumors.
- Lesion biopsy is of utmost importance in confirming a histologic diagnosis and in helping determine appropriate therapy.
- The preoperative differentiation of different types of spinal tumors, specifically primary and secondary tumors, is crucial in determining the surgical approach (en bloc vs interalesional resection) and the ultimate management of these tumors.
- The role of surgery for patients with metastatic disease is still being defined because the goal of this intervention is palliation.
- A multidisciplinary approach is crucial for optimal disease management.

SUGGESTED READINGS

Algra PR, Heimans JJ, Valk J, et al. Do metastases in vertebrae begin in the body or pedicles? Imaging study in 45 patients. *AJR Am J Roentgenol* 1992;158: 1275–1279.

Bilsky MH, Boland PJ, Panageas KS, Woodruff JM, Brennan MF, Healey JH. Intralesional resection of primary and metastatic sarcoma involving the spine: outcome analysis of 59 patients. *Neurosurgery* 2001;49:1277–1286; discussion 1286–1287.

Bradway JK, Pritchard DJ. Ewing's tumor of the spine. In: Sundaresan N, Schmidek HH, Schiller AL, Rosenthal DI, eds. *Tumors of the Spine: Diagnosis and Clinical Management*. Philadelphia, PA: WB Saunders; 1990:235–239.

Camins MB, Rosenblum BR. Osseous lesions of the cervical spine. *Clin Neurosurg* 1991;37:722–739.

Camins MB, Rosenblum BR. Osseous lesions of the vertebral axis. In: Lewis MM, ed. *Musculoskeletal Oncology*. Philadelphia, PA: WB Saunders; 1992.

Dahlin DC. *Bone Tumors: General Aspects and Data on 6221 Cases*. 3d ed. Springfield, IL: Charles C. Thomas; 1978.

Dahlin DC, Coventry MB. Osteogenic sarcoma. A study of six hundred cases. *J Bone Joint Surg Am* 1967;49:101–110.

Dehdashti F, Siegel BA, Griffeth LK, et al. Benign versus malignant intraosseous lesions: discrimination by means of PET with 2-[F-18]fluoro-2-deoxy-D-glucose. *Radiology* 1996;200:243–247.

Djindjian M. Vertebral hemangiomas with neurologic symptoms: summary. [in French] *Neurochirurgie* 1989;35:264.

Frank JA, Ling A, Patronas NJ, et al. Detection of malignant bone tumors: MR imaging vs scintigraphy. *AJR Am J Roentgenol* 1990;155:1043–1048.

Gosfield E 3rd, Alavi A, Kneeland B. Comparison of radionuclide bone scans and magnetic resonance imaging in detecting spinal metastases. *J Nucl Med* 1993;34:2191–2198.

Grubb MR, Currier BL, Pritchard DJ, Ebersold MJ. Primary Ewing's sarcoma of the spine. *Spine* 1994;19:309–313.

Karparov M, Kitov D. Aneurysmal bone cyst of the spine. *Acta Neurochir (Wien)* 1977;39:101–113.

MacCarty CS, Waugh JM, Mayo CW, Coventry MB. The surgical treatment of pre-sacral tumor: a combined problem. *Mayo Clin Proc* 1952;27:73–84.

Mohan V, Arora MM, Gupta RP, Izzat F. Aneurysmal bone cysts of the dorsal spine. *Arch Orthop Trauma Surg* 1989;108:390–393.

Nguyen JP, Djindjian M, Pavlovitch JM, Badiane S. Vertebral hemangioma with neurologic signs. Therapeutic results. Survey of the French Society of Neurosurgery. [in French] *Neurochirurgie* 1989;35:299–303, 305–308.

O'Mara RE. Bone scanning in osseous metastatic disease. *JAMA* 1974;229: 1915–1917.

Patchell RA, Tibbs PA, Regine WF, et al. A randomized trial of direct decompressive surgical resection in the treatment of spinal cord compression caused by metastasis. [Abstract] *Proc Am Soc Clin Oncol* 2003;22:1.

Poor MM, Hitchon PW, Riggs CE Jr. Solitary spinal plasmacytomas: management and outcome. *J Spinal Disord* 1988;1:295–300.

Rosenblum BR, Camins MB. Bony lesions of the cervical spine. In: Camins MB, O'Leary P, eds. *Disorders of the Cervical Spine*. Baltimore, MD: Williams & Wilkins; 1992;519–529.

Sailer SL, Harmon DC, Mankin HJ, Truman JT, Suit HD. Ewing's sarcoma: surgical resection as a prognostic factor. *Int J Radiat Oncol Biol Phys* 1988;15:43–52.

Sanerkin NG. The diagnosis and grading of chondrosarcoma of bone: a combined cytologic and histologic approach. *Cancer* 1980;45:582–594.

Sharafuddin MJ, Haddad FS, Hitchon PW, Haddad SF, el-Khoury GY. Treatment options in primary Ewing's sarcoma of the spine: report of seven cases and review of the literature. [Review] *Neurosurgery* 1992;30:610–618; discussion 618–619.

Shires JL, Wold LE, Dahlin DC. Chondrosarcoma and its variants. In: *Diagnosis and Treatment of Bone Tumors*. Mayo Clinic Monograph. Thorofare, NJ: Charles B. Slack; 1983.

Sundaresan N, Krol G, DiGiacinto, et al. Metastatic tumors of the spine. In: Sundaresan N, Schmidek HH, Schiller AL, Rosenthal DI, eds. *Tumors of the Spine: Diagnosis and Clinical Management*. Philadelphia, PA: WB Saunders; 1990a:279–304.

Sundaresan N, Krol G, Hughes JEO. Primary malignant tumors of the spine. In: Youmans JR, ed. *Neurological Surgery*. 3d ed. Philadelphia, PA: WB Saunders; 1990b:3548–3573.

Sundaresan N, Rosen G, Huvos AG, Krol G. Combined treatment of osteosarcoma of the spine. *Neurosurgery* 1988;23:714–719.

Weinstein JN: Differential diagnosis and surgical treatment of primary benign and malignant neoplasms. In: Frymoyer JW, ed. *The Adult Spine: Principles and Practice*. New York, NY: Raven Press; 1991:829–860.

Weinstein JN. Surgical approach to spine tumors. *Orthopedics* 1989;12:897–905.

15   Tumors of the Spinal Cord and Intradural Space

Laurence D. Rhines and Morris D. Groves

Chapter Overview 296
Introduction 296
Spinal Cord and Intradural Lesions 297
    Patient History and Physical Examination 299
    Diagnostic Imaging 304
    Serum and CSF Tests 305
    Other Diagnostic Tests 306
    Therapeutic Interventions 306
Intramedullary Tumors 307
    Incidence and Etiology 307
        Astrocytomas 307
        Ependymomas 307
        Hemangioblastomas 308
        Other Intramedullary Tumors 308
    Clinical Presentation 308
    Diagnostic Imaging 308
    Surgical Treatment 309
        General Considerations 309
        Astrocytomas 311
        Ependymomas 311
        Hemangioblastomas 313
        General Postresection Technique 313
        Outcomes 313
Extramedullary Tumors 316
    Incidence and Etiology 316
        Nerve Sheath Tumors 316
            Neurofibromas 317
            Schwannomas 317
        Meningiomas 317
        Myxopapillary Ependymomas of the Filum Terminale 317
        Other Extramedullary Tumors 318
    Clinical Presentation 318
    Diagnostic Imaging 319

Surgical Treatment 319
   General Considerations 319
   Nerve Sheath Tumors 320
   Meningiomas 321
   Myxopapillary Ependymomas of the Filum Terminale 321
   Outcomes 323
Cauda Equina Lesions 324
Conclusion 326
Key Practice Points 326
Suggested Readings 327

CHAPTER OVERVIEW

Intradural spinal tumors are a rare but critically important subset of tumors affecting the central nervous system. Most of these tumors are benign or of low biologic grade. Surgical excision therefore has a vital role in the management of these tumors. Because numerous pathologic processes can mimic spinal cord neoplasia, the initial focus of management is the pursuit of an accurate diagnosis. Advances in imaging, surgical techniques, and intraoperative electrophysiologic monitoring have improved the safety and efficacy of surgery and have improved patient outcome and survival. This chapter outlines the diagnostic evaluation of patients who have intradural lesions and describes the management of the most common intramedullary, extramedullary, and cauda equina neoplasms.

INTRODUCTION

Intradural spinal tumors represent 10% to 15% of central nervous system (CNS) neoplasms. These tumors are generally classified by their relationship to the dura mater and spinal cord parenchyma: within the spinal cord parenchyma (intramedullary), outside the spinal cord parenchyma (extramedullary), or in the cauda equina. In adults, two thirds of these tumors are extramedullary and the remaining third are intramedullary. Tumors of the spinal cord and intradural space encompass a wide variety of histologic types, and their optimal management depends on accurate identification of the pathologic process. Whereas many of the neoplastic processes that occur within the intradural space may be addressed surgically, a nonsurgical approach is usually more appropriate for inflammatory, infectious, and vascular processes. The different entities may be difficult to distinguish radiographically. At M. D. Anderson Cancer Center, when a patient presents with an abnormality in the spinal cord or intradural space, the bulk of our initial efforts is focused on establishing a most likely diagnosis. Given the inherent risks of surgery in and around the spinal cord, our goal is to eliminate the possibility of operating on a pathologic process that will not benefit from surgical intervention. This goal is best approached in a multidisciplinary fashion, and all patients are seen by both a neurosurgeon and a neuro-oncologist for extensive diagnostic workup. We begin by discussing the general approach at M. D. Anderson to the evaluation and diagnosis of patients with spinal cord and intradural lesions and then review the common neoplastic entities that arise in the intramedullary and extramedullary intradural compartments.

SPINAL CORD AND INTRADURAL LESIONS

In this section, we explain the framework to assist in the diagnosis of patients who present with spinal cord or intradural lesions, especially lesions that resemble tumors or defy immediate classification. Typical clinical scenarios can be segregated anatomically as lesions affecting the spinal cord (either intramedullary or extramedullary) and lesions below the level of the conus medullaris. Because of the common use of high-sensitivity diagnostic magnetic resonance imaging (MRI), many patients are now referred for evaluation on the basis of imaging findings before the development of clinical symptoms or signs that would help point to a diagnosis. This situation creates the opportunity for early diagnosis and treatment, but it also creates the potential for iatrogenic injury if overzealous diagnostic or therapeutic actions are taken.

We focus on outpatient evaluation targeted toward preventing unnecessary surgical procedures. Acute, fulminant encephalomyelitis or myelitis or rapidly progressive paralysis is an emergency and is not the focus of this discussion.

Most broad etiologic categories of human illness include diseases that can result in spinal cord or nerve root lesions. These diseases include those that are neoplastic, inflammatory or demyelining, infectious, postinfectious, toxic or metabolic, nutritional, developmental, traumatic, or vascular. Determining the etiology of gradual, progressive lesions is often difficult but is critical for appropriate treatment. Establishing an accurate diagnosis requires a detailed and precise patient history and physical examination, high-quality neuroimaging, and often blood and cerebrospinal fluid (CSF) testing. Even with "positive" test results, one must exercise caution and avoid the tunnel vision that can prematurely exclude potential diagnoses. Many tests lack specificity and can be interpreted as positive even though the indicated cause may not be responsible for a patient's neurologic disorder. For example, many persons will test positive for antibody titers to herpes simplex virus or Epstein-Barr virus, but beginning antiviral drug therapy solely on the basis of serology or CSF analysis could expose a patient to potentially dangerous and unwarranted therapy.

Intramedullary spinal cord lesions usually present the most challenging diagnostic scenarios. One reason is the indirect nature of the diagnostic evaluation, since biopsy samples of these tumors are infrequently taken because of the potential risk. Establishing the ultimate diagnosis in these cases requires tenacity and a willingness to simultaneously consider multiple alternative diagnoses for a prolonged time. The coexistence of 2 diseases causing myelopathy, such as cervical spondylarthropathy and multiple sclerosis or an intrinsic cervical spinal cord tumor, can be particularly challenging. Seeking the opinions of internists, rheumatologists, neuroradiologists, and other consultants can be helpful. The algorithm shown in Figure 15–1 and the details in Tables 15–1 through 15–4 may help

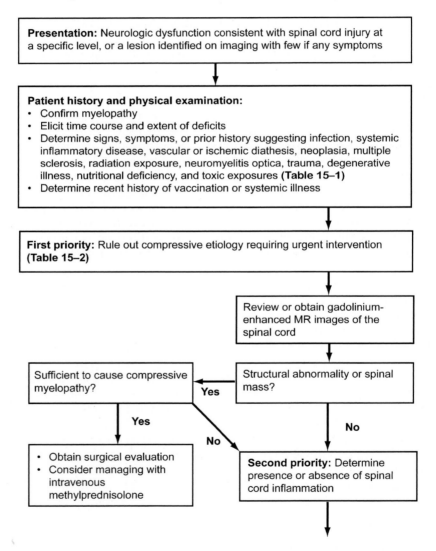

Figure 15–1. Diagnostic workup of tumors of the spinal cord and intradural space.

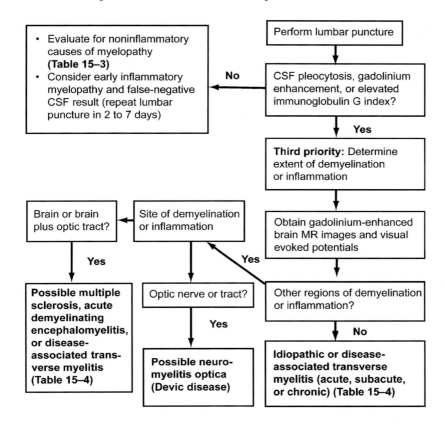

Figure 15–1. *(continued)*

with sequencing the diagnostic workup and suggest specific diagnostic tests that may be useful.

Patient History and Physical Examination

Historical information such as the patient's age, race, and sex can be useful in diagnosis. For instance, compared with other groups, women are more likely to develop demyelinating or autoimmune illnesses such as multiple sclerosis, African Americans are more likely to suffer sarcoidosis, and men in their fifties and sixties with a history of cardiovascular disease are more likely to develop spinal dural arteriovenous fistulas. Simple information such as a history of fever, night sweats, or weight loss can help in solving the diagnostic puzzle. Night sweats may indicate an underlying lymphoma or bacterial infection; weight loss might support the search for an underlying systemic malignancy. Details of the history or physical examination that can help elucidate the cause of the symptomatic lesion can include travel and environmental or toxic exposures. Travel to areas where tuberculosis is

**Table 15–1. Signs, Symptoms, and Useful Non-CSF Diagnostic Tests
for Evaluating Myelopathy**

Cause of Myelopathy (Indicative Signs and Symptoms)	Non-CSF Tests To Be Considered
Infection (fever, meningismus, rash, concurrent systemic infection, immunocompromised state, recurrent genital infection, symptoms of zoster radiculopathy, adenopathy, travel/residence in area endemic for parasitic infections)	Complete blood cell count; C-reactive protein; chest radiography; Lyme antibody titer; ESR; HIV; rapid plasma reagin; antibodies to HSV, HTLV-1, VZV; *Borrelia burgdorferi*; hepatitis A, B, and C; *Mycoplasma*; parasites
Systemic inflammatory disease (rash, oral or genital ulcers, adenopathy, livedo reticularis, serositis, photosensitivity, inflammatory arthritis, erythema nodosum, xerostomia, keratitis, conjunctivitis, contractures or thickening of the skin, anemia, leukopenia, thrombocytopenia, Raynaud's phenomena, history of arterial or venous thrombosis, history of miscarriage)	Serum angiotensin-converting enzyme; complement levels; urinalysis for microscopic hematuria; lip or salivary gland biopsy; chest radiography; chest CT; Schrimer's test; anti-phospholipid antibodies (anti-cardiolipin antibodies, Russel viper venom time, partial thromboplastin time); auto-antibodies: ANA, double-stranded DNA, SS-A (Ro), SS-B (La), Sm (Smith), ribonucleoprotein
Vascular or ischemic cause (middle aged and male, history of vascular disease)	CT myelography, spinal arteriogram
Neoplasia (history of systemic cancer, weight loss, anorexia, adenopathy)	Positron emission tomography, body imaging with CT or MRI, serum markers for cancer, prostate-specific antigen, carcinoembryonic antigen, CA125, CA29.27
Multiple sclerosis or neuromyelitis optica (previous demyelinating event, incomplete deficit clinically with MRI abnormality ≤2 spinal segments and <50% of cord diameter)	Brain MRI, evoked potentials
Radiation exposure (patchy neurologic deficits in path of radiation beam)	MRI for enhancement
Trauma (history of spine injury)	MRI
Degenerative disease (history of arthritis, degenerative joint disease)	MRI
Nutritional or toxic metabolic cause (history of starvation, alcoholism, unusual dietary habits [e.g., zinc overconsumption], history of poisoning)	Serum vitamin B12, methylmalonic acid, homocysteine, copper, and ceruloplasmin levels; urine heavy metal screen

Table 15–1. *(continued)* **Signs, Symptoms, and Useful Non-CSF Diagnostic Tests for Evaluating Myelopathy**

Cause of Myelopathy (Indicative Signs and Symptoms)	*Non-CSF Tests To Be Considered*
Idiopathic transverse myelitis (no clinical or paraclinical features suggestive of another diagnostic category)	Evoked potentials, electromyography/nerve conduction velocity

Abbreviations: ANA, anti-nuclear antibody; CT, computed tomography; ESR, erythrocyte sedimentation rate; HIV, human immunodeficiency virus; HSV, herpes simplex virus; HTLV-1, human T-cell leukemia virus type 1; MRI, magnetic resonance imaging; SS, Sjögren's syndrome; VZV, varicella zoster virus.

Table 15–2. **Causes of Myelopathy Requiring Urgent Intervention or Potential Biopsy or Resection**

Type of Myelopathy	*Cause*
Infectious	Epidural abscess, Pott's disease
Systemic inflammatory	Cervical spine subluxations in rheumatoid arthritis
Neoplastic	
Metastatic	Bone metastasis with fracture, instability, or epidural metastasis
Primary	Astrocytoma, ependymoma, hemangioblastoma, oligodendroglioma, or meningioma
Traumatic	Fracture with instability, severe cord contusion, or epidural hematoma
Degenerative	Critical spinal cord compression from progressive spinal stenosis, osteophyte overgrowth, or syringomyelia

Table 15–3. **Further Evaluation for Noninflammatory Causes of Myelopathy**

Noninflammatory Cause	*Evaluation*
Ischemic (arterial, venous, watershed, or arteriovenous) malformation	High-resolution MRI through region of interest, computed tomographic myelography, or spinal arteriography
Epidural lipomatosis	High-resolution MRI through region of interest
Fibrocartilaginous embolism	High-resolution MRI through region of interest
Radiation damage	High-resolution MRI through region of interest

Table 15–4. **Disease-Associated Causes of Transverse Myelopathy and Suggested CSF and Other Evaluations**

Type of Myelopathy, and Signs and Symptoms	Suggested Evaluations	Specific Illness Implicated
Infectious		
Fever, meningism, rash, concurrent systemic infection, immuno-compromised state, adenopathy	CSF Gram's stain and bacterial culture; CSF viral cultures; CSF PCR: CMV, EBV, HSV-1, HSV-2, HHV-6, VZV, enteroviruses; HIV	Bacterial and viral meningomyelitides
	HTLV-1 IgG antibodies	Tropical spastic paraparesis
	CSF acid-fast bacteria smear and culture; CSF PCR for tuberculosis, skin test for tuberculosis and controls	Tuberculous meningitis
	Fungal smear and culture, India Ink preparation	Fungal infections, cryptococcosis
Recurrent genital infection	CSF VDRL, serum rapid plasma reagin	Tabes dorsalis
Vesicular rash in dermatomal pattern	CSF PCR for VZV	VZV-associated myelopathy
Migrating rash, history of tick bite	CSF and serum anti-*Borrelia burgdorferi* antibodies	Lyme disease
Travel to area endemic for parasitic infections	CSF eosinophil count	CNS parasitic infections
Demyelinating	CSF myelin basic protein, oligoclonal bands, IgG index	Multiple sclerosis
	Serum NMO-IgG, CSF with polymorphonuclear pleocytosis, absent oligoclonal bands	Neuromyelitis optica
Autoimmune, inflammatory, or vasculitic	Serum and CSF angiotensin-converting enzyme	Sarcoidosis
	ANA, serum anti-Ro and anti-La antibodies	Sjögren's syndrome
	ANA, RF, serum p-ANCA, c-ANCA, otorhinolaryn-gologic evaluation	Wegener's granulomatosis
	RF, ANA	Rheumatoid arthritis
	Mycoplasma antibody titers, IgM, IgG, chest radiography	Mycoplasma-associated myelitis

Table 15–4. *(continued)* **Disease-Associated Causes of Transverse Myelopathy and Suggested CSF and Other Evaluations**

Type of Myelopathy, and Signs and Symptoms	Suggested Evaluations	Specific Illness Implicated
Autoimmune, inflammatory, or vasculitic *(continued)*	ANA, ESR, RF, anti-double stranded-DNA, serum anti-phospholipid antibodies	Systemic lupus erythematosus
	HLA-B51	Behçet's syndrome
	Serum anti-phospholipid antibodies	Antiphospholipid antibody syndrome
	Serum IgA	Henoch-Schönlein purpura
	Dermatology evaluation	Kohlmeier-Degos syndrome
	Serum cryoglobulins, hepatitis panel, serum protein electrophoresis	Mixed cryoglobulinemia
	ANA, RF, anti-SCL 70, anti-centromere antibodies	Progressive systemic sclerosis
	ESR, arteriography, arterial biopsy	Takayasu's arteritis
	ESR, arterial biopsy	Temporal arteritis
	ANA, ESR, RF, angiography, brain and spine, biopsy	Isolated CNS angiitis
	Hepatitis panel HIV titer, p-ANCA	Polyarteritis nodosa
	History of asthma, eosinophilia, p-ANCA	Churg-Strauss syndrome
Nutritional	Serum vitamin B12 level, methylmalonic acid, homocysteine	Subacute combined degeneration
	Serum copper, ceruloplasmin	Copper deficiency, zinc overconsumption
Drug induced		Treatment with sulfasalazine, intrathecal methotrexate, cytosine arabinoside, or thiotepa

Abbreviations: ANA, anti-nuclear antibody; c-ANCA and p-ANCA, antibodies directed to neutrophil cytoplasmic antigens, cytoplasmic type and perinuclear type; CMV, cytomegalovirus; CNS, central nervous system; CSF, cerebrospinal fluid; EBV, Epstein-Barr virus; ESR, erythrocyte sedimentation rate; HHV, human herpesvirus; HIV, human immunodeficiency virus; HLA, human leukocyte antigen; HSV, herpes simplex virus; HTLV-1, human T-cell leukemia virus type 1; IgA, IgG, and IgM, immunoglobulin A, G, and M; PCR, polymerase chain reaction; RF, rheumatoid factor; VDRL, Venereal Disease Research Laboratory; VZV, varicella zoster virus.

endemic or a history of swimming in a body of water potentially contaminated with schistosomiasis would be of interest. Symptoms or signs of an underlying inflammatory diathesis can be helpful. A history of unexplained rashes, dry eyes, joint pain, and symptoms of hypothyroidism (which is often an autoimmune disease) is useful information. A known history of rheumatoid arthritis, Sjögren's syndrome, or Crohn's disease should intensify the search for an inflammatory cause of the patient's problem. A family history of autoimmune disease such as hypothyroidism can also be used to narrow the diagnostic focus. A history of prior or ongoing cancer greatly influences the diagnostic considerations. Multifocal neuraxis symptoms such as bladder retention combined with diplopia and seizure may indicate leptomeningeal tumor dissemination (see chapter 12). Details of the neurologic symptom complex are helpful. For example, symptoms of morning back pain or back pain when supine often predict an intradural tumor. The cadence of development of a patient's symptoms can help with the diagnosis as well: a slow insidious course over a few months suggests a slowly growing intramedullary primary spinal cord tumor, whereas a more rapid course might suggest a metastatic focus of tumor in the CNS or an inflammatory disorder. The history and physical examination help narrow the diagnostic considerations in these challenging cases, but further objective data are almost always needed.

Diagnostic Imaging

High-quality, high-resolution, T1-weighted contrast-enhanced and T2-weighted MRI is critical in the diagnostic evaluation. MRI of the entire neuraxis is often needed to search for multifocal lesions. A complete imaging search of the nervous system can identify asymptomatic lesions, which can also help focus the diagnosis. Occasionally, contrast-enhanced computed tomographic (CT) myelography is useful in confirming spinal vascular malformations. Spinal angiography may be needed for diagnostic confirmation and treatment planning. Nuclear imaging studies such as gallium scanning can be useful in searching for systemic sarcoidosis, particularly the hilar adenopathy or parotid gland tracer uptake seen as the "panda bear" sign. After high-quality MRI, an extensive serum and CSF workup may not be necessary in fairly straightforward cases, such as a woman with widely metastatic breast cancer who develops a contrast-enhanced epidural spinal cord mass extending from a previous site of bone metastasis. Lesions found in such a setting may not require additional workup other than screening images of the rest of the spine to look for subtle, subclinical lesions to be tracked or irradiated to prevent later morbidity.

Intramedullary contrast-enhanced masses can sometimes be diagnosed based on images if typical features are seen. For example, in hemangioblastomas, vessels and prior hemorrhage may be evident. Ependymomas tend to have sharp margins with central edema or cystic areas above and below the contrast-enhanced lesions. Primary astrocytic tumors of the spinal cord can be contrast enhanced (usually portending a higher grade) but are more often diffuse and infiltrating in appearance and may have an eccentric location within the spinal cord. Distinguishing various lower-grade intramedullary spinal cord lesions can be difficult, and many ultimately require biopsy.

Neoplastic extramedullary lesions can be metastatic or primary. When an enhanced mass results in myelopathy and there is no prior history of cancer, then an appropriate systemic primary cancer evaluation should be carried out. Evaluation should include CT of the chest, abdomen, and pelvis; mammography; and positron emission tomography if indicated.

In evaluating lesions below the conus medullaris, myxopapillary ependymoma, schwannoma, metastatic cancer, radiation injury, and inflammatory disorders should all be considered. By far, MRI is the most useful diagnostic radiologic procedure for evaluating myelopathy or cauda equina lesions. Expert neuroradiologic opinion is useful in interpreting the images and can help guide further workup and therapy.

Serum and CSF Tests

Many patients with a spinal cord or nerve root lesion do not have pathognomonic imaging features, and the diagnosis is not immediately evident based on other patient history or physical examination data. These patients require additional serum and CSF testing. Peripheral blood counts are usually not helpful in the diagnosis, but they may reveal a leukocytosis or leukopenia with underlying infection. Patients with myelitis or encephalomyelitis will often show CSF abnormalities. CSF glucose, protein, cell count, differential, and cytologic analyses should be performed. Viral causes of myelitis and chronic fungal infections can result in a CSF pleocytosis of 10 to 2,000 cells/mm^3, often mononuclear early in the illness. CSF protein levels rise nonspecifically in most cases of myelopathy and can be quite high when CSF flow is blocked by an enlarged, swollen spinal cord. When a specific inflammatory cause of myelitis is suspected, CSF-to-serum immunoglobulin G ratios can help identify CSF production of antibodies. Specific immunoglobulin Gs should be tested. Testing with acute and convalescent serum antibodies can be helpful in the diagnosis. The presence of oligoclonal bands supports the diagnosis of multiple sclerosis. Specific CSF immunoglobulin M levels of particular pathogens can also help with an early diagnosis.

CSF glucose levels are often normal in viral infections of the CNS, whereas hypoglycorrhachia is often seen in malignant meningitis as well as bacterial, tuberculous, and fungal infections. In all patients with undiagnosed myelopathies, standard CSF testing with Gram stain and acid-fast bacteria should be performed. India ink testing can identify cryptococcal infection. Cultures for viruses and fungi should also be performed when these pathogens are considered possible causes of the clinical presentation. CSF testing for nucleic acids from herpesvirus, enterovirus, and polyomavirus can be carried out using polymerase chain reaction.

In the setting of an underlying cancer and immunocompromise, special consideration should be given to less common causes of myelopathy or radiculopathy, including herpesvirus infection, measles, adenovirus infection, toxoplasmosis, pneumocystis, cryptococcus, histoplasmosis, cytomegalovirus infection, and papovavirus infection.

Myelopathy due to vasculitis can have an infectious etiology if the infection interferes with the patency of the anterior spinal artery. Potential infectious conditions in such a setting can include varicella zoster virus infection, tuberculosis, syphilis, and schistosomiasis. A number of infections that may not directly injure the spinal cord can cause postinfectious myelopathy: vaccinia, measles, rubella, mumps, and other respiratory tract infections. The spinal cord can be directly infected by varicella zoster virus, Borrelia, or human T-lymphotropic virus type 1, the latter of which usually affects the thoracic spinal cord. Human immunodeficiency virus infection can cause spastic paraparesis and sensory ataxia. Lower motor neuron manifestations of infectious myelitis can be due to enterovirus (e.g., poliovirus and enterovirus 71) infection, arbovirus infection, and rabies.

Rheumatologic diseases can result in myelopathy, but spinal cord injury is not often the presenting feature of the illness. When a rheumatologic disease is high on the list of differential diagnoses, the focus should be on systemic lupus erythematosus, sarcoidosis, Sjögren's syndrome, and vasculitis.

Other Diagnostic Tests

Patients with a history or examination that suggests CNS or optic nerve involvement should have visual evoked potential tests performed to look for subtle or subclinical optic nerve damage suggestive of optic neuritis or neuromyelitis optica.

Therapeutic Interventions

Because many of the infectious causes of myelitis or radiculitis can be treated, these pathogens must be identified as soon as possible. Effective antibiotic therapy is available for nearly all bacterial infections. Effective antiviral therapy is available to treat herpes simplex virus infection, varicella zoster virus infection, and cytomegalovirus-associated radiculomyelitis. If extensive diagnostic workup excludes infection and still no diagnosis is evident, relief provided by systemic corticosteroids can support a diagnosis of an inflammatory or autoimmune cause for myelopathy or radiculopathy. At M. D. Anderson, we often use a short course of corticosteroids not only as therapeutic intervention before definitive treatment but also for its potential diagnostic benefit. An abnormality that resolves on imaging studies after steroid administration points to an inflammatory or autoimmune etiology. However, lymphoma in the spinal cord or CSF may also respond to systemic steroids, so follow-up and repeat evaluation are mandatory if this is a consideration.

In patients for whom no precise diagnosis can be established and no evidence of ongoing clinical or radiographic progression is apparent, watchful waiting with serial imaging and examination is a reasonable course of action. If these patients are stable radiographically and clinically, continued observation may be the safest course of action. Imaging, preferably MRI every 3 to 4 months and gradually decreasing in frequency over time, is the most useful tool with which to track such patients.

INTRAMEDULLARY TUMORS

Incidence and Etiology

A wide variety of pathologic processes can arise within the spinal cord. Glial tumors account for at least 80% of intramedullary tumors in most series. These tumors are predominantly astrocytomas and ependymomas; the latter are slightly more common. Hemangioblastomas are the third most common type of intramedullary tumors, and the remaining include inclusion tumors and cysts, nerve sheath tumors, other vascular abnormalities, and metastases (Neumann et al, 1989; Olindo et al, 2006). Nonneoplastic processes can present as intramedullary mass lesions. These processes include inflammatory, autoimmune, and infectious conditions. The lesions may be difficult to distinguish radiographically from neoplastic processes, and a careful history with particular attention to the time course and severity of symptoms as well as additional laboratory testing may be required to narrow the diagnosis.

Astrocytomas

Approximately 3% of CNS astrocytomas arise within the spinal cord (Sloof, et al, 1964). These can occur at any age but seem to be most prevalent during the first 3 decades of life. They are by far the most common pediatric intramedullary spinal cord tumor. They seem to be most common in the cervical and cervical thoracic regions of the spine. As in the brain, astrocytomas have heterogeneous histologic features and natural histories. They include low-grade and pilocytic astrocytomas, anaplastic astrocytomas, glioblastomas, and rare oligodendrogliomas (Baptiste and Fehlings, 2006).

Ependymomas

Ependymomas are the most common intramedullary tumors in adults. They occur throughout life but are most common in the middle adult years and equally affect men and women. Approximately 65% of patients will have associated syrinxes, particularly when the tumor occupies a cervical or cervicothoracic location. There are a number of histologic subtypes, but the most common is the cellular ependymoma. Almost all ependymomas are benign. These tumors are usually well circumscribed and do not infiltrate into the adjacent spinal cord, as astrocytomas do (McCormick and Stein, 1990).

Hemangioblastomas

Hemangioblastomas account for 3% to 8% of intramedullary tumors, and 15% to 25% of these are associated with von Hippel-Lindau disease, which is an autosomal dominant trait with incomplete penetrance and incomplete expression (Neumann et al, 1989; Salvi et al, 2006). Hemangioblastomas are benign tumors of vascular origin that are sharply circumscribed but not encapsulated. Almost all have a pial attachment, which is typically dorsally situated on the spinal cord.

Other Intramedullary Tumors

Rounding out the list of neoplasms are the inclusion tumors, vascular lesions, and metastases. Lipomas are the most common of the inclusion tumors and account for about 1% of the intramedullary tumors. They enlarge because of increased fat deposition in metabolically normal fat cells in the subpial space. Metastases account for fewer than 5% of intramedullary tumors and should prompt a search for evidence of leptomeningeal disease. The lung and breast are the most common primary sites that give rise to intramedullary metastases.

Clinical Presentation

The clinical presentation of patients with intramedullary spinal cord tumors is somewhat variable. Early symptoms are often vague, and the progression of these tumors may be slow and subtle. In many cases, symptoms will be present for several years before the correct diagnosis is made. Pain, weakness, and numbness are the most frequent presenting symptoms. Pain usually localizes to the level of the tumor, and the distribution of the numbness and weakness corresponds to the location of the tumor within the spinal cord. Bowel and bladder dysfunction may also occur, but these tend to occur later. It is important that these symptoms be recognized as soon as possible to make the correct diagnosis and initiate the appropriate treatment, as patients with milder symptoms at the time of treatment tend to have a better overall outcome.

In some cases, a more rapid progression of symptoms can be observed. For example, the growth of a metastatic or highly malignant neoplasm may cause a more rapid onset and development of symptoms than more benign pathologic types do. Furthermore, tumors such as ependymomas may hemorrhage, thereby causing sudden development of symptoms. The presence of fairly acute or subacute symptoms should increase suspicion for a nonneoplastic process such as infection or myelitis.

Diagnostic Imaging

Gadolinium-enhanced MRI is the gold standard imaging modality for preoperative evaluation of intramedullary tumors. Not only can such imaging studies help define the location of the tumor within the spinal cord and rule out the presence of multiple lesions, but the tumor's appearance on the MR images can give diagnostic clues. Most spinal cord tumors are isointense or slightly hypointense relative to the spinal cord on T1-weighted images without contrast and are typically hyperintense to the spinal cord on T2-weighted images. T2-weighted images are also ideal for detecting the degree of edema and the presence of related syrinx formation. Often the spinal cord is swollen and enlarged at the location of the neoplasm. Nearly all of the intramedullary tumors demonstrate contrast enhancement, but the degree of enhancement is somewhat variable. Ependymomas typically demonstrate uniform contrast enhancement and tend to be symmetrically located within the central portion of the spinal cord, whereas heterogeneous contrast enhancement is usually observed with intratumoral cysts, calcification, or necrosis. Astrocytomas tend to be less well defined than ependymomas and their margins more irregular; the contrast enhancement is also typically less uniform, and an eccentric position in the spinal cord is not uncommon. Irregular, unclearly demarcated margins and an eccentric location in the spinal cord ought to raise suspicion for an astrocytoma. Finally, hemangioblastomas tend to be very brightly enhanced and sharply demarcated, and they usually abut the dorsal surface of the spinal cord. Associated vessels may be apparent on the T2-weighted or contrast-enhanced images. Because the radiographic appearance of nonneoplastic lesions and that of intramedullary neoplasms may overlap significantly, a wide differential diagnosis must always be kept in mind when a patient with an intramedullary lesion is being evaluated.

Surgical Treatment

General Considerations

Advances in imaging, surgical technique, and intraoperative sensory and motor electrophysiologic monitoring and the widespread use of the operative microscope have steadily improved the safety and efficacy of surgery for intramedullary spinal cord tumors. Most intramedullary tumors are low-grade neoplasms, and most authors agree that surgery now represents the most effective treatment for these benign, well-circumscribed tumors (Cooper, 1989; Epstein et al, 1993).

Perhaps the single most important factor that dictates the surgeon's ability to resect an intramedullary tumor is the quality of the plane between the tumor and the surrounding spinal cord. This issue can be resolved only at the time of surgery once an adequate myelotomy has been performed. For noninfiltrative tumors such as ependymomas and hemangioblastomas, the border between the tumor and the surrounding spinal cord is often distinct in both texture and color, and the tumor can be satisfactorily resected without extending the dissection into functioning spinal cord. The situation is far more variable for astrocytomas: some will seem relatively well circumscribed, and others will have a very indistinct plane where the tumor seems to merge with the surrounding spinal cord. In fact, the infiltration of the tumor into the surrounding spinal cord is often signified by a gradual loss of the plane between the 2. These tumors are therefore seldom curable, and extending the dissection into possibly functioning spinal cord can have deleterious consequences for the patient without any clinical benefit. Even for some of the less common neoplasms, the tumor–spinal cord interface is a strong determinant of the degree to which the lesion can be treated surgically. As in the brain, metastases within the spinal cord tend to be fairly well demarcated with respect to the surrounding spinal cord, and often gross total resection can be achieved. Lipomas, on the other hand, tend to insinuate themselves into the nearby spinal cord, making complete surgical resection typically impossible.

Regardless of the degree of resection, one of the most important goals of surgery is to establish the diagnosis. In fact, making this determination can greatly affect surgical treatment. For example, if the plane seems indistinct when the tumor is being resected but the biopsy reveals an ependymoma, additional effort should be spent trying to find a plane, as it is likely to be present.

For all suspected intramedullary tumors, after general endotracheal intubation and administration of the appropriate antibiotics and steroids, the patient is placed in the prone position on the operating table to allow maximal decompression of the chest and abdomen. By relieving pressure on these structures, venous pressures are decreased and epidural venous bleeding is potentially lessened during a surgical procedure that antici-pates operating with this space exposed and with evacuation of signifi-cant amounts of spinal fluid. Rigorous radiographic interrogation is used to determine the appropriate levels for the incision, and after sterile preparation, an incision and subperiosteal dissection are performed to expose the posterior elements of the spine.

A wide laminectomy is performed with care taken to preserve the facet joints so as to avoid causing iatrogenic instability. Once the laminectomy is performed, gel foam and cottonoid patties are placed in the lateral recesses to control any epidural bleeding. Ultrasonography is used to con-firm the presence of the tumor within the operative field with adequate access to the cephalad and caudal poles of the lesion.

The dura mater is opened in the midline by using sharp dissection, and the dural leaves are held out of the way with 4–0 braided nylon sutures tacked to the muscle laterally. The operating microscope is brought into the operating field. Strict hemostasis must be obtained before the dura mater is opened, as any blood in the spinal fluid will obstruct the view. With use of the operating microscope, the arachnoid is opened with microscissors and can be tacked to the retracted dural edges with small microvascular clips. The spinal cord is carefully inspected to help reveal the presence of the underlying abnormality and, in the case of hemangioblastomas, the site of pial attachment and to help localize the posterior median septum (the midline dorsal raphe), where the midline myelotomy is typically performed. The presence of an intrinsic spinal cord tumor can cause rotation of the spinal cord, thereby making local-ization of the midline challenging. Small veins exiting from the midline septum can help establish the location of the midline; moreover, the dor-sal midline can typically be estimated by noting the midpoint between the dorsal nerve root entry zones bilaterally. Once the small vessels crossing the midline septum are cauterized, sharp dissection with microscissors or an 11-blade knife is used to incise the pia mater, and microdissectors can then be used to deepen the midline myelotomy until the dorsal surface of the tumor is encountered. This midline myelotomy must extend over the entire rostrocaudal extent of the tumor to facilitate satisfactory resection and minimize damage to the spinal cord. At M. D. Anderson, we use 6–0 prolene pial tack-up sutures to hold the dorsal spinal cord open during the surgery, which facilitates intramedullary dissection. The tumor dis-section is typically initiated at the point of maximum diameter (generally at the midpoint of its rostrocaudal extent). With the use of microdissec-tors, the dorsal surface of the tumor is dissected away from the adjacent spinal cord, and this process is extended both rostrally and caudally. Again, the pial tack-up sutures are placed as the dorsal surface of the tumor is exposed, rostrally and caudally, to hold the spinal cord open and facilitate the subsequent dissection. As dissection proceeds around the tumor laterally, gentle traction on the tumor opposed by countertraction from the pial tack-up sutures allows the planes to be developed. This process is continued toward the poles of the tumor. Ventrally, the plane is established by gently lifting the tumor away from the cord while the small feeding blood vessels and fibrous adhesions are cauterized and then cut sharply. The degree to which the tumor can be completely removed directly relates to the plane between the tumor and the spinal cord. The identification and surgical treatment of a cervical intradural intramedullary ependymoma are illustrated in Figure 15–2.

Astrocytomas

For astrocytomas, the plane of dissection is usually less distinct that that for ependymomas. It is critical to remove sufficient tumor to establish the diagnosis, but the ability to achieve a complete resection is generally lim-ited. As the planes between tumor and spinal cord become obscure, the risks of additional resection begin to outweigh the benefits. For this reason, the primary goal is to establish the diagnosis while preserving function.

Ependymomas

The reddish grey tumor surface of ependymomas is generally quite distinct from the surrounding spinal cord, and typically a plane can be established

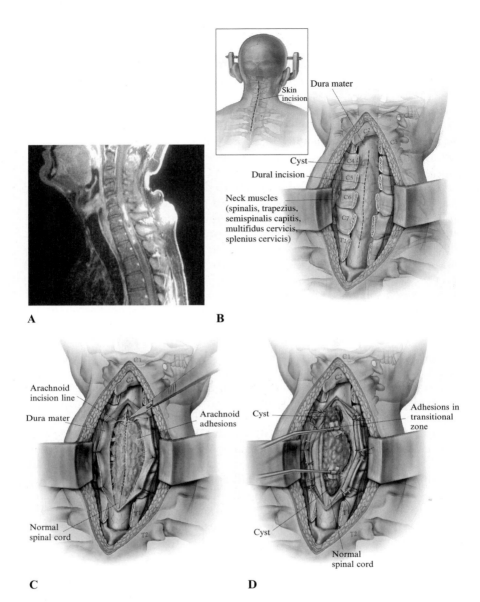

Figure 15–2. (A) Sagittal gadolinium-enhanced T1-weighted image of a patient with a cervical intradural intramedullary ependymoma. (B) Artist's rendering of the initial step in resection of an intramedullary ependymoma of the spinal cord. A wide laminectomy is performed while avoiding injury to the facet joints. Bone removal must be sufficient to access both the cephalad and caudal poles of the tumor. This can be confirmed before the dura mater is opened by using intraoperative ultrasonography. (C) After laminectomy, the dura mater is opened in the midline and the dural edges are held out of the way with 4-0 Neurolon sutures. Sharp dissection is used to lyse arachnoid adhesions and provide access to the dorsal surface of the spinal cord. The pia-arachnoid on the dorsal surface of the spinal cord is divided sharply over the midline septum, thereby allowing dissection down to the dorsal tumor surface.

completely around the tumor and the lesion removed in 1 piece. Occasionally, for large tumors, internal debulking may be required to facilitate dissection around the outer limits of the tumor.

Hemangioblastomas

Hemangioblastomas may have a dorsal pial attachment that is separate from the midline. Because they are highly vascular, these tumors ought to be resected without being violated. This resection is facilitated by removing the pial attachment as part of the tumor mass. After the overlying surface vessels have been coagulated, the pial attachment is sharply circumscribed to allow access to the portion of the tumor buried within the spinal cord. Hemangioblastomas generally have a sharp plane of demarcation with the spinal cord, and by bipolar coagulation of the tumor surface and the subsequent shrinking of the lesion, this plane can be established circumferentially and the tumor removed in 1 piece.

General Postresection Technique

After removal of the spinal cord tumor, the resection cavity is inspected and meticulous hemostasis is obtained. The pial tack-up sutures are released, the thecal sac is irrigated copiously with saline, and the dura mater is closed meticulously with a primary closure. When the dura mater cannot be closed this way, a dural patch may be used. The use of dural sealants after primary closure is a matter of the surgeon's preference. After the operation, the patient is mobilized as rapidly as possible; at M. D. Anderson, we use physical and occupational therapy for both evaluation and treatment. If possible, MRI is performed within 48 hours of the surgical resection to assess the extent of resection. Serial imaging is then obtained during subsequent clinic visits, as radiographic recurrence will typically precede clinical symptoms of recurrence.

Outcomes

The preservation rather than restoration of neurologic function is the reasonable expectation for patients undergoing surgery for intramedullary spinal cord tumors. The surgical outcome is most directly related to the patient's preoperative status and tumor location. Virtually all patients will note significant sensory loss soon after surgery, which may be quite

---

Figure 15–2. *(continued)* (D) Once the dorsal tumor surface is exposed from its cephalad to caudal pole, pial tack-up sutures are placed to facilitate the subsequent dissection around the lateral aspects of the tumor. A combination of blunt and sharp dissections is used beginning at the mid-portion of the tumor (where it is typically widest) and then working toward the poles. As shown in the artist's rendering, gentle traction on the tumor helps to reveal adhesions and small feeding vessels requiring cauterization and division.

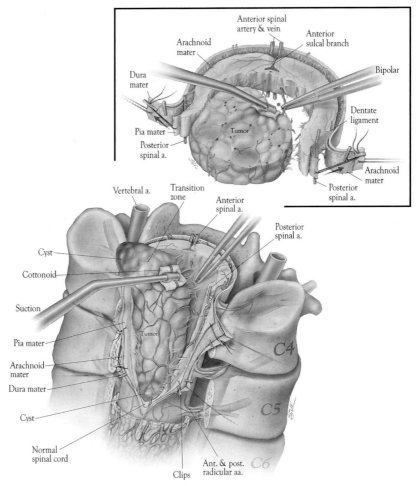

Anterior spinal
artery & vein

Anterior
sulcal branch

Arachnoid
mater

Bipolar

Dura
mater

Dentate
ligament

Pia mater

Tumor

Posterior
spinal a.

Arachnoid
mater

Posterior
spinal a.

Vertebral a.

Transition
zone

Anterior
spinal a.

Posterior
spinal a.

Cyst

Cottonoid

Suction

Tumor

C4

Pia mater

Arachnoid
mater

Dura mater

Cyst

C5

Normal
spinal cord

Clips

Ant. & post.
radicular aa.

C6

E

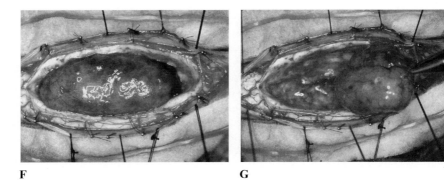

F   **G**

profound and limit their functional ability even though motor power may remain intact. These deficits generally improve over the ensuing weeks and months. Patients with major or long-standing preoperative deficits are less likely to make a significant recovery. The tumor location may also affect the outcome. Tumors in the cervical spine can affect the functioning of both the upper and lower extremities and thus have implications for patient function after surgery. Moreover, the blood supply may be more tenuous in the thoracic spine than in other areas of the spinal cord, so surgery may be less forgiving in the thoracic spine than in other locations (Cooper, 1989; McCormick and Stein, 1990; Hoshimaru et al, 1999).

The risk of recurrence exists after the resection of any spinal cord tumor, and serial imaging and follow-up must be performed. The likelihood of tumor recurrence depends predominantly on the histology of the tumor and the completeness of the original resection. For benign intramedullary ependymomas, gross total resection is often curative without adjuvant therapy. However, careful follow-up is necessary because these tumors can recur. If a recurrence is noted and the patient is in clinically good condition, we will frequently offer repeat resection (McCormick et al, 1990b; Hoshimaru et al, 1999).

The use of radiotherapy after a subtotal resection is more controversial, and it is difficult to provide a clear answer based on the small populations, lack of suitable controls, and limited follow-up in most studies. It may be that radiotherapy provides additional tumor control after a subtotal resection. At M. D. Anderson, we generally reserve adjuvant radiotherapy for malignant variants of ependymomas or for when a tumor simply cannot be resected completely.

The ideal treatment strategy for astrocytomas is less clear partly because of the rarity of these tumors and the clinical and biologic variability of their

---

Figure 15–2. *(continued)* (E) After dissection around the lateral aspects and poles of the tumor, the remaining ventral attachments can then be divided. Gentle traction using a cottonoid patty can be used to lift the tumor and expose ventral adhesions and feeding vessels arising from the anterior spinal artery. These vessels must be cauterized and cut sharply. If they are torn or avulsed, they can withdraw into the ventral substance of the cord and the bleeding can be difficult to stop without causing injury. (F) Intraoperative photo during resection of an intramedullary ependymoma. The dorsal and lateral surfaces of the tumor have been exposed. The pial tack-up sutures help to maintain exposure during the resection. (G) Once the lateral surfaces and poles of the tumor have been dissected, gentle traction is used to lift the tumor out of the spinal cord. This places ventral adhesions and feeding vessels under light stretch, facilitating safe cauterization and division. Note the distinct margin between this ependymoma and the surrounding spinal cord. (Panels B–E are reprinted from Hanbali F, Fourney DR, Marmor E, et al. Spinal cord ependymoma: radical surgical resection and outcome. *Neurosurgery* 2002;51:1162–1174 with permission from Lippincott, Williams, and Wilkins.)

behavior. Most authors agree that high-grade gliomas do not benefit from aggressive surgical resection and that radiotherapy is an important adjuvant treatment once the diagnosis has been made. The influence of the extent of resection on outcome has not been determined for low-grade intramedullary spinal cord astrocytomas. In the relatively rare case of a gross total resection, close observation may be warranted. But in most cases, resection is subtotal and postoperative radiotherapy is given, although the data on its efficacy for low-grade tumors are not conclusive. Because of the unclear benefit of postoperative radiotherapy, its potentially adverse effect on future surgical efforts, and the increased risk of subsequent deformity, some clinicians follow patients clinically and radiographically after subtotal resection and even offer surgery at the time of clinical recurrence if the patient is a surgical candidate. Again, the small numbers of patients and the high degree of biologic variability limit our ability to create conclusive treatment algorithms.

EXTRAMEDULLARY TUMORS

Incidence and Etiology

Approximately two thirds of intradural spinal tumors in adults are extramedullary. Nerve sheath tumors (schwannomas and neurofibromas), meningiomas, and myxopapillary ependymomas of the filum terminale account for more than 95% of extramedullary tumors. Metastases, inclusion tumors and cysts, and paragangliomas make up the rest of these cases. With few exceptions, extramedullary tumors are benign and may be amenable to complete surgical excision.

Nerve Sheath Tumors

In adults, nerve sheath tumors represent approximately 25% of intradural tumors and 40% of extramedullary tumors. Patients with a solitary lesion consistent with a neurofibroma or schwannoma undergo imaging of the entire neuraxis, and once the diagnosis is confirmed, they are evaluated for other manifestations of the disease. If the tumor is arising from the ventral or motor root, it is more likely to be a neurofibroma. While most nerve sheath tumors tend to be intradural, approximately 30% do extend through the nerve root sleeve as a dumbbell-shaped tumor with both intradural and extradural components. Approximately 10% of nerve sheath tumors are epidural or even paraspinal in location, and many of these paraspinal tumors are picked up as incidental findings on other imaging studies. Rarely, these tumors grow in the intramedullary compartment. Approximately 2.5% of intradural nerve sheath tumors are malignant, and at least half of these occur in patients with neurofibromatosis. These tumors carry a poor prognosis, and adjuvant therapy is typically used in addition to surgery. Although frequently grouped together, neurofibromas and schwannomas are distinct demographically, histologically, and biologically.

Neurofibromas. Neurofibromas tend to predominate in neurofibromatosis 1. Neurofibromas produce fusiform enlargement of the involved nerve with the presence of nerve fibers within the tumor stroma, thereby making it impossible to dissect tumor from nerve tissue. This arrangement makes surgical resection more difficult and creates a higher risk of neurologic injury (Russell and Rubenstein, 1989). The presence of multiple neurofibromas establishes the diagnosis of neurofibromatosis.

Schwannomas. Most nerve sheath tumors occur as solitary schwannomas and arise proportionally throughout the spinal canal. These tumors most commonly present in the fourth through sixth decades of life, and men and women are equally affected (de Seze et al, 2005). Unlike neurofibromas, schwannomas are more common in neurofibromatosis 2, and rather than enlarging the nerve from which they originate, schwannomas tend to be suspended eccentrically from the nerve with a discrete point of attachment. While the parent nerve may be quite effaced and splayed by the tumor, there is often a discrete plane between tumor and nerve, which may make surgical resection easier. The fact that schwannomas most commonly arise from a dorsal or sensory nerve root facilitates surgical resection because sectioning of a sensory root can generally be performed without significant morbidity.

Meningiomas

Meningiomas typically arise from arachnoid cap cells in the dura mater near the region of the nerve root sleeve. They may also originate from meningothelial cells making up the arachnoid villi near the dorsal root ganglia. This anatomic arrangement explains why these tumors frequently arise in a lateral location within the spinal canal. These tumors occur with approximately equal frequency as the nerve sheath tumors, representing approximately 40% of intradural extramedullary tumors. Most meningiomas occur after the fourth decade of life and have a significant predilection for females (approximately 75% to 85% of cases). Meningiomas arise primarily in the thoracic region (approximately 80%); the cervical region is affected less often, and lumbar and sacral tumors are relatively rare. These tumors typically grow in a globoid configuration with a region of dural attachment. Rarely, they can grow as a carpet-like plaque (the so-called en plaque meningiomas). Meningiomas tend not to invade the pia mater, which improves the ability to resect them safely.

Myxopapillary Ependymomas of the Filum Terminale

Myxopapillary ependymomas of the filum terminale represent approximately 15% of intradural extramedullary tumors. They typically occur in adults and are the most common tumors to arise in the filum terminale. These tumors are benign, and their classic appearance is a papillary arrangement of cuboid or columnar epithelial cells with rich mucin content. Although these tumors arise from the filum terminale, they can secondarily involve the nerve roots of the cauda equina. They can also seed the spinal fluid compartment with "drop metastases," which necessitates adjuvant treatment.

Other Extramedullary Tumors

A wide variety of neoplastic and nonneoplastic processes round out the list of the intradural extramedullary pathologies. Inclusion tumors and cysts (e.g., dermoids, epidermoids, lipomas, and neurenteric cysts) can occur in the extramedullary intradural space and in conjunction with other evidence of disordered embryogenesis. Paragangliomas, which occur mostly in adults, are uncommon tumors originating from the neural crest. They typically arise from the filum terminale and less commonly from a nerve root. Identification of dense core neurosecretory granules on electron microscopy confirms the diagnosis. Paragangliomas are typically completely resectable. Metastases can also occur in the intradural extramedullary compartment, and if it is noted in a patient with a known cancer diagnosis, evidence for leptomeningeal disease should be sought. Vascular lesions (e.g., cavernous malformations and hemangioblastomas) can also occur in an extramedullary location along the cauda equina. Finally, inflammatory pathologic processes such as sarcoidosis, tuberculosis, and infection can also present as intradural mass lesions.

Clinical Presentation

As with intramedullary tumors, the clinical presentation of intradural extramedullary tumors can be quite variable. The location of the tumor can significantly affect the clinical presentation. Lateral location, as is common with the extramedullary tumors, can cause pressure on the exiting nerve roots, leading to local or radicular pain as well as segmental numbness or weakness. Once the spinal cord is compressed, a Brown-Séquard type of syndrome (i.e., ipsilateral weakness and loss of tactile discrimination, vibratory and position sensation, and contralateral pain and temperature sensory loss) can also occur. Ventrally located tumors, which are more common in the upper cervical spine, can cause a pattern of weakness affecting predominantly the distal upper extremities. Radicular symptoms can occur in the thoracic spine but long tract signs, including difficulty with ambulation and spasticity, are a common presentation. Although patients with tumors of the filum terminale and nerve roots of the cauda equina can certainly present with lower extremity symptoms or bowel and bladder dysfunction, the most common presenting complaint of patients with tumors in these locations is pain associated with recumbency. Back pain exacerbated with recumbency ought to prompt a search for a tumor in the cauda equina.

Diagnostic Imaging

Gadolinium-enhanced MRI is the gold standard for the evaluation of intradural tumors. Not only is MRI exquisitely sensitive with respect to finding even small tumors within the intradural space, but the signal characteristics on MR images can be very helpful in establishing the diagnosis for certain types of lesions, particularly lipomas, inclusion tumors such as dermoids or epidermoids, arachnoid cysts, and vascular anomalies. Nerve sheath tumors, meningiomas, and myxopapillary ependymomas tend to be enhanced after the administration of intravenous contrast. Meningiomas may be the most uniformly enhanced of the group, although nonenhanced areas of calcium deposition may be present. Meningiomas typically will have a more obvious area of dural attachment, the so-called dural tail, which distinguishes these tumors from schwannomas. Compared with meningiomas, schwannomas tend to be hyperintense on T2-weighted images. In the region of the conus medullaris and cauda equina, nerve sheath tumors and myxopapillary ependymomas may be difficult to distinguish radiologically. Both tend to be enhanced, but the pattern of enhancement may not be uniform because of the presence of intratumoral cysts, hemorrhage, or necrosis. Although myelographic and postmyelographic CT are not frequently used in the evaluation of intradural pathology, the high resolution of those studies may be helpful in determining whether a lesion is intramedullary or extramedullary.

Surgical Treatment

General Considerations

Because most intradural extramedullary tumors are benign and may be cured with gross total surgical excision, surgical efforts should be directed at achieving this goal. Thus, adequate access is one of the most important tenets of planning a surgical resection of an intradural extramedullary tumor. Most of these tumors can be accessed through a standard midline approach via laminectomy to gain access to the spinal canal and intradural space. The need to add unilateral or bilateral facetectomy is dictated by the extent of the tumor. Adding an anterior approach for lesions that extend beyond the spine ventrally may also be necessary. The more extensive the bone and ligament resection, the more likely that supplemental spinal stabilization will be required. Once the intradural space is entered, dorsal and dorsolaterally situated tumors tend to be well within the field of view. Ventral tumors situated anterior to the spinal cord may require sectioning of the dentate ligament in order to facilitate adequate visualization. Although ventrally situated lumbar tumors may be obscured by the cauda equina, meticulous dissection and sharp sectioning of the arachnoid will generally allow sufficient mobilization of the roots to provide adequate visualization of the tumor.

Nerve Sheath Tumors

The treatment for benign nerve sheath tumors is complete surgical excision (McCormick et al, 1990a). For tumors contained within the spinal canal, excision is almost always possible through a standard laminectomy approach. Most of these tumors are dorsally situated, as they arise from the sensory nerve roots and are therefore fairly accessible from a standard posterior approach. Ventral tumors may require additional lateral bone exposure with sectioning of the dentate ligament or dissection of the lumbar nerve roots to achieve satisfactory ventral access. Sharp division of the arachnoid generally reveals the tumor. Subsequent tumor removal then requires identification of the nerve root giving rise to the tumor. Depending on the size of the tumor, multiple nerve roots may be stretched over the surface of the tumor as they pass by, and these roots can very often be dissected free of the tumor. Sometimes internal debulking to shrink the size of the tumor can help facilitate this procedure, although the bleeding that results may obscure the surgical field. In general, the nerve root of origin must be sacrificed in order to resect the tumor, and identifying this nerve root proximal and distal to the tumor is the key to the resection. At M. D. Anderson, we generally use electromyographic recordings in the cauda equina and stimulate the perceived nerve of origin before sacrifice to ensure that this nerve does not perform a critical motor function. It is our experience that the functional loss from sacrifice of the nerve root is generally minimal, probably because over time the functions of that nerve have been assumed by neighboring roots. Because of their slow growth, it may be reasonable to stop after a subtotal resection if performing a gross total resection exposes the patient to significant neurologic risks (Seppala et al, 1995a).

Larger nerve sheath tumors may present additional challenges. A tumor that originates very proximally may be partially embedded in the pial surface of the spinal cord and require additional dissection to separate it from the spinal cord itself. More commonly, the added difficulty comes from extension of the tumor beyond the spine and into the paraspinal region. This growth pattern is common for dumbbell-shaped lesions. A variety of extended spinal approaches are available to help manage these larger tumors. Facetectomy can be added to standard laminectomy to gain additional width of exposure throughout the spine. In the thoracic and lumbar regions, this procedure can be further extended via a lateral extracavitary approach to allow for simultaneous exposure of the midline posterior structures and the anterolateral compartment of the spine (Steck et al, 1994; McCormick, 1996). An advantage of the lateral extracavitary approach in the thoracic spine is the ability to stay outside of the pleural cavity. If the dura mater has been opened, this approach can help prevent the possibility of a CSF-pleural fistula. Occasionally, however, the anterior component of the tumor is so large that a ventral approach is also required, particularly when the tumor is abutting vital organs anterior to the spine, including aerodigestive and vascular structures. In this case, the tumor may need to be dissected under direct visualization, and staged posterior/anterior procedures or simultaneous combined procedures may be necessary. Again, when one is working in the chest, great care must be taken to prevent a CSF fistula, and we do not hesitate to use local pedicled muscle flaps to cover areas that are at risk for a CSF leak and isolate them from the negative intrathoracic pressures that drive fistula formation. As the surgical approach gains magnitude and complexity, the likelihood of iatrogenic spinal instability increases and preparations may be needed for spinal stabilization.

Meningiomas

As is the case for nerve sheath tumors, the goal for meningiomas is gross total surgical excision with the intention of cure. Gross total excision can be achieved in most cases, largely because these tumors tend not to invade the spinal cord or the bone surrounding the dura mater. Even so, the recurrence rate may be as high 10% to 15%. Simple posterior laminectomy provides adequate exposure in almost all cases. The addition of facetectomy, a lateral extracavitary approach, or an extreme lateral approach in the region of the foramen magnum may be required to gain access to ventral meningiomas. Sectioning of the dentate ligament and suture retraction to rotate the cord may also help. Even with these extended approaches, it may be difficult to visualize the entire margin of a ventrally situated tumor. Fortunately, there is usually a protective layer of arachnoid between these tumors and the ventral surface of the spinal cord. While dorsal and dorsolaterally situated meningiomas may be removed en bloc (including the site of dural attachment), for ventrally situated tumors, the resection is generally piecemeal and resection of the dura mater may not be possible. When the tumor and dura mater can be resected, a variety of dural patch materials (both natural and synthetic) are available for dural reconstruction.

At M. D. Anderson, our preferred technique of piecemeal resection is to try to identify the caudal and cephalad poles of the meningioma, use cottonoid patties to prevent spillage of debris into the CSF, and cauterize the surface of the tumor. After this, the tumor capsule is incised and the tumor is debulked internally by using either suction and bipolar cautery or an ultrasonic aspirator. As this process proceeds, the tumor can be further coagulated and incised down to its dural base. Once the tumor has been reduced to the dural base, we extensively cauterize the dural base to eradicate any residual tumor cells.

Myxopapillary Ependymomas of the Filum Terminale

The surgical treatment of a myxopapillary ependymoma of the filum terminale depends significantly on the extent of the tumor and its involvement of the cauda equina. All patients suspected of having myxopapillary ependymomas should undergo imaging of the entire neuraxis to look for signs of CSF dissemination, which may alter the decision for a surgical approach. Ideally, a solitary lesion is identified in the region of the filum terminale without obvious involvement of the adjacent cauda equina. In these cases, the goal of surgery is gross total excision, which, if possible, should be performed en bloc to limit the dissemination of the tumor within the CSF. In these cases, the filum terminale can be identified both above and below the tumor. Electromyographic stimulation can be performed to confirm that there is no neurologic activity, and then the filum can be sectioned above and below the tumor, thereby allowing the tumor to be removed en bloc. Again, if possible, an intralesional approach should be avoided to limit CSF dissemination. The identification and surgical treatment of a myxopapillary ependymoma of the filum terminale are illustrated in Figure 15–3.

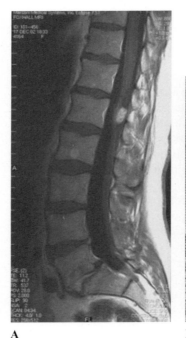

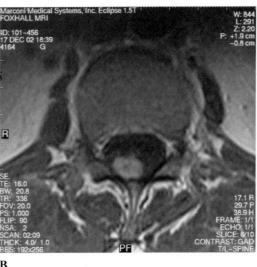

A   B

Figure 15–3. (A) Sagittal gadolinium-enhanced T1-weighted MR image reveals an ovoid enhanced mass in the proximal cauda equina. Myxopapillary ependymoma and benign nerve sheath tumor lead the differential diagnosis. (B) Axial gadolinium-enhanced T1-weighted MR image of the same lesion.

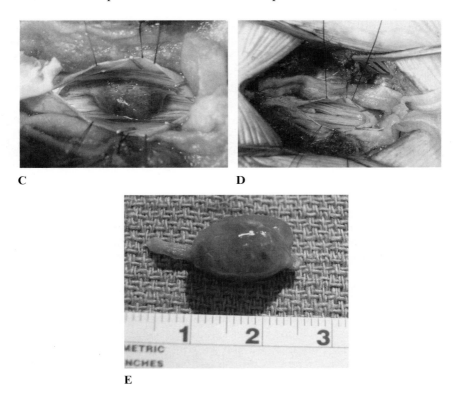

Figure 15–3. *(continued)* (C) Intradural exploration reveals a well-circumscribed, reddish-gray mass originating from the filum terminale. (D) Electrical stimulation of the filum terminale above and below the mass reveals no neurologic activity. The filum is then cauterized and cut above and below the mass. Note the cut end of the filum, which is apparent in this photo following removal of the mass. (E) Pathologic evaluation confirms the diagnosis of myxopapillary ependymoma.

Larger myxopapillary ependymomas with insinuation among the roots of the cauda equina present a much more challenging problem. These tumors can become quite large, and they tend to be unencapsulated and insinuated among the nerve roots. CSF seeding is a significant risk. Tumor resection in these cases is piecemeal, and gross total resection is rarely achieved. Although surgery may not be curative, it can confirm the histologic diagnosis and potentially improve symptoms in patients with large tumors.

Outcomes

Severe, long-term adverse effects after surgical excision of benign nerve sheath tumors are rare. These tumors are generally cured by gross total excision, and patients with this diagnosis have an excellent life expectancy. Recurrence is quite rare after gross total resection, and it occurs at a rate of approximately 50% after subtotal resection (Seppala et al, 1995b). Adjuvant focused radiation may be considered for the very rare patient who has failed multiple surgical procedures and in whom additional surgery carries a prohibitive risk.

After complete resection of a spinal meningioma, the long-term recurrence rate ranges from 3% to 23%. Solero and colleagues (1989) found no significant difference in recurrence rates of meningiomas when the dural base was resected versus extensively cauterized. We generally favor repeat resection should recurrence occur and would consider adjuvant treatment such as radiation only when resection is not feasible.

Recurrence is rare after successful en bloc resection of a myxopapillary ependymoma of the filum terminale. However, if gross total resection is achieved in a piecemeal fashion, local recurrence becomes a much more significant risk (Sonneland et al, 1985). Because the natural history and biologic behavior of these lesions vary from patient to patient, as does their response to radiotherapy, there are no hard and fast treatment algorithms to be applied in these cases. In general, if a gross total or nearly total piecemeal removal can be achieved, it is reasonable to follow the patient with serial imaging and consider reoperating or irradiating at the time of local recurrence or progression. This approach offers the benefit of gaining insight into the natural history of the patient's tumor, and it may be that reoperation is less complicated if the patient has not received radiotherapy. In cases of significant residual tumor or CSF dissemination, adjuvant therapy with radiation is typically used (Whitaker et al, 1991).

CAUDA EQUINA LESIONS

The diagnostic considerations and tests for patients with cauda equina lesions are similar to those used for patients with spinal cord lesions. Neoplastic lesions affecting the cauda equina can be primary or metastatic as well as inflammatory. These inflammatory processes may be local or systemic. Primary tumors of the cauda equina include myxopapillary ependymomas originating from the filum terminale as well as benign schwannomas or neurofibromas originating from the nerve roots. A slowly progressive course of lumbosacral symptoms consisting of weakness or sensory changes is typical in such patients. Occasionally, imaging of the entire neuraxis is necessary to help in the diagnosis and to establish the extent of disease. Potential causes of leptomeningeal and pachymeningeal nerve root enhancements and lesions and corresponding helpful diagnostic tests are listed in Table 15–5.

**Table 15–5.   Types of Leptomeningeal and Pachymeningeal Nerve Root
Enhancements and Lesions and Useful Diagnostic Tests**

Type of Enhancement or Lesion, *and Potential Diagnoses*	*Diagnostic Tests*
Infectious	
Viral infection (CMV, HSV-1, HSV-2, HTLV-1, EBV, VZV, human orphan virus, enteric cytopathogenic virus)	Appropriate viral cultures and PCR for viral DNA
Fungal infection (Candida, aspergillus)	Fungal smears and culture
Tuberculosis	Acid-fast bacteria smears and culture
Syphilis	CSF VDRL
Lyme disease	CSF Borrelia titers
Cysticercosis	Serum and CSF cysticercosis enzyme-linked immunosorbent assay
Autoimmune or inflammatory	
Sarcoidosis	Serum and CSF angiotensin-converting enzyme, gallium scan, bone marrow biopsy
Rheumatoid arthritis	ANA, RF, biopsy
Wegener's granulomatosis	Serum p-ANCA, c-ANCA
Behçet's syndrome	Pathergy test
Sjögren's syndrome	Anti-Ro and anti-La antibodies
Temporal arteritis	ESR
Guillain-Barré syndrome or chronic inflammatory demyelinating polyradiculopathy	CSF albuminocytologic dissociation, electromyography/nerve conduction velocity
Idiopathic hypertrophic pachymeningitis	Biopsy
Isolated CNS angiitis	ANA, RF, arteriography
Systemic lupus erythematosus	ANA, RF, anti-phospholipid antibodies
Vascular	
Spinal dural arteriovenous fistula	MRI, MR angiogram, CT myelogram, spinal arteriogram
Radiation injury	MRI
Neoplastic	
Carcinomatous meningitis	CSF protein, glucose, cytology
Lymphomatous meningitis	CSF cytology, CSF β2 microglobulin (also elevated in bacterial or viral meningitis)
Leukemic meningitis	CSF cytology, CSF for flow cytometry
Plasmacytoma	CSF cytology, protein electrophoresis
En plaque meningioma	Imaging, biopsy
Solitary fibrous tumor	Imaging, biopsy
Schwannoma	Imaging
Vertebral metastases	Imaging

(continued)

Table 15–5. *(continued)* **Types of Leptomeningeal and Pachymeningeal Nerve Root Enhancements and Lesions and Useful Diagnostic Tests**

Type of Enhancement or Lesion, and Potential Diagnoses	*Diagnostic Tests*
Paraneoplastic disease (lymphoma, leukemia, lung cancer*)	Anti-Hu antibodies*
Traumatic or iatrogenic	
Spinal stenosis	Imaging
Herniated nucleus pulposus	Imaging
Post-lumbar puncture dural venous engorgement	History, imaging
Spontaneous intracranial hypotension	History, imaging

Abbreviations: ANA, anti-nuclear antibody; c-ANCA and p-ANCA, antibodies directed to neutrophil cytoplasmic antigens, cytoplasmic type and perinuclear type; CMV, cytomegalovirus; CNS, central nervous system; CSF, cerebrospinal fluid; CT, computed tomography; EBV, Epstein-Barr virus; ESR, erythrocyte sedimentation rate; HSV, herpes simplex virus; HTLV-1, human T-cell leukemia virus type 1; MRI, magnetic resonance imaging; PCR, polymerase chain reaction; RF, rheumatoid factor; VDRL, Venereal Disease Research Laboratory; VZV, varicella zoster virus.

CONCLUSION

A wide variety of pathologic processes can arise within the intradural spinal compartment. Before surgical interventions are considered, the patient's history, presenting symptoms, physical examination results, imaging studies, and blood and CSF analyses data should be carefully assessed. At M. D. Anderson, to exclude nonsurgical pathologic processes, we use a multidisciplinary approach so that a complete differential diagnosis can be considered and evaluated. The advances in imaging and surgical techniques that have improved our ability to treat the neoplasms that arise in the intradural space have been gratifying because most of these tumors are benign.

KEY PRACTICE POINTS

- Intradural spinal tumors represent 10% to 15% of CNS neoplasms and are classified as intramedullary, extramedullary, or cauda equina tumors.
- An extensive multidisciplinary diagnostic evaluation is necessary to eliminate the possibility of operating on a process that will not benefit from surgical intervention. However, extensive diagnostic testing can be misleading because of false-positive results. When spinal cord lesions are being evaluated, an open mind is needed about the diagnosis until one is proved or the condition remits.

KEY PRACTICE POINTS *(continued)*

- Arteriovenous malformations of the spinal cord or dura mater can be extremely difficult to diagnose and should be considered in older men with a history of cardiovascular disease.

- High-quality, high-resolution, T1-weighted contrast-enhanced and T2-weighted MRI of the entire neuraxis is a critical part of the diagnostic evaluation. Expert neuroradiologic opinion is needed to obtain the best interpretation of an imaging series.

- In the setting of an underlying cancer or immunocompromise, consideration must be given to less common causes of myelopathy or radiculopathy, such as viral, fungal, and parasitic infections or infestations.

- Glial tumors account for 80% of intramedullary tumors. Ependymoma is the most common type of intramedullary tumor, astrocytoma the second most common, and hemangioblastoma the third most common.

- Most intramedullary tumors are low-grade neoplasms. Surgery represents the most effective treatment option for these tumors.

- Most extramedullary tumors are benign and are potentially curable with total surgical excision. All efforts should be directed at achieving this goal.

- The surgical outcome is most directly related to the patient's preoperative neurologic status and the tumor's location.

SUGGESTED READINGS

Baptiste DC, Fehlings MG. Pathophysiology of cervical myelopathy. *Spine J* 2006;6(Suppl):S190–S197.

Cooper PR. Outcome after operative treatment of intramedullary spinal cord tumors in adults: intermediate and long-term results in 51 patients. *Neurosurgery* 1989;25:855–859.

de Seze J, Lanctin C, Lebrun C, et al. Idiopathic acute transverse myelitis: application of the recent diagnostic criteria. *Neurology* 2005;65:1950–1953.

Epstein FJ, Farmer JP, Freed D. Adult intramedullary astrocytomas of the spinal cord. *J Neurosurg* 1992;77:355–359.

Epstein FJ, Farmer JP, Freed D. Adult intramedullary spinal cord ependymomas: the result of surgery in 38 patients. *J Neurosurg* 1993;79:204–209.

Garcia DM. Primary spinal cord tumors treated with surgery and postoperative irradiation. *Int J Radiat Oncol Biol Phys* 1985;11:1933–1939.

Hoshimaru M, Koyama T, Hashimoto N, Kikuchi H. Results of microsurgical treatment for intramedullary spinal cord ependymomas: analysis of 36 cases. *Neurosurgery* 1999;44:264–269.

Lee M, Epstein FJ, Rezai AR, Zagzag D. Nonneoplastic intramedullary spinal cord lesions mimicking tumors. *Neurosurgery* 1998;43:788–795.

McCormick PC. Surgical management of dumbbell and paraspinal tumors of the thoracic and lumbar spine. *Neurosurgery* 1996;38:67–75.

McCormick PC, Post KD, Stein BM. Intradural extramedullary tumors in adults. *Neurosurg Clin N Am* 1990a;1:591–608.

McCormick PC, Stein BM. Intramedullary tumors in adults. [Review] *Neurosurg Clin N Am* 1990;1:609–630.

McCormick PC, Torres R, Post KD, Stein BM. Intramedullary ependymomas of the spinal cord. *J Neurosurg* 1990b;72:523–532.

Neumann HP, Eggert HR, Weigel K, Freidburg H, Wiestler OD, Schollmeyer P. Hemangioblastomas of the central nervous system. A 10-year study with special reference to von Hippel-Lindau syndrome. *J Neurosurg* 1989;70:24–30.

Olindo S, Cabre P, Lezin A, et al. Natural history of human T-lymphotropic virus 1-associated myelopathy: a 14-year follow-up study. *Arch Neurol* 2006;63: 1560–1566.

O'Sullivan C, Jenkin RD, Doherty MA, Hoffman HJ, Greenberg ML. Spinal cord tumors in children: long-term results of combined surgical and radiation treatment. *J Neurosurg* 1994;81:507–512.

Burger PC, Scheithauer BW, Vogel FS. *Surgical Pathology of the Nervous System and Its Coverings.* New York, NY: Churchill Livingstone, 2002.

Russell DS, Rubenstein LJ. *Pathology of Tumors of the Nervous System.* Baltimore, MD: Williams & Wilkins, 1989.

Salvi F, Jones J, Weigert B. The assessment of cervical myelopathy. *Spine J* 2006;6:S182–S189.

Seppala MT, Haltia MJ, Sankila RJ, Jaaskelainen JE, Heiskanen O. Long-term outcome after removal of spinal schwannoma: a clinicopathological study of 187 cases. *J Neurosurg* 1995a;83:621–626.

Seppala MT, Haltia MJ, Sankila RJ, Jaaskelainen JE, Heiskanen O. Long-term outcome after removal of spinal neurofibroma. *J Neurosurg* 1995b;82:572–577.

Sloof JL, Kernohan JW, MacCarty CS. *Primary Intramedullary Tumors of the Spinal Cord and Filum Terminale.* Philadelphia, PA: W.B. Saunders, 1964.

Solero CL, Fornari M, Giombini S, et al. Spinal meningiomas: review of 174 operated cases. *Neurosurgery* 1989;25:153–160.

Sonneland PR, Scheithauer BW, Onofrio BM. Myxopapillary ependymoma: a clinicopathologic and immunocytochemical study of 77 cases. *Cancer* 1985;56: 883–893.

Steck JC, Dietze DD, Fessler RG. Posterolateral approach to intradural extramedullary thoracic tumors. *J Neurosurg* 1994;81:202–205.

Whitaker SJ, Bessell EM, Ashley SE, Bloom HJ, Bell BA, Brada M. Postoperative radiotherapy in the management of spinal cord ependymoma. *J Neurosurg* 1991;74:720–728.

16 SYMPTOM MANAGEMENT FOR PATIENTS WITH BRAIN TUMORS: IMPROVING QUALITY OF LIFE

Allen W. Burton, Tracy L. Veramonti,
Phillip C. Phan, and Jeffrey S. Wefel

Chapter Overview 330
Introduction 330
Neurocognitive Dysfunction 331
   Variables Contributing to Neurocognitive Dysfunction 331
      Disease Factors 331
      Patient Factors 333
      Treatment Factors 333
         Radiotherapy 334
         Chemotherapy 334
         Supportive Agents 335
   Assessment of Quality of Life and Neurocognitive Functioning 335
      Quality of Life 336
      Neurocognitive Functioning 337
   Pharmacologic and Psychologic Management of
      Neurocognitive Sequelae 338
      Pharmacologic Interventions 339
      Neurocognitive Rehabilitation Strategies 340
      Fatigue Management and Other Behavioral Strategies 341
Pain Management 341
   Assessment of Pain 341
      Chief Complaint 344
      Oncologic History 344
      Pain History 345
      Review of Medical Record and Radiologic Studies 345
      Psychologic and Social History 345
      Medical History 345
      Physical Examination 345
   Cancer Pain Management 346
      Continuous Subcutaneous Infusion of Opioids 347
      Continuous Intravenous Infusion of Opioids 347

Intraspinal Analgesia 347
Nerve Blocks 348
Vertebroplasty 348
Neuromodulation 348
Neurosurgery 348
Key Practice Points 349
Suggested Readings 349

CHAPTER OVERVIEW

Patients with brain tumors who have progressive disease are often highly symptomatic. This multisymptom burden can include cognitive impairment, fatigue, pain (usually in the form of headache), and mood disturbance and can result in loss of independence. Often, the symptom burden at the time of diagnosis is related to the histologic grade, location, and size of the brain tumor. Treatment of the tumor frequently leads to symptomatic stabilization or improvement. Numerous palliative treatments also exist primarily for symptom control. Pharmacologic and behavioral interventions are increasingly being used to manage the adverse effects of neurocognitive dysfunction among patients with brain tumors. The art of neuro-oncology involves optimizing a patient's quality of life through collaborative care among neuro-oncologists, radiation oncologists, neurosurgeons, neuropsychologists, and supportive care specialists. Regardless of the tumor type and stage, the basic tenet of supportive care applies: the quality and quantity of life should be optimized whenever possible in accordance with the wishes of the patient. Multidisciplinary care should guide patient care with the available expertise to carefully balance aggressive treatment and symptom control.

INTRODUCTION

Primary and metastatic brain tumors are among the most symptomatic of all cancers. For primary malignant brain tumors, long-term cure remains elusive, and even "benign" brain tumors often cause significant debility and a profound symptom burden. Metastatic tumors of the brain are seen in up to 30% of patients with solid tumors of the lung, breast, skin, kidney, and other sites. The treatment of metastatic brain tumors is complicated by the different tumor types involved, whether there are solitary or multiple metastases, the extent of systemic disease, the patient's age, and medical comorbidities. The most common symptoms seen in brain tumor patients are cognitive dysfunction, headache, ataxia, focal weakness, and seizure. For example, Tucha and associates (2000) demonstrated that cognitive dysfunction is evident at the time of diagnosis in more than 90% of brain tumor patients. Headache is a presenting symptom in up to 55% of brain tumor patients, and seizure develops in 30% to 50%. The identification and optimal treatment of these symptoms will improve the quality of life (QOL) of brain cancer patients.

NEUROCOGNITIVE DYSFUNCTION

It is generally recognized that neurocognitive dysfunction can develop in cancer patients as a direct result of cancer affecting the central nervous system (CNS), as an unfortunate consequence of therapeutic modalities (e.g., radiotherapy, chemotherapy, and bioimmunotherapy) used as primary or prophylactic treatment for CNS tumors as well as systemic disease, or as a side effect of adjuvant medications (e.g., corticosteroids, antiepileptic drugs, immunosuppressive agents, antiemetics, and drugs used to treat infection or pain) used to prevent or limit medical complications. Patient survival and time to tumor progression have served as traditional outcomes in clinical trials of new anticancer agents, but such end points fail to capture other important aspects of patient functioning, including QOL. The routine functional assessment of variables that affect QOL, including neurocognitive status, physical symptoms, ability to perform activities of daily living, and psychosocial functioning, was deemed a research priority and recommended as the standard of care for patients with primary brain tumors by the Brain Tumor Progress Review Group (2000), which was cosponsored by the National Cancer Institute and the National Institute of Neurologic Disorders and Stroke. In addition, the integrity of neurocognitive functioning has been demonstrated to have prognostic significance even after well-established predictors of survival such as patient age, patient performance status, and tumor histologic type are controlled for. Because of the poor prognosis and significant morbidity associated with cancers of the CNS and primary brain tumors in particular, QOL may be one of the most important areas that the clinician can significantly influence. Evaluation of the cognitive, behavioral, and emotional sequelae that may occur in these patients can assist in the development of appropriate intervention strategies, thereby improving the quality of care, and ultimately the QOL, of these patients.

Variables Contributing to Neurocognitive Dysfunction

Disease Factors

In adult patients with primary malignant brain cancer, tumor location, tumor-related epilepsy, tumor pathology, tumor momentum (i.e., speed of growth), and tumor volume can all contribute to the presentation of cognitive deficits, which vary significantly across patients. Depending on the site of the tumor, there can be profound disturbances in neurocognitive functioning, personality, and psychologic well-being. Changes in the ability to perform daily activities are common and can lead to increased dependence on others, decreased productivity, and impaired social functioning. Depending on its location, size, or type, a tumor can also cause seizure, alter endocrine patterns, or disrupt afferent or efferent pathways between functional systems, thereby leading to neurocognitive and motor dysfunction.

Although they may arise in the brainstem and cerebellum, primary brain tumors in adults tend to occur supratentorially, often compromising the association cortex and resulting in predictable, location-specific patterns of impairment. For instance, tumors in the left hemisphere tend to compromise language abilities, whereas tumors in the right hemisphere may produce disturbances in visuospatial perception and scanning. Regardless of the specific site of the lesion, memory impairment and changes in executive functioning (the capacity for intentional behavior, planning and organization skills, mental flexibility, abstraction, accurate self-awareness, self-regulation, personality, etc.) as a result of frontal lobe disruption are common neurocognitive sequelae. Notably, while lesions in the frontal lobe can directly lead to impairment of executive functions, lesions in other parts of the brain can also contribute to "frontal" deficits because they disrupt the frontal subcortical or frontal limbic circuitry. Executive functions are considered "necessary for appropriate, socially responsible, and effectively self-serving adult conduct" (Lezak et al, 2004, p. 611), and marked changes in personality characterized by deficits in social functioning and judgment have been documented after surgical removal of tumors. Finally, neurobehavioral slowing and fatigue are ubiquitous in patients with brain tumors. Fatigue can adversely affect cognitive functioning and mood, and the reverse is also true: impaired cognitive functioning and mood disorders can lead to fatigue.

Certain tumors are well circumscribed, grow slowly, result in very little compromise of the adjacent cortex, and are quite amenable to surgical resection. Other, usually highly malignant, tumors may grow more rapidly and diffusely infiltrate or displace adjacent tissue. Such tumors can result in significant disruption of brain function. As they grow in size and block the flow of cerebrospinal fluid, larger tumors can lead to increased intracranial pressure and to a progressive, generalized decline in neurocognitive functioning. However, even seemingly benign brain tumors, such as meningiomas, can grow and "crowd" viable brain tissue, resulting in significant disability and, in some cases, life-threatening conditions.

Even after lesion volume is controlled for, the rate of tumor growth can be a significant factor in the presentation of neurocognitive deficits. For example, a patient initially diagnosed with a low-grade astrocytoma that undergoes histologic transformation into a glioblastoma multiforme over several years may have cognitive difficulties that are less severe than those of a newly diagnosed patient with glioblastoma multiforme who presented with rapidly progressive symptoms.

Patient Factors

Knowledge of the relevant patient-related factors that can contribute to changes in neurocognitive functioning in those with CNS cancer is essential for the interpretation of neuropsychologic test results, functional prognostication, and treatment recommendation. Age is perhaps one of the most pertinent variables to be considered. Older patients tend to present with both biologically and histologically more malignant tumors; even low-grade tumors tend to behave more aggressively in older patients. In addition, the toxicities associated with treatment (e.g., radiotherapy and chemotherapy) tend to be more devastating in older patients. Moreover, one must consider the dynamic nature of the aging brain. A number of studies have documented modest age-related changes in specific brain regions, particularly the temporal lobe, hippocampus, and basilar subcortical regions, that may be associated with age-related changes in cognition. Changes in white matter integrity with age that are common in nondemented, asymptomatic individuals may contribute to poorer performance on tests of processing speed, memory, and executive functions. Older adults are at higher risk for having concurrent neurodegenerative diseases, such as Alzheimer's disease or Parkinson's disease, which may contribute to a poor cognitive status at baseline (i.e., before surgery or before adjuvant treatment). Finally, infection, concurrent or chronic illness, and side effects of medication must be considered in evaluating the test results for any patient. In summary, validated and reliable measures for which normative data exist are crucial in distinguishing between "normal neurocognitive aging" and neurodegenerative changes in the context of cancer-related neurocognitive impairments.

Numerous other patient-related factors inherent in any assessment of cognitive functioning should also be considered. These factors include education, sex, handedness, race, sociocultural variables, language preference, mental health history and current psychologic status (e.g., depression, anxiety, or fatigue), and premorbid personality and social adjustment. The relevant medical history, a history of head trauma, epilepsy, and developmental disorders should likewise be considered in any neuropsychologic investigation. A full discussion of these variables is beyond the scope of this chapter, and the reader is referred to Lezak and associates (2004) for a more complete description.

Treatment Factors

Often, the nature and extent of neurocognitive dysfunction in patients with brain tumors are more generalized than what are expected for a focal lesion. Microscopic tumor infiltration, adverse distal effects on the brain (e.g., diaschisis), or the adverse effects of treatment on "normal tissue" have all been hypothesized to be factors that contribute to cognitive dysfunction. Unfortunately, cancer treatments place normal tissues and organs at risk, and the CNS is particularly vulnerable to systemic cancer treatments, those directed specifically at brain malignancies, and adjuvant medications used to treat medical complications. An overview of the neurocognitive effects of radiotherapy, chemotherapy, and common supportive agents used to manage medical complications follows.

Radiotherapy. Preferential disruption of frontal subcortical networks in the brain is a common consequence of radiotherapy. This effect is perhaps due to the toxic effects of radiation on white matter tracts, which are particularly dense in frontal and subcortical areas. Encephalopathy secondary to radiotherapy has been described to occur in 3 stages: acute, early delayed, and late delayed. Within the first 2 weeks of treatment, patients frequently develop fatigue and exacerbation of preexisting neurologic deficits. They may also develop new focal deficits and experience headache, seizure, nausea, or vomiting. Early-delayed effects develop 1 to 4 months after completion of radiotherapy and include slowed information-processing speed, executive dysfunction, diminished memory function, and motor deficits. These symptoms are believed to result from transient demyelination; subsequent remyelination is associated with variable symptom improvement. Some patients experience late-delayed encephalopathy (from 6 months to years after completing radiotherapy) that can involve progressive neurologic decline, dementia, leukoencephalopathy, or brain necrosis.

Neuropsychologic studies of patients before and after radiotherapy have documented neurocognitive impairments consistent with dysfunction of frontal network systems, including impaired information-processing speed, attention (e.g., working memory), mental flexibility, learning, memory, and motor functioning. Several factors that contribute to the occurrence of radiation encephalopathy have been identified, including age 60 years or older, a higher total radiation dose, a dose per fraction of 2 Gy or larger, a greater irradiated brain volume, hyperfractionated schedules, a shorter overall treatment time, concomitant or subsequent use of chemotherapy, and comorbid vascular risk factors. For a more comprehensive review of the neurobehavioral effects of radiotherapy in brain tumor patients, the reader is referred to Crossen and associates (1994).

Chemotherapy. Neurotoxicities affecting both the CNS and the peripheral nervous system have been associated with adjuvant treatment with chemotherapy. Numerous complications, including encephalopathy (acute and chronic), neuropathy (central and peripheral), and cerebellar symptoms, have been described. Neuropsychologic deficits include memory loss, reduced information-processing speed, executive dysfunction, decreased attention, anxiety, depression, and fatigue. Some chemotherapeutic drugs may have relatively specific mechanisms of action and thereby place specific neurocognitive functions at risk (e.g., memory) (Meyers, 1997), whereas other drugs have more diffuse effects on the brain with a pattern suggestive of frontal subcortical system dysfunction.

Studying the effects of chemotherapy in patients with brain tumors is challenging because most treatment schedules administer chemotherapy after radiotherapy, thereby confounding the measurement of chemotherapeutic drug-specific adverse effects. However, neuropsychologic investigation of patients with other types of cancer has provided proof-of-principle evidence that some chemotherapeutic agents are associated with neurocognitive toxicity. These investigations have also demonstrated that patient-reported measures of neurocognitive dysfunction fail to adequately capture the changes observed on objective measurements of neurocognitive function. The correlation between mood and patient-reported neurocognitive function has been quite robust, but mood has not been found to be highly correlated with objectively assessed neurocognitive function. Finally, the long-term effects of chemotherapeutic agents on cognition are not well understood.

Supportive Agents.   The use of corticosteroids, especially in high doses or when taken chronically, is associated with a number of neuropsychiatric and neurocognitive sequelae, including anxiety, depression, mania, insomnia, restlessness, increased motor activity, memory dysfunction, and delirium. Side effects of antiepileptic medications commonly include sedation, distractibility, somnolence, and dizziness; these symptoms tend to increase in frequency and intensity with the use of multiple agents and with elevated serum levels of these agents. In patients with brain tumors, the use of phenytoin, carbamazepine, and valproic acid has been associated with impaired attention, processing speed, and memory. The newer anticonvulsant agents, including lamotrigine, oxcarbazepine, and gabapentin, appear to induce less severe side effects, including fewer neurocognitive side effects. Finally, pharmacologic agents prescribed to manage pain, particularly opioids, have been associated with impaired performance on cognitive tasks. Nonetheless, the effects may be modest if the medication regimen is stable, and performance could improve if the severity of the pain is reduced.

Assessment of Quality of Life and Neurocognitive Functioning

The endpoints of survival and disease-free survival, which traditionally have been used to assess outcome in patients with cancer, fall painfully short as measures of success in treating brain tumors. From the perspective of patients and families, "outcome" is a multidimensional, daily reality, and quality of life can be at least as important as survival. So, too, assessment of quality of life is increasingly used to evaluate the risks and benefits of new treatments. . . . Because the current treatment armamentarium has little to offer many patients with brain tumors, saving a life can be a considerable achievement. Saving a life without considering future constraints on how life can be lived, however, may offer an unacceptable outcome (Brain Tumor Progress Review Group, 2000, p. 30).

Quality of Life

Evaluating QOL in a patient with a brain tumor is not always straightforward because the patient's neurocognitive impairments may compromise his or her ability to provide accurate self-reported information. For example, impaired awareness of one's neurocognitive deficits and their effect on functioning is a common consequence of frontal lobe dysfunction. Even in the case of profound cognitive impairments, patients with frontal lobe impairment may grossly underestimate or outright deny problems. Performance-based measures, such as tests of neuropsychologic functioning, may be necessary to capture changes in patients who are experiencing neurologic deterioration, regardless of whether the patients can understand and respond to questions on a self-report QOL measure.

Historically, QOL has been a difficult term to define. Discrepancies across research findings have been attributed to differences in methods of data collection and to the nature of the QOL instrument. The Karnofsky performance scale has been the most widely used outcome measure, and commonly the primary assessment of QOL, in many neuro-oncologic studies. This tool is used to assess a patient's performance status on a scale ranging from 0 (dead) to 100 (normal, no evidence of disease). However, it does not address the domains considered crucial for measuring QOL or for evaluating neurocognitive status, and as a measure, it suffers from a lack of reliability and validity. An appropriate instrument for assessing QOL in a neuro-oncology setting should address the unique physical, emotional, and social consequences of cancer affecting the CNS, including the specific neurologic and neurocognitive difficulties commonly encountered as a consequence of the cancer and its treatment. Both the Functional Assessment of Cancer Therapy–Brain (FACT-Br) questionnaire, which was developed by Weitzner and colleagues (1995), and the European Organization for Research and Treatment of Cancer's Quality of Life Questionnaire–Brain Module (QOQ-BCM) questionnaire were developed for patients with brain tumors. Each of these questionnaires addresses the patient's physical, familial, social, emotional, and functional well-being.

Depression, anxiety, reduced tolerance for frustration, increased emotional reactivity, and familial stress have all been reported in studies of the QOL of brain tumor patients that used similar measures. Patients' personality characteristics, current availability and use of social supports, and access to community services were more strongly associated with overall QOL than were histologic diagnosis, prognosis, or age. Additional characteristics that have been found to place a patient with a brain tumor at risk for a poor QOL include being female, being divorced, having finished chemotherapy, having a tumor in both hemispheres, and having a poor performance status.

Increased attention to symptoms of affective distress in patients with CNS cancer through appropriate assessment and referral to skilled professionals for psychotherapy, pharmacotherapy, or both is clearly warranted.

Recent data from the Glioma Outcomes Project conducted with the support of the Joint Section on Tumors of the American Association of Neurological Surgeons and the Congress of Neurological Surgeons documented self-reported symptoms suggesting depression in approximately 93% of brain tumor patients before and up to 6 months after surgery; in contrast, physicians detected depression in approximately 22% of patients (Litofsky et al, 2004). Thus, many patients did not receive potentially efficacious therapy for their affective distress. This situation was unfortunate, as patient-reported depression was associated with shorter survival times and more complications.

Neurocognitive Functioning

The assessment of neurocognitive functioning in both clinical and research settings has routinely been limited to a brief screening of global neurocognitive functioning, such as the Mini-Mental Status Examination (MMSE). Although markedly impaired MMSE scores certainly distinguish between subjects with severe impairment and neurocognitively intact subjects, the MMSE is much less effective in distinguishing those with mild impairments. Among patients with brain tumors, the sensitivity of the MMSE is poor partly because this instrument does not measure many of the neurocognitive functions known to be impaired in brain tumor patients. To elucidate this point, Meyers and colleagues (1997) presented data from a phase II study examining the neurotoxicity of a novel mitotic inhibitor in brain tumor patients. In this trial, 67% of patients showed a clinically and statistically significant decline in memory functioning on neuropsychologic testing after each infusion of the drug, whereas no patients demonstrated a change on cognitive screening instruments, including the MMSE. Had the researchers limited their conclusions to the MMSE results, they might have decided that the drug produced no neurotoxic side effects—a conclusion that is not only incorrect but potentially dangerous. In summary, the MMSE cannot substitute for a formal evaluation of neurocognitive functioning in clinical settings or research endeavors that seek to monitor the neurotoxicity of anticancer treatments, assist with differential diagnostic decisions, and ultimately contribute to treatment recommendations.

Comprehensive neuropsychologic assessment of neurocognitive dysfunction in patients with brain tumors has been demonstrated to be both feasible and well tolerated by patients in research trials and clinical settings. Neuropsychologic assessments have been useful in identifying both the risks and benefits of a variety of anticancer treatments on neurocognitive functioning and have been shown to predict survival better than clinical prognostic factors alone in patients with primary brain tumors, leptomeningeal disease, or parenchymal brain metastases. Moreover, understanding the constellation of neurocognitive symptoms before surgery or initiation of anticancer treatment can serve as a useful baseline from which to judge the effect of treatment, and it may help to develop a plan for early intervention. Serial evaluation at regular intervals, either in conjunction with sentinel events (i.e., when the risk for cognitive decline or affective distress increases) or with clinical data (e.g., neuroimaging results), allows for monitoring of neurotoxicity, assists with differential diagnosis (e.g., depression vs dementia), and can be used to refer patients for appropriate pharmacologic or behavior management.

Neuropsychologic assessment is a complex undertaking that requires knowledge, skill, and clinical sensitivity. The competent neuropsychologist considers the patient's performance in light of normative standards and interprets the pattern of test scores across a battery assessing multiple neurocognitive abilities to arrive at a unified conceptualization of the patient's strengths and weaknesses that is coherent with established brain-behavior relationships and consistent with the patient's history.

Pharmacologic and Psychologic Management of Neurocognitive Sequelae

Most patients with brain tumors succumb to neurocognitive, emotional, and behavioral impairments that compromise their ability to independently carry out routine activities of daily living. Return to full-time or part-time work after diagnosis and treatment for a brain tumor is the exception, not the rule. However, promising advances in neurocognitive rehabilitation for neurologically impaired individuals and our growing knowledge regarding the benefits of pharmacologic agents could reduce the morbidity associated with this disease and its treatment. It is likely that brain tumor patients represent a "niche" rehabilitation population, as the types of problems they experience and the progressive nature of their disease are different from those of traditional rehabilitation patients (e.g., those with stroke or traumatic brain injury). Nevertheless, rehabilitation-related disciplines have contributed a wealth of knowledge about effective behavioral practices and psychopharmacologic interventions for other neurologically compromised patients, and the success of these practices and interventions in brain tumor patients warrants investigation (Brain Tumor Progress Review Group, 2000). Moreover, brain tumor patients often experience patterns of impairment that follow a somewhat predictable course based on the tumor characteristics (e.g., lesion location, volume, and momentum) and the treatment plan (e.g., surgery followed by adjuvant therapy, which may include chemotherapy, radiotherapy, or both). The possibility of intervening *before* the emergence of neurocognitive disabilities offers exciting potential for prophylactic behavioral rehabilitation and pharmacologic strategies. The goal of such interventions would be to protect the brain from further neurocognitive compromise associated with disease progression and cancer treatment or to implement compensatory strategies designed to circumvent problems before they progress to life-limiting disabilities.

Pharmacologic Interventions

As has already been stated, frontal lobe dysfunction is a common problem in brain tumor patients as an adverse effect of both the tumor and the treatment. The hallmarks of frontal lobe dysfunction, including neurobehavioral slowing and impairments in attention and working memory, are likely due to disruption of the monoamine pathways of the frontal brainstem reticular system. Attention and working memory are also modulated by catecholamines. Consequently, the benefit of stimulant therapy, specifically methylphenidate, for reducing frontally mediated neurocognitive dysfunction and fatigue has been investigated as a possible treatment in neuro-oncology settings. Methylphenidate hydrochloride is a mixed dopaminergic-noradrenergic agonist and is pharmacologically similar to amphetamines. A phase I trial using a single treatment group and a dose-escalating design demonstrated that treatment with this drug was associated with significant improvements in psychomotor speed, memory, visuomotor skill, executive functions, and manual dexterity in a group of 30 patients with malignant gliomas. Seventy-eight percent of the patients who received a 10-mg (twice daily) dose experienced subjective improvement in their ability to function (e.g., increased energy, improved concentration, brighter mood, and improved ambulation), and 100% of the patients who received a 30-mg (twice daily) dose experienced improvement (Meyers et al, 1998). Adverse effects such as irritability and "shakiness" were minimal and resolved immediately when the drug was discontinued. The results obtained could not simply be attributed to improved mood and were particularly powerful in light of evidence of tumor progression or progressive radiation injury in half of the study participants.

The novel vigilance-promoting agent modafinil is commonly used to treat excessive daytime somnolence associated with narcolepsy and idiopathic hypersomnia. Its effectiveness in alleviating fatigue in patients with brain tumors was recently examined in a pilot study of 15 subjects. Roughly two thirds of the patients reported moderate to significant improvement in cancer-related fatigue after 10 weeks of treatment with modafinil (200 mg daily, increased to 300 mg after 4 weeks in nonresponders) (Nasir, 2003). Adverse effects such as anxiety and dizziness were mild except in 1 patient, who required discontinuation of medication secondary to encephalopathy. Further study of modafinil for managing symptoms of brain cancer is clearly warranted.

Pharmacotherapies used to treat Alzheimer's disease have also been examined for their possible benefit in patients with brain tumors. Donepezil, an acetylcholinesterase inhibitor commonly used to treat Alzheimer's disease-related dementia, was recently examined in a phase II trial. Rapp and colleagues (2004) reported improvements in neurocognitive function (e.g., attention, memory, and verbal fluency) and QOL after 6 months of treatment with donepezil (5 to 10 mg daily) in a group of long-term survivors of partial or whole-brain radiotherapy. Further investigation into donepezil and other agents used to treat dementia (e.g., memantine) is on the horizon.

Temporal lobe radionecrosis is an unfortunate but common side effect of unilateral or bilateral temporal lobe radiotherapy and is characterized most significantly by memory impairment. Vitamin E has been demonstrated in studies of nonhumans to inhibit lipid peroxidation, reduce cell death in hypoxic neurons, and decrease the degeneration of hippocampal cells after ischemia (Yoshida et al, 1985; Hara et al, 1990). A recent study by Chan and colleagues (2003) examined the effect of megadose vitamin E (1,000 IU twice daily) in a group of patients with nasopharyngeal carcinomas who had undergone standard treatment with unilateral or bilateral temporal lobe radiotherapy. Using an open-label, nonrandomized, treatment-versus-control design, the researchers demonstrated improved memory and executive functions in patients with temporal lobe radionecrosis after 1 year of dietary supplementation with vitamin E.

Neurocognitive Rehabilitation Strategies

Inpatient and outpatient rehabilitation has the potential to decrease the morbidity associated with brain tumors and their treatment by limiting the effect of symptoms on QOL. At present, there is no established model for inpatient or outpatient rehabilitation of brain tumor patients. Moreover, clinical practice patterns reveal a general lack of physician knowledge about the benefits of rehabilitative services for this population. Nevertheless, some data regarding the effectiveness of rehabilitation programs designed primarily for survivors of stroke or traumatic brain injury have emerged for brain tumor patients. Such studies have generally revealed that persons with brain tumors who participate in a comprehensive, interdisciplinary inpatient rehabilitation program achieve significant gains in functional status. (Interdisciplinary rehabilitation programs often involve a combination of specialty care providers, including physicians, psychologists, neuropsychologists, social workers, physical therapists, occupational therapists, and speech and language therapists.) Furthermore, brain tumor patients who participate in a postacute, outpatient, comprehensive, interdisciplinary treatment program demonstrate increased independence and productivity, and these gains are maintained after discharge. In addition, brain tumor patients make gains in functional status that are comparable to gains made by other rehabilitation populations (e.g., patients with stroke or traumatic brain injury) often despite a shorter length of stay, thereby lowering the overall cost of care. Finally, after discharge from an inpatient or outpatient rehabilitation program, brain tumor patients enjoy improved QOL, even in the face of a disease that is often progressive.

For patients for whom comprehensive rehabilitation programs are not necessary or feasible, goal-focused compensatory interventions and behavioral strategies are often quite helpful. While there are numerous anecdotal reports of individualized rehabilitation approaches being useful for these patients, there is a dearth of evidence from prospective, randomized, controlled experimental trials. Individualized, targeted interventions involve making accommodations to the patient's primary environment, changing a daily routine, or teaching new skills. The goals of such strategies may include maximizing the patient's function, improving the level of independence, and compensating for neurocognitive inefficiencies. For example, external memory aids such as memory notebooks, medication reminder systems, personal digital assistants, and even user-programmable paging systems have all been used to help neurologically impaired patients compensate for forgetfulness. Systematic, explicit instruction improves a patient's success in using these types of external aids. In lower-functioning patients who may be confused or disoriented, environmental modifications that serve to increase structure, reduce distraction, and decrease demands for decision making can be quite comforting.

Fatigue Management and Other Behavioral Strategies

The National Comprehensive Cancer Network defines cancer-related fatigue as "a distressing, persistent, subjective sense of tiredness or exhaustion related to cancer or cancer treatment that is not proportional to recent activity and interferes with usual functioning" (National Comprehensive Cancer Network, 2006, p. FT-1). Cella and colleagues (1998) emphasized the persistent and interfering quality of this fatigue, highlighting the sufferer's sense of exhaustion, which is not relieved by rest. It is well accepted that physical, psychologic, and medical factors such as anemia, cachexia, systemic illness, pain, and medication use can contribute to fatigue. There is sufficient evidence to support the correction of anemia and the use of aerobic exercise programs to manage fatigue. As an example of an adaptive coping strategy to manage fatigue, Lovely (2004) recommends developing an "energy conservation plan" (p. 280). The plan involves taking an inventory of energy levels throughout the day and then scheduling important activities at times when energy levels are highest, resting when energy levels are lowest, and determining which tasks can be deleted or delegated to other people. The plan also stresses a good night's sleep. Another behavioral strategy is to instruct patients in progressive muscle relaxation to decrease the physiologic and psychologic tension associated with affective distress. Further research is needed to determine the efficacy of psychostimulants, psychosocial intervention to decrease affective distress, sleep intervention, and energy conservation to combat cancer-related fatigue.

PAIN MANAGEMENT

Assessment of Pain

Pain is a common complaint of patients who have brain tumors. More than 70% of patients with advanced cancers rate pain as moderate to severe. Many pain clinics use a questionnaire to aid in and standardize

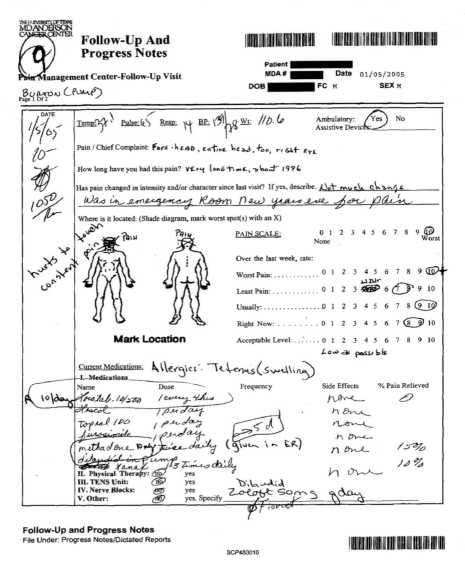

Figure 16–1. The modified BPI used by the M. D. Anderson Pain Clinic for follow-up assessment of pain in patients with brain tumors.

assessment. The Wisconsin Brief Pain Inventory (BPI) is a well accepted and standard tool for assessing cancer pain. At M. D. Anderson Cancer Center, an institutionally approved 2-page questionnaire (a modified BPI) is used for the initial and follow-up assessments of patients (Figure 16–1). This modified BPI is a 15-minute questionnaire that can be self-administered.

THE UNIVERSITY OF TEXAS
MD ANDERSON
CANCER CENTER

**Follow-Up And
Progress Notes**

Pain Management Center-Follow-up Visit

Page 2 Of 2

Patient	
MDA #	**Date** 01/05/2005
DOB	**FC** M **SEX** M

DATE	

Other Symptoms:

Bowel Patterns: Usual Frequency: _2-3 days_   Consistency: _med_

Last B M: _2 days ago_   Bowel Regimen: ✓ No _____ Yes

Sexual Disfunction: No _____   Yes ✓

Other Symptoms:

	NONE (Best)										Worst
Fatigue	0	1	2	3	4	5	⑥	7	8	9	10
Nausea	⓪	1	2	3	4	5	6	7	8	9	10
Depression	0	1	2	3	4	5	6	⑦	8	9	10
Anxiety	0	1	2	3	4	5	6	7	⑧	9	10
Drowsiness	0	1	2	3	4	⑤	6	7	8	9	10
Difficulty Thinking Clearly	0	1	2	3	4	⑤	6	7	8	9	10
Shortness of Breathe	0	1	2	3	4	5	6	7	⑧	9	10
Poor Appetite	0	1	2	3	4	⑤	6	7	8	9	10
Insomnia	0	1	2	3	4	5	⑥	7	8	9	10
Feeling of Well-Being	0	1	2	3	4	5	6	7	⑧	9	10

Anything Else We Can Help You With Today?

Needs refill on Zoloft & Lortab

IT pump refill done in clinic

Plan Of Care:

Teaching: see ITPR _____→ see IPOCTR

Treatment Plan of Care: see IPTP _____

Other: _RTC- 6/6/05 for IT pump refill_

Signature: _Mel Mayer RN_ ,R.N.

Follow-Up and Progress Notes
File Under: Progress Notes/Dictated Reports

SCP483010

Figure 16–1.   *(continued)*

It includes several questions about the characteristics of the pain, including its origin and the effect of prior treatments, and it incorporates 2 valuable features of the McGill Pain Questionnaire: a graphic representation of the location of pain, and groups of qualitative descriptors. The severity of pain is assessed by a series of visual analog scales that allow the patient to indicate the worst, least, and usual pain levels. The perceived level of

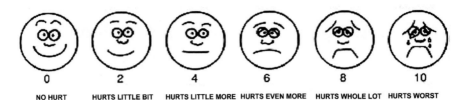

0	2	4	6	8	10
NO HURT	HURTS LITTLE BIT	HURTS LITTLE MORE	HURTS EVEN MORE	HURTS WHOLE LOT	HURTS WORST

Brief word instructions: Point to each face using the words to describe the pain intensity. Ask the child to choose face the best describes own pain and record the appropriate number.

Original instructions: Explain to the person that each face is for a person who feels happy because he has no pain (hurt) or sad because he has some or a lot of pain. **Face 0** is very happy because he doesn't hurt at all. **Face 2** hurts just a little bit. **Face 4** hurts a little more. **Face 6** hurts even more. **Face 8** hurts a whole lot. **Face 10** hurts as much as you can imagine, although you don't have to be crying to feel this bad. Ask the person to choose the face that best describes how he is feeling.

Figure 16–2. The Wong–Baker FACES pain rating scale. This scale can be used with young children (sometimes as young as 3 years of age). It also works well for many older children and adults as well as for those who speak a different language. From Hockenberry MJ, Wilson D, Winkelstein ML: *Wong's Essentials of Pediatric Nursing,* ed. 7, St. Louis, 2005, p. 1259. Used with permission, Copyright, Mosby.

interference with normal function is also quantified with visual analog scales. Preliminary evidence suggests that the modified BPI is cross-culturally valid and is useful, particularly when patients are not fit to complete a more thorough or comprehensive questionnaire.

At M. D. Anderson, pediatric cancer pain assessment includes the use of Beyer's "The Oucher," Eland's color scale body outline, Hester's poker chip tool, the Wong–Baker FACES pain rating scale (Figure 16–2), and other tools.

Pain evaluation should be integrated with a detailed oncologic, medical, and psychologic assessment. The initial evaluation should include evaluation of the patient's feelings and attitudes about the pain and disease, family concerns, and the premorbid psychologic history. A comprehensive but objective approach to assessment instills confidence in the patients and family, which will be valuable throughout treatment. The comprehensive evaluation of patients with cancer pain involves 7 aspects, as described below.

Chief Complaint

The chief complaint is obtained to ensure appropriate triage. For example, a patient with severe pain and bowel obstruction may need to be sent to the emergency center for urgent treatment.

Oncologic History

The oncologic history is then obtained to gain the context of the pain problem. This history includes the diagnosis and stage of the disease, the therapy and outcome (including side effects), and the patient's understanding of the disease process and prognosis.

Pain History

For each new pain site, the pain history should include premorbid chronic pain; onset and evolution; site and radiation; pattern (constant, intermittent, or unpredictable); worst, least, usual, and current intensity (on scales from 0 to 10); quality; exacerbating and relieving factors; interference with usual activities; neurologic and motor abnormalities, including bowel and bladder continence; and vasomotor changes. Current and past analgesic use, its efficacy, and its side effects should be cataloged. Prior treatments for pain such as radiotherapy, nerve block, and physiotherapy should be noted.

Review of Medical Record and Radiologic Studies

Many specific cancers cause well-established pain patterns. For example, brain tumors can cause headache, facial pain, or other cranial and neck pain syndromes. Many of the treatments for cancer can cause pain themselves. For example, chemotherapy and radiotherapy can induce neuropathies.

Psychologic and Social History

The psychologic and social history should include marital and residential status, employment history and status, educational background, functional status, activities of daily living, recreational activities, support systems, the health and capabilities of the spouse or significant other, and the history of or current drug or alcohol abuse.

Medical History

A medical history independent of oncologic history is obtained to assess coexisting systemic disease, exercise intolerance, allergies to medications, medication use, and prior illness and surgery. The medical history also provides a thorough review of the systems: general (anorexia, weight loss, cachexia, fatigue, weakness, insomnia, etc.), neurologic (pre-existing cognitive deficit, sedation, confusion, hallucination, headache, motor weakness, altered sensation, incontinence, etc.), respiratory (dyspnea, cough, pneumonia, etc.), gastrointestinal (dysphagia, nausea, vomiting, dehydration, constipation, diarrhea, etc.), psychologic (irritability, anxiety, depression, dementia, suicidal ideation, etc.), and genitourinary (urgency, hesitancy, hematuria, etc.).

Physical Examination

The physical examination must be thorough, although at times it is appropriate to perform a focused examination. For patients with brain tumors, a complete neurologic exam is mandatory.

Cancer Pain Management

The basic tenets of cancer pain control include taking the context of the disease into account. For example, a patient with residual chronic headache and cognitive dysfunction after surgical resection and radiotherapy will be managed in a similar fashion as a patient with chronic headache, whereas a patient with a progressive tumor should be treated with analgesics (in addition to treatments directed at the tumor such as radiotherapy and steroids) in accord with the World Health Organization's pain relief ladder for cancer pain management. When a comprehensive trial of pharmacologic therapy fails to provide adequate analgesia or leads to unacceptable side effects, alternative modalities should be considered, although for most CNS tumors, effective control is attainable through pharmacologic manipulation. These other modalities include parenteral opioid infusions, neuraxial medication infusion, neurolytic blockade, and other procedures such as vertebroplasty when appropriate. If one applies the World Health Organization ladder approach to cancer pain management, interventional therapies may be considered the fourth step (Figure 16–3).

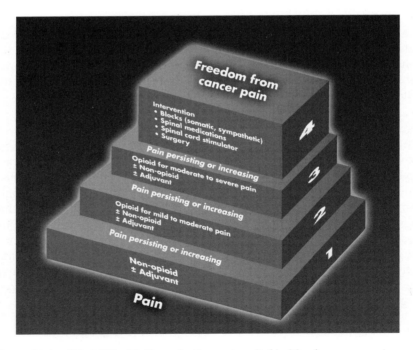

Figure 16–3. World Health Organization pain relief ladder for cancer pain management modified to include a fourth step for interventional pain management modalities. Adapted with permission from World Health Organization.

Continuous Subcutaneous Infusion of Opioids

Continuous subcutaneous infusion (CSCI) of opioids is an excellent option for patients whose medical condition precludes the use of the oral route or whose pain is poorly controlled despite large doses of oral opioids. Starting doses are calculated using a conversion table in which the 24-hour dose requirement of intravenous morphine is divided by 24, which provides the hourly rate. Tissue irritation is minimized when volumes less than 1 to 2 mL per hour are prescribed (which can be achieved by concentrating the mixture). A 27-gauge butterfly needle is inserted subcutaneously anywhere, but preferred sites include the subclavian fossa and the chest wall to allow for ease of ambulation. Absorption of subcutaneously administered opioids is rapid, and steady-state plasma levels are generally approached within 1 hour. Morphine and hydromorphone are the most commonly used opioids for CSCI, although most parenteral opioids are suitable.

Continuous Intravenous Infusion of Opioids

Continuous intravenous infusion of opioids is indicated for patients who cannot tolerate the oral route because of gastrointestinal obstruction, malabsorption, opioid-induced vomiting, dysphagia, or the requirement of large numbers of pills. It is also indicated for patients who have a prominent bolus effect with intermittent injection, when rapid titration may be needed, or when bolus injections that exceed nursing capabilities are required. This type of infusion is very similar to CSCI, although CSCI is preferred in the home care setting unless a permanent vascular access device is already in place. Patient-controlled analgesia is a similar version and an excellent option, but its use is reserved for patients who can understand and use this modification correctly. The dose should be adjusted upward until pain relief is adequate or side effects become intolerable.

Intraspinal Analgesia

Neuraxial analgesia is achieved by the epidural, intrathecal, or intraventricular administration of opioids alone or with other agents. This modality is useful for patients who have intolerable opioid-related side effects or who have unrelieved pain despite escalating doses of opioids and adjuvants. The principle of neuraxial opioid therapy is that introducing minute quantities of opioids close to their receptors (i.e., in the substantia gelatinosa of the spinal cord) achieves a high local concentration. With this therapy, analgesia may be superior to that achieved with opioids administered by other routes, and because the absolute amount of drug administered is reduced, side effects should be minimized. Local anesthetics and other analgesic medications can enhance the analgesic effect of opioids, although the success in treating headache and craniofacial pain is anecdotal.

The most important aspects of intraspinal analgesia are its reversibility and the reliability and simplicity of screening measures to confirm its efficacy. Screening can generally be accomplished on an outpatient basis by observing the patient's response to a morphine infusion via a temporary percutaneous epidural catheter or to a single intrathecal injection. If the improved pain control and the reduced side effects are sufficient to warrant more prolonged therapy, a temporary catheter for delivering the medication may be used for days to weeks and then a catheter and pump may be permanently implanted.

Neuraxial analgesia is suitable for patients with any stage of cancer, including cured patients. This technique is contraindicated in patients with infections or coagulopathy.

Nerve Blocks

Many cancer patients in search of a "nerve block" to alleviate their pain are referred to pain specialists. Some focal syndromes are amenable to these procedures, but many are not. Neoplastic head and neck pain is extremely difficult to control because of the rich sensory innervations of the involved structures. For selected patients, blockade of the involved cranial or upper cervical nerves can be very helpful. Blockade of the trigeminal nerve within the foramen ovale at the base of skull or its branches may reduce facial pain. However, most facial cancer pain lies outside of the distribution of a single nerve and thus is not amenable to neural blockade.

Vertebroplasty

Many cancer patients with metastatic or osteoporotic vertebral compression fractures present with movement-related back pain. Percutaneous vertebroplasty is a minimally invasive procedure that involves injecting an opacified bone cement (usually polymethyl methacrylate) into the fractured vertebral body to alleviate the pain and perhaps enhance its structural stability. Percutaneous vertebroplasty is highly efficacious in treating vertebral compression fracture-related pain in cancer patients, and it has a low complication rate.

Neuromodulation

Spinal cord stimulation is a nonpharmacologic method used to treat refractory chronic neuropathic pain. At M. D. Anderson, spinal cord stimulation has been successfully used to treat chemotherapy-induced neuropathic pain.

Neurosurgery

Neurosurgical techniques such as tumor resection, stereotactic radiosurgery, and cerebrospinal fluid shunting reduce intracranial pressure and may palliate symptoms. Reversible, titratable, lower-risk techniques have largely replaced the older, neurosurgical, destructive palliative techniques. The latter techniques, which include pituitary ablation, myelotomy, and cordotomy, should be used in patients for whom more conservative pharmacologic and interventional approaches have failed.

KEY PRACTICE POINTS

- The principles of symptom control in patients with CNS tumors are in most respects similar to those that apply to good medical practice. Patients should be carefully examined and their neurocognitive status and painful syndromes carefully assessed.

- Although rarely eliminated altogether, symptoms (including pain) can be controlled in the vast majority of patients, usually with careful diagnostic acumen and application of straightforward pharmacologic and other measures. For patients whose pain is not readily controlled with noninvasive analgesics, carefully selected alternative measures are also associated with a high degree of success.

- Comprehensive cancer care is best regarded as a continuum that commences with prevention and early detection, focuses intensely on curative therapy, and ideally is rendered complete by a seamless transition to palliation and attention to QOL.

- The future of cancer pain relief is bright. Much mechanistic research is looking into different groups of specifically targeted medications, including tumor necrosis factor α receptor antagonists, osteoclast inhibitors, inhibitors of glutamate release, substance P inhibitors, and nitric oxide synthetase inhibitors.

SUGGESTED READINGS

Anderson SW, Damasio H, Tranel D. Neuropsychological impairments associated with lesions caused by tumor or stroke. *Arch Neurol* 1990;47:397–405.

Brain Tumor Progress Review Group. *Report of the Brain Tumor Progress Review Group*. NIH Publication No. 01–4902. National Cancer Institute and National Institute of Neurological Disorders and Stroke; 2000. Available at: http://planning.cancer.gov/pdfprgreports/2000braintumor.pdf.

Burton AW, Rajagopal A, Shah HN, et al. Epidural and intrathecal analgesia is effective in treating refractory cancer pain. *Pain Med* 2004;5:239–247.

Cella D, Peterman A, Passik S, Jacobsen P, Breitbart W. Progress toward guidelines for the management of fatigue. [Review] *Oncology (Huntingt)* 1998;12:369–377.

Chan AS, Cheung M, Law SC, Chan JH. Phase II study of alpha-tocopherol in improving the cognitive function of patients with temporal lobe radionecrosis. *Cancer* 2003;100:398–404.

Cicerone KD, Dahlberg C, Kalmar K, et al. Evidence-based cognitive rehabilitation: recommendations for clinical practice. *Arch Phys Med Rehab* 2000;81: 1596–1615.

Clohisy DR, Mantyh PW. Bone cancer pain. *Cancer* 2003;97:866S–873S.

Crossen JR, Garwood D, Glatstein E, Neuwalt EA. Neurobehavioral sequelae of cranial irradiation in adults: a review of radiation-induced encephalopathy. *J Clin Oncol* 1994;12:627–642.

Fourney DR, Schomer DF, Nader R, et al. Percutaneous vertebroplasty and kyphoplasty for painful vertebral body fractures in cancer patients. *J Neurosurg* 2003;98:21–30.

Gregor A, Cull A, Traynor E, Stewart M, Lander F, Love S. Neuropsychometric evaluation of long-term survivors of adult brain tumours: relationship with tumour and treatment parameters. *Radiother Oncol* 1996;41:55–59.

Hara H, Kato H, Kogure K. Protective effect of α-tocopherol on ischemic neuronal damage in the gerbil hippocampus. *Brain Res* 1990;510:335–338.

Huang ME, Cifu DX, Keyser-Marcus L. Functional outcome after brain tumor and acute stroke: a comparative analysis. *Arch Phys Med Rehab* 1998;79:1386–1390.

Huang ME, Wartella JE, Kreutzer JS. Functional outcomes and quality of life in patients with brain tumors: a preliminary report. *Arch Phys Med Rehab* 2001;82: 1540–1546.

Lezak MD, Howieson DB, Loring DW. *Neuropsychological Assessment.* New York, NY: Oxford University Press, 2004.

Litofsky NS, Farace E, Anderson F, et al. Depression in patients with high-grade glioma: results of the Glioma Outcomes Project. *Neurosurgery* 2004;54:358–367.

Lovely MP. Symptom management of brain tumor patients. *Semin Oncol Nurs* 2004;20:273–283.

Meyers CA. Issues of quality of life in neuro-oncology. In: Vecht CJ, ed. *Handbook of Clinical Neurology, Neuro-Oncology, Part I. Brain Tumors: Principles of Biology, Diagnosis and Therapy.* Vol. 23. Amsterdam, The Netherlands: Elsevier Science BV; 1997:389–409.

Meyers CA. Neuropsychological deficits in brain tumor patients: effects of location, chronicity, and treatment. *Cancer Bull* 1986;38:30–32.

Meyers CA, Abbruzzese JL. Cognitive functioning in cancer patients: effect of previous treatment. *Neurology* 1992;42:434–436.

Meyers CA, Hess KR, Yunk WKA, Levin VA. Cognitive function as a predictor of survival in patients with recurrent malignant glioma. *J Clin Oncol* 2000;18: 646–650.

Meyers CA, Kudelka AP, Conrad CA, Gelke CK, Grove W, Pazdur R. Neurotoxicity of CI-980, a novel mitotic inhibitor. *Clin Cancer Res* 1997;3: 419–422.

Meyers CA, Wefel JS. The use of the Mini-Mental State Examination to assess cognitive functioning in cancer trials: no ifs, ands, buts, or sensitivity. *J Clin Oncol* 2003;21:3557–3558.

Meyers CA, Weitzner MA, Valentine AD, Levin VA. Methylphenidate therapy improves cognition, mood, and function of brain tumor patients. *J Clin Oncol* 1998;16:2522–2527.

Nasir S. Modafinil improves fatigue in primary brain tumor patients. [Abstract] *Neuro-oncol* 2003;5:335.

National Comprehensive Cancer Network. *Cancer-Related Fatigue.* NCCN Practice Guidelines in Oncology version 1.2006. National Comprehensive

Cancer Network; 2006. Available at: http://www.nccn.org/professionals/physician_gls/PDF/fatigue.pdf.

O'Dell MW, Barr K, Spanier D, Warnick RE. Functional outcome of inpatient rehabilitation in persons with brain tumors. *Arch Phys Med Rehab* 1998;79: 1530–1534.

Rapp SR, Rosdhal R, D'Agostino RB, et al. Improving cognitive function in brain irradiated patients: a phase II trial of an acetylcholinesterase inhibitor (donepezil). [Abstract] *Neuro-oncol* 2004;6:357.

Scheibel RS, Meyers CA, Levin VA. Cognitive dysfunction following surgery for intracerebral glioma: influence of histopathology, lesion location, and treatment. *J Neurooncol* 1996;30:61–69.

Sherer M, Meyers CA, Bergloff P. Efficacy of postacute brain injury rehabilitation for patients with primary malignant brain tumors. *Cancer* 1997;80:250–257.

Sherman AM, Jaeckle K, Meyers CA. Pretreatment cognitive performance predicts survival in patients with leptomeningeal disease. *Cancer* 2002;15:1311–1316.

Taphoorn MJ, Klein M. Cognitive deficits in adult patients with brain tumours. [Review] *Lancet Neurol* 2004;3:159–168.

Tucha O, Smely C, Preier M, Lange KW. Cognitive deficits before treatment among patients with brain tumors. *Neurosurgery* 2000;47:324–333.

Wefel JS, Kayl AE, Meyers CA. Neuropsychological dysfunction associated with cancer and cancer therapies: a conceptual review of an emerging target. *Br J Cancer* 2004;90:1691–1696.

Weitzner MA, Meyers CA, Gelke CK, Byrne KS, Cella DF, Levin VA. The Functional Assessment of Cancer Therapy (FACT) scale. Development of a brain subscale and revalidation of the general version (FACT-G) in patients with primary brain tumors. *Cancer* 1995;75:1151–1161.

Yoshida S, Busto R, Watson BD, Santiso M, Ginsberg MD. Postischemic cerebral lipid peroxidation in vitro: modification by dietary vitamin E. *J Neurochem* 1985;44:1593–1601.

INDEX

A

Abdominal striae, 195
ACNU, *See* Nimustine
ACTIVATE trial, 185–186
Adamantinomatous
    craniopharyngiomas, 78, 80
Addisonian crisis, 194
Adenocarcinomas, 233, 234, 246, 287
Adenovirus infection, 306
Adrenocorticotropic hormone
    (ACTH), 148, 193–194,
    197–199, 207–208, 221
Adrenocorticotropic hormone-
    secreting adenomas, 195,
    206–209, 211f, 214
AEE788 compound, use in treating
    gliomas, 176–177
Aneurysmal bone cysts, 278–279
Angiitis, 303t, 325t
Angiography, 87, 277, 279, 288, 304
    catheter, 50
    cerebral, 50
    CT, 38–40
    MRI, 42
    spinal, 277
Antibody-guided therapy, 184–185
Anti-CD68 antibody, 33
Anti-HAM56 antibody, 33
Antihistamines, as cause of
    meningiomas, 14, 20
Anti-phosphohistone H3 (pHH3)
    antibody, 29, 29f
Antiphospholipid antibody
    syndrome, 303t
Antiprogesterone agents, 57
Ara-C, *See* Cytarabine

Arachnoiditis, 81, 257
Ashkenazi Jews, incidence of
    breast cancer brain metastases
    in, 235
Astrocytomas, 97f, 143, 145–146,
    307, 309, 311
    anaplastic, 45f, 163–165, 173
    pilocytic, 7t, 32, 94, 109–116,
    109–111f, 145, 307
    pilomyxoid, 30
Astroglial variants of gliomas
    clinical features, 109–110
    histopathologic characteristics,
    112–113
    neuroimaging features, 111–112
    therapeutic options, 114–116

B

B-cell antigens, 265
BCNU, *See* Carmustine
Beevor's sign, 275
Behçet' syndrome, 303t, 325t
Bevacizumab, use in treating
    glioblastomas, 163
Biopsy tissue, handling of
    cytologic specimens, 26–27
    formalin-fixed, paraffin-
    embedded tissue sections, 28
    frozen tissue sections, 27
    tissue for ultrastructural
    examination, 28
Blood-brain barrier, 41–42, 155–156,
    181, 199, 237, 247, 267
Blood transfusion, during
    surgery, 288
Bracing, of spine after surgery, 292

Bragg peak, 141
BRCA gene, 235
Broca's motor speech area, 128
Bromocriptine, 202, 204, 210, 212
Brown-Séquard syndrome, 275, 318
Busulfan, use in treating PCNSL, 269–270

C
Cabergoline, 202, 204, 212
Capecitabine, 163, 174
Carbamazepine, 156, 335
Carboplatin, 161–163, 165, 174, 233
Carcinoembryonic antigen, 253, 300t
Carmustine (BCNU), 142, 160–164, 173, 179, *See also* Gliadel wafers
Cauda equina lesions, 305, 324
 causes of, 325–326t
 diagnostic tests for, 325–326t
Cauda equina syndrome, 275
CCNU, *See* Lomustine
CDKN2 tumor suppressor gene, 56, 172
Cell saving, during surgery, 288
Cellular immunotherapy, 182–184
Cellular telephone use, and brain tumors, 16–17
Central Brain Tumor Registry of the United States (CBTRUS), 3–6
Central nervous system (CNS) neoplasms, *See* Intradural spinal tumors
Central neurocytomas, 30, 32
c-erb oncogene, 56–57
Cerebrospinal fluid (CSF) analysis, 250, 252–253
Cervical spondylarthropathy, 298
Chemotherapy, 106–108, 116, 125, 132, 144, 156, 214, 217, 281, 292
 adjuvant, 66, 107, 292, 334–335

for anaplastic astrocytomas, 163–166, 173
for anaplastic oligodendrogliomas, 165–166
for astroglial variants, 116
for glioblastomas, 159–163
for high-grade gliomas, 173–174
with immunotherapy, 186
intrathecal (IT), 255–257, 270
for low-grade gliomas, 106–108, 108t, 166–167
methotrexate-based, 267–268, 303t
for neoplastic meningitis, 257
for oligodendrogliomas, 30, 99
for PNETs, 143–144
for SLCL metastases, 233
Choline-to-creatine ratio, 45–46, 45–46f
Chondrosarcomas, 282–284, 283f
Chordoid gliomas, 30, 32
Chordomas, 12, 281–282
Choroid plexus papillomas
 clinical presentation, 84–85
 diagnostic imaging, 85, 85f
 epidemiology, 84
 etiology, 84
 management, 86
Churg-Strauss syndrome, 303t
Cisplatin, 116, 160, 162, 164, 233
Clinically nonfunctional adenomas, 193–194, 196, 199, 210–212, 214
Collimators, 136–139, 137f, 139f
Computed tomography (CT)
 angiography and venography, 38–40, 39–40f
 of astroglial variants, 111–112
 CT-guided needle biopsy, 276
 as diagnostic tool, 279–280, 300t, 304–305, 325t
 of epidermoid and dermoid cysts, 83
 of hemangioblastomas, 87
 information bias of, 155

of low-grade gliomas, 96, 100
for lung cancer, 232
of meningiomas, 59, 64
of metastatic brain
    tumors, 227
of PCNSL, 264
perfusion, 40–41, 41f
of schwannomas, 68–71
of spinal tumors, 276–278
vs MRI, 96, 251–252
Conus medullaris syndrome, 275
Corticotropin, *See*
    Adrenocorticotropic hormone
Cranial nerve dysfunctions, 73–77,
    213
Craniopharyngiomas, 218–219
clinical presentation of, 78
cystic, 80
diagnostic imaging of, 79, 79f
epidemiology of, 77
etiology of, 77–78
management of, 80–81
pathology of, 80
squamous-papillary, 80
Cranioplasty, 63
Crohn's disease, 304
Cryptococcosis, 302t
Cryptococcus, as cause of
    myelopathy, 306
CTP-11, *See* Irinotecan
Cushing's disease, 193, 195,
    198–199, 207–209, 221
Cyclophosphamide, use in treating
    PCNSL, 266, 269–270
Cyclophosphamide, doxorubicin,
    vincristine, and
    dexamethasone (CHOD), 267
Cytarabine (Ara-C), 255–257, 267,
    269–270
Cytochrome p450, 13t, 156
Cytochrome p450 (*CYP2D6*) gene,
    15
Cytologic techniques,
    intraoperative, 27t
Cytomegalovirus, 303t, 306, 326

D
Dacarbazine, use in treating
    meningiomas, 66
Deep vein thrombosis prophylaxis
    and anticoagulation, use of
    after sugery, 292
DepoCyt, *See* Cytarabine
Dermoid cysts, *See* Epidermoid
    and dermoid cysts
Diabetes insipidus, 78, 80–81, 195,
    198, 215, 249t
Diabetes mellitus, 125, 195,
    198, 206
Diagnosis, of CNS tumors
errors in, 31–33, 32t
tools for, 6, 26, 38–50, 59–61,
    68–70, 79, 85, 87, 250–253
Diaziquone, use in treating
    neoplastic meningitis, 256
Diffuse low-grade gliomas, 33, 116
clinical features, 95
histopathologic characteristics,
    96–98
molecular profiles, 98–99
neuroimaging features, 96
prognostic factors, 99–100
therapeutic options, 100–108
Diplopia, 59, 74, 77, 196–197, 215,
    247, 304
Distal sacral tumors, 291
Diuretics, effect on cancer
    incidence, 14, 20
Doxorubicin, 66, 266–267
Dysembryoplastic neuroepithelial
    tumors, 30, 32

E
Eastern Cooperative Oncology
    Group (ECOG), 142, 160, 165
EGFRvIII antigen, 174, 176, 182,
    185–186
Electromagnetic fields, effect on
    cancer incidence, 13t, 16
Electrophysiologic monitoring, use
    during surgery, 288

Embolization, 50, 87, 277–279,
    281–282, 287–288
Encephalopathy, 258, 269, 334, 339
Endocrinopathy, 78–81, 148
Endoscopy, use in resecting
    pituitary tumors, 200
Ependymomas, 11, 247, 304, 307,
    309, 311–313, 315
Epidemiology, of brain tumors
  age differences, 4–7f, 6–8, 7t
  ethnicity, 8–9, 9f
  genetic susceptibility and
      familial aggregation, 12–15, 13t
  geographic variations, 8–10
  incidence rates, 3–6, 6–7f, 8–10, 9f
  infectious agents and
      immunologic response, 14t,
      20–21
  ionizing and non-ionizing
      radiation, 13t, 15–17
  lifestyle factors, 13t, 14, 18–19
  medical history and medication
      use, 14, 14t, 19–20
  mortality and survival rates,
      4–6, 4–6f, 158t
  occupational exposure, 13t,
      17–18
  sex differences, 8
Epidermal growth factor receptor
    (*EGFR*) allele, 10–11, 30–31
Epidermal growth factor receptor
    (HER2), 236–237
Epidermoid and dermoid cysts
  clinical presentation, 82
  diagnostic imaging, 83–84
  epidemiology, 81–82
  etiology and pathogenesis, 82
  management, 84
Epidural lipomatosis, 301t
Epstein-Barr virus, 264, 297,
    303t, 326
Erlotinib, use in treating GBM,
    163, 176
Etoposide, 160–161, 163–165, 233,
    269–270

European Organization for
    Research and Treatment of
    Cancer (EORTC), 99–100, 104,
    106–108, 108t, 161, 165, 173
Ewing's sarcomas, 282
Extradural spinal tumors
  adjuvant therapies for, 291–292
  bony spinal lesions, 277–284
  clinical presentation of, 275
  diagnostic tests for, 275–277
  indications for surgery, 287
  metastatic spinal lesions,
      284–287, 285–286f
  postoperative care for, 292
  surgical adjuncts for, 288
  surgical techniques for, 288–291
Extramedullary tumors
  clinical presentation, 318
  diagnostic imaging, 319
  incidence and etiology, 316–318
  surgical treatment, 319–324

F

Facetectomy, 319–321
Fertility, effect of excess hormone
    secretion on, 194–196, 199
α-Fetoprotein, as marker of
    neoplastic meningitis, 253
Fibrocartilaginous embolism, 301t
Fluoroscopy, during surgery, 288
Folinic acid, 256–257
Follicle-stimulating hormone
    (FSH), 193–194, 196, 210, 212
Foster–Kennedy syndrome, 59
Fried egg cytologic appearance, 97
Fungal infections, 302t, 305, 325t

G

Gadolinium enhancement, *See*
    Magnetic resonance imaging
Gangliogliomas, 11, 95,
    109–110, 113
Gefitinib, use in treating
    gliomas, 176
Germinomas, 144

Giant cell tumors, 280–281
Gliadel wafers, 161–162, 179, *See also* Carmustine
Glial fibrillary acidic protein (GFAP), 28, 97, 113
Glioblastoma multiforme (GBM), 48f, 123–124, 123–124t, 126f, 156–159, 172, 191, 252f, 332
  chemotherapy for, 159–163, 173
  immunotherapy for, 182, 184–185
  signal transduction inhibitors for, 175–177
Glioblastomas, 7t, 25, 31, 112–113, 124, 130f, 184, 332
  chemotherapy for, 108, 159–163, 160–161t, 163t
  epidemiology of, 4–7, 10
Gliomas, 10, 14, 20, 33, 129f, 304, *See also* Diffuse low-grade gliomas; High-grade gliomas; Low-grade gliomas
Glutathione transferase θ (*GSTT1*) gene, effect on tumor incidence, 15
Gonadotropin-secreting tumors, 195, 210, 212, 214
GP240 antigen, use in treating gliomas, 172
Growth hormone (GH), 148, 193, 195, 199, 214
Growth hormone-secreting adenomas, 204–207, 213–214, 219

H
Headache, 78, 87, 95, 147, 197, 215, 228, 236, 239, 247, 256, 331, 344–347
Hemangioblastomas, 32, 50, 307–309, 311, 313
  clinical presentation, 87
  diagnostic imaging, 87
  epidemiology and genetics, 86–87
  management, 87–89

Hemangiomas, 278
Hemorrhage, 38, 42, 59, 197, 230–231, 239–240, 278–279, 304, 308, 319
Hemostasis, during surgery, 129, 310, 313
Henoch-Schönlein purpura, 303t
Herpesvirus infection, as cause of brain tumors, 264, 300t, 302t, 305–306
High-grade gliomas
  chemotherapy for, 173–174
  classification and characteristics of, 121–122
  decision to resect, 122–125
  diagnostic imaging of, 178f
  drug delivery techniques for, 179
  immunotherapy for, 179–186, 180t, 183t
  signal transduction inhibitors for, 174–179
  survival after surgery, 124t
  surgical approaches for, 125–132
  targets of, 174
Histology, of brain tumors, *See* individual tumor types and WHO classification system
Histoplasmosis, 306
β-Human chorionic gonadotropin, as marker of neoplastic meningitis, 253
Human immunodeficiency virus infection, 306
Hydroxyurea, 66, 163–165, 176
Hypertension, 77, 125, 195, 206
Hyperthyroidism, 195, 209–210
Hypopituitarism, 147, 192, 203, 208–211, 215
Hypothyroidism, 78, 80, 210, 304
Hypoxia-inducible factor-1 (HIF-1), effect on brain tumor incidence, 86–87

I

Idiopathic transverse myelitis, 301t
Immunoglobulin, 180, 265, 281,
    303t, 305
Immunohistochemical markers, of
    brain tumors, 28–29
Insulin-like growth factor I (IGF-I),
    58, 195, 197, 204–206, 221
Interleukin, use in cancer therapy,
    179, 182, 184, 257
Intracranial germ cell tumors, 144
Intradural spinal tumors, *See also*
    Extramedullary tumors
    diagnostic imaging, 304–305
    diagnostic workup, 298–299,
        298–299f, 300–303t
    incidence and mortality
        rates, 3–5
    patient history and physical
        examination, 299–304
    serum and CSF tests, 305–306
    therapeutic interventions,
        306–307
Intramedullary tumors
    clinical presentation, 308
    diagnostic imaging, 308–309,
        312f
    incidence and etiology, 307–308
    surgical treatment, 309–316, 312f
Intraoperative fluoroscopy, 288,
    314f
Irinotecan (CPT-11), use in treating
    recurrent tumors, 162–163,
    165, 174

J

Janus kinase (Jak)/STAT pathway,
    174, 175f
Juvenile nasal angiofibromas, 50

K

Karnofsky performance scale
    (KPS), 123, 158, 158t, 185, 228,
    234, 240–241, 254, 258, 336
Ki-67 antigen, 29, 67

Kohlmeier-Degos syndrome, 303t
Kyphoplasty, 289–290

L

Laryngeal mask intubation, 127
Leptomeningeal disease, 236, 254,
    270, 318, 337
Leptomeninges, 54, 113, 246–247,
    255, 264, 270
Leukoencephalopathy, 147–148,
    257, 334
Lhermitte's sign, 147
Li-Fraumeni syndrome, 13t, 14
Lipomas, 308, 310
Lomustine (CCNU), 107, 116,
    162–163, 165, 173, 177, 214, 270
Loss of heterozygosity (LOH),
    10–12, 30, 56–57, 68, 94, 96f,
    98–101, 106–108, 156, 159,
    165–167, 172
Low-grade gliomas
    astroglial variants
        (circumscribed), 108–116
    chemotherapy for, 108t, 166–167
    classification and
        characterization of, 94, 94t
Luteinizing hormone (LH),
    193–194, 196–197, 210, 212
Lyme disease, 302t, 325t

M

Mafosfamide, use in treating
    neoplastic meningitis, 256
Magnetic resonance imaging (MRI)
    advantages of, 6, 41, 102, 102f,
        193, 198–199, 226, 251, 264,
        297, 305
    angiography and venography,
        42, 43f
    of astroglial variants, 111–112
    as diagnostic tool, 276–277, 300t,
        304, 325t
    fluid-attenuated inversion
        recovery (FLAIR), 41–42, 83,
        83f, 129f, 228

functional, 47, 49f
gadolinium enhancement, use
    of, 41–42, 47, 70, 96, 112, 177,
    178f, 199, 228, 239, 251–253f,
    264, 277, 308, 319
information bias of, 155
of low-grade gliomas, 95
maximum intensity projection
    and volume rendering, 42
of meningiomas, 59–61, 59–60f,
    64, 146
of PCNSL, 264
perfusion imaging, 47, 48f
of radiation necrosis, 149
relaxation time, 41
of schwannomas, 68–71
spectroscopy, 44–47, 44–46f
of spinal tumors, 276–277
of tumor vascular perfusion,
    177–178
T1-weighted images, 41–42,
    59–60, 87, 228, 309
T2-weighted images, 41–42,
    60–61, 228, 309
vs CT, 79, 251–252
Major histocompatibility complex
    (MHC), 180
Marimastat, 162, 176
McCune-Albright syndrome,
    220
McGill Pain Questionnaire, 343
Medulloblastomas, 7–8, 7t, 11,
    64f, 143–144
Meningiomas, 7t, 11, 16, 20, 25, 50,
    54, 146, 317, 319, 321
clinical presentation, 58–59
common sites and incidence in
    adults, 55, 55t
diagnostic imaging, 39–40f,
    59–61, 64, 146
epidemiology, 55
etiology, 55–58
management, 62–66
pathologic subtypes, 61–62
recurrence, 66–67

Meningitis, 82, 256, 302t, 305, 325t,
    See also Neoplastic meningitis
Meningomyelitides, 302t
MERLIN protein, 56, 68
Metaplastic theory, 78
Metastases to the brain, 144–145
from breast cancer, 235–238, 286
from lung cancer, 232–235
from malignant melanoma,
    238–240, 239f, 288
from renal cell carcinoma, 231,
    287–288
from thyroid carcinoma, 288
Metastases to the spine, 145, 253f
Methotrexate (MTX), 148, 255–257,
    267–271, 303t
Methyl methacrylate injections,
    285f, 289
MGMT, *See* O^6-methylguanine-
    DNA methyltransferase
MIB-1 labeling index, 213
β_2-Microglobulin, 180, 253,
    265, 325t
Mifepristone, use in treating
    meningiomas, 57, 66
Mixed cryoglobulinemias, 303t
Monoclonal antibody 81C6,
    184–185
Monomorphous angiocentric
    bipolar gliomas, 30
Multidrug resistance (*MDR*) gene,
    155
Multifocal neuraxis symptoms, 304
Multiple endocrine neoplasia type 1
    (MEN1), 219–221
Mutliple sclerosis, 298, 300t,
    302t, 305
Mycoplasma-associated
    myelitis, 302t
Myelopathy, 305–306
disease-associated causes and
    evaluations, 301–303t
signs, symptoms, and diagnostic
    tests, 300–301t
Myxedema, 194

Myxopapillary ependymomas of
    the filum terminale, 25, 32,
    317–318, 321–323, 322–323f

N
N-Acetylaspartate (NAA), 44–45,
    44f, 61
National Association of Brain
    Tumor Consortium (NABTC),
    174, 176, 178
Neoplasia, 300t
Neoplastic meningitis (NM)
    diagnosis, 247–253, 248f, 249t
    epidemiology, 246–247
    management, 253–258
    pathophysiology, 247
    prognosis, 258–259, 258–259t
    treatment, 259
Nerve block, for pain
    management, 348
Nerve sheath tumors, 7t, 67,
    316–317, 319–321
Neuraxial analgesia, for pain
    management, 347–348
Neurocognitive deficit, due to
    radiotherapy, 148
Neurocognitive dysfunction
    assessment of, 335–338
    pharmacologic and psychologic
        management of, 338–341
    variables contributing to, 331–335
Neurocognitive functioning
    assessment of, 335, 337
    variables contributing to,
        333–334, 339
Neuroendocrine dysfunction, due
    to radiotherapy, 148
Neurofibromas, 317
Neurofibromatosis (NF), 13t, 14,
    55, 68, 317
    type 1 (NF1), 13t, 14, 317
    type 2 (NF2), 13t, 14, 55, 67–68,
        317
Neuromodulation, for pain
    management, 348

Neuromyelitis optica, 302t, 306
Nevoid basal cell carcinoma
    syndrome, 13t, 14
Nimustine (ACNU), 256
Nitrosourea, use in treating
    glioblastomas, 162–165
N-Nitroso compounds, effect on
    cancer incidence, 13t, 18–19
Non-small cell lung carcinoma
    (NSCLC), 232–234
North American Brain Tumor
    Consortium (NABTC), 157, 162
North Central Cancer Treatment
    Group (NCCTG), 104, 157,
    164–165
Null cell adenomas, 194, 210

O
Octreotide, use in treating
    hormone-secreting tumors,
    204, 210
Oligodendrogliomas, 10–11, 46f,
    49f, 94–99, 96f, 101, 107–108,
    173
    anaplastic, 98–99, 107, 165–166
O^6-Methylguanine-DNA
    methyltransferase (MGMT),
    31, 157, 159
Oncostatin M, expression in
    meningiomas, 58
Opioids, use in pain management,
    347
Osteoblastic lesions, 279–280
Osteoblastomas, 279–280
Osteochondromas, 280
Osteoid osteomas, 279–280
Osteoporosis, 195, 199
Osteoporotic fractures, 277, 348
Osteosarcomas, 282

P
p16 gene, 10, 13t, 15, 172
$p16^{ink4a}$ gene, 9, 30
p53 gene, 9–14, 56, 99, 156,
    176, 213

Pain
  assessment of, 341–345
  management of, 346–349, 346f
  WHO ladder approach to pain
    relief, 346
Papillary glioneuronal tumors, 30
Papovavirus infection, 306
Paragangliomas, 25, 32, 50,
  316, 318
Parasitic infections, 300t, 302t
Pars intermedia cysts, 218
Pediculectomy, use during
  surgery, 291
Pegvisomant, 57, 205
PEP-3 vaccination, 185
Percutaneous needle vertebral
  augmentation, 289
Perfusion imaging, 40–41, 47
P-glycoprotein, 155
Phenobarbital, 156
Phenytoin, 156, 335
Phosphatase and tensin homolog
  (PTEN) gene, 10, 30, 156, 159,
  174, 177
PI3K/AKT axis, 174, 175f, 177
Pituitary adenomas, 39f, 146–147,
  192–194, 194t, 201f, 205f, 210,
  211f, 215, 216f, 218
Pituitary gland, 196, 203, 205,
  208–209, 212, 218–220
  compression of, 194–195,
    210, 218
  enlargement of, 210
  metastases to, from systemic
    cancer, 215–218
Pituitary metastases, 215, 216
Pituitary tumors, 7
  clinical presentation of, 194–197
  laboratory investigation of,
    197–198
  malignant, 212–215
  pathology of, 193–194
  radiologic evaluation of, 198–199
  syndromes of, 219–220
  treatment for, 146–147, 199–212

Plasma cell neoplasms, 281
Plasmacytomas, 281
Platelet-derived growth factor
  (PDGF), 57–58, 86, 172, 174,
  176–177
Pleomorphic xanthoastrocytomas
  (PXAs), 30, 32, 94–95, 109–110,
  113, 115
Pneumocystis, 306
Polyarteritis nodosa, 303t
Poly-ICLC vaccination, 185
Positron emission tomography,
  48–49, 67, 149, 227, 277, 305
PRECISE trial, 162
Prednisone, use in treating
  PCNSL, 266
Primary central nervous system
  lymphoma (PCNSL)
  AIDS-related, 264–265
  diagnosis and staging of,
    264–265, 265t, 266f
  salvage treatment for, 270–271
  treatment for, 266–270, 268f
Primitive neuroectodermal tumors
  (PNETs), 7t, 8, 19, 143–144
Procarbazine, 107, 163, 165, 173,
  267–270
Procarbazine, CCNU, and
  vincristine (PCV), 107–108,
  116, 161, 163–166, 173
Progressive systemic sclerosis, 303t
Prolactin, 193–197, 214
Prolactin-secreting adenomas, 196,
  199, 202–204, 212–213, 219
Proliferation markers, 29
Prophylactic cranial irradiation
  (PCI), use in treating lung
  cancer brain metastases, 233
Prostate cancer, 286–287
Pseudomonas exotoxin, use in
  treating gliomas, 179
PTEN/MMAC tumor suppressor,
  177
PTK787 compound, use in treating
  gliomas, 177

Q

Quality of life
  assessment of, 336
  variables contributing to, 106,
    187, 254, 259, 285

R

RAD001, *See* Rapamycin
Radiation, effect on tumor
    incidence, 13t, 15–17, 56
Radiation Therapy Oncology Group
    (RTOG), 107–108, 108t, 142t,
    157, 164–166, 228, 266–267
Radionuclide bone scanning, 277,
    280
Radiotherapy, 63–66, 81, 86,
    115–116, 125, 132, 141–145,
    173, 203–206, 209–210, 214,
    254, 266, 282, 285, 291
  adjuvant, 63–66, 86, 88, 145, 291,
    315, 324
  adverse effects of, 147–149
  benign tumors, role in, 145–147
  brachytherapy, 140, 141f,
    142–143
  classic 3-dimensional, 137
  conformal, 136–137, 196
  CyberKnife radiosurgery, 138
  external-beam, 64–65, 80–81,
    125, 160, 165, 203, 217,
    254–255, 291
  fractionated sterotactic, 72–73,
    146
  Gamma Knife radiosurgery, 65,
    71–72, 74, 88, 138, 203, 234
  intensity-modulated (IMRT),
    65–66, 141, 139
  linear accelerator (LINAC)-
    based radiosurgery, 65, 88, 138
  of low-grade gliomas, 104–106,
    105t
  malignant tumors, role in,
    141–145
  proton therapy, 138, 140–141,
    144, 147

radiosurgery, 65, 71–73, 76,
    88–89, 138–139, 144–145, 203
  stereotactic radiosurgery (SRS),
    65, 71–73, 138–139, 203, 226
  tomotherapy system, 139
  whole-brain (WBRT), 226,
    230–235, 237, 240, 266–268, 339
Rapamycin (RAD001), use in
    treating gliomas, 177
ras gene, 58
Ras/MEK/ERK pathway, 174, 175f
Response Evaluation Criteria in
    Solid Tumors (RECIST), 157
Retinoblastoma (*Rb*) gene, 13t, 238
Rheumatoid arthritis, 301–302t,
    304, 325t
Rituximab, use in treating PCNSL,
    268, 270–271
Rosetted glioneuronal tumors, 30

S

Sacrectomy, 280, 291
Sarcoidosis, 79, 299, 302t, 304, 306,
    318, 325t
Schistosomiasis, 304, 306
Schwannomas, 11–12, 25, 75f,
    317, 319
  of the cranial nerves, 73–77
  facial nerve, 74, 75f
  jugular foramen, 75–77, 76f, 76t
  trigeminal, 73–74, 73f
  vestibular, 67–73, 69–70f, 72f
Sella turcica, cystic lesions of,
    217–219
Signal transducers and activators
    of transcription (STAT), 174,
    178
Sjögren's syndrome, 301–302t, 304,
    306, 325t
Small cell lung carcinoma (SCLC),
    232–233, 236, 246, 251f, 259,
    286, 291
SMARCB2 gene, 56
Southwest Oncology Group
    (SWOG), 160, 165–166

Spastic paraparesis, 302t, 306
Squamous cell carcinoma, 233, 287
Steroids, 80, 147, 207, 226, 228,
    230–233, 236, 264, 287, 306,
    346
Subependymal giant cell
    astrocytomas (SEGAs), 32,
    94–95, 109–110, 113, 115
Surgical resection, 227–228,
    230–232, 234–235, 240
Surveillance, Epidemiology, and
    End Results (SEER) program,
    3–6
SV40-contaminated polio vaccine,
    effect on cancer incidence, 20
SV-40 virus, role in choroid plexus
    papillomas, 84
Syphilis, 306, 325t
Systemic lupus erythematosus,
    303t, 306, 325t

T
Tabes dorsalis, 302t
Takayasu's arteritis, 303t
Tamoxifen, 57, 66, 160
Temozolomide, 108, 160–166, 173,
    175–177, 240, 256, 268,
    270–271
Temporal arteritis, 303t, 325t
Tenascin, use in treating gliomas,
    172, 184
Teniposide, 161, 233
Thiotepa (triethylenethiophos-
    phoramide), 255–257, 269–270
Thoracic kyphotic deformities,
    287
Thyrotropin (TSH), 193, 197, 213
Thyrotropin-secreting tumors,
    194–195, 199, 209–210
Tinea capitis, 15, 56
Tinnitus, 68, 74, 249t
Topotecan, 161, 233, 256, 268, 270
Toxoplasma gondii, as cause of
    meningiomas, 14, 20
TP53 gene, 30, 84, 159, 172

Transsphenoidal surgery, 80, 200,
    201f, 204, 205f, 208–210, 211f,
    216f, 217–218, 217f
Trastuzumab, use in treating
    breast cancer brain
    metastases, 236–237
Trigeminal nerve deficits, 74
Tuberculosis, 299, 302t, 306, 318,
    325t
Tuberous sclerosis, 13t, 14, 109
Tuberous sclerosis 2 (TSC2) gene,
    effect on ganglioglioma
    incidence, 11
Tumor, node, metastases (TNM)
    schema, 236

U
Ultrasonography, intraoperative,
    102, 104, 126, 128–129, 230, 310
Ultraviolet light and malignant
    melanoma, 238

V
Vaccination, 185–186
Valsalva maneuver, use during
    surgery, 129
Varicella zoster virus (VZV), 14,
    20, 301–302t, 306, 325t
Vascular endothelial growth factor
    (VEGF), 58, 86–87, 176–177
Vasculitis, 40, 306
Venography, 38–40, 42
Vertebrectomy, 290–291
Vertebroplasty, 281, 289–290,
    289f, 348
Vertigo, 68, 74, 249t
Vincristine, use in treating PCNSL,
    266–267, 269–270
von Hippel-Lindau (VHL) disease,
    86–89, 308

W
Warburg effect, 179
Wegener's granulomatosis, 302t,
    325t

Wernicke's speech area, 128
Wisconsin Brief Pain Inventory
    (BPI), 342
Wong-Baker FACES pain rating
    scale, 344, 344f
World Health Organization
    (WHO) classification system,
    25, 158t, 346f

and astrocytomas, 141, 143, 145
and choroid plexus papillomas,
    84
and gliomas, 94–95, 98–99, 101,
    107–108, 113, 154, 158, 166
and meningiomas, 58, 61–62, 64
WP1066 compound, use in treating
    gliomas, 178